169+ Lose It Or Else

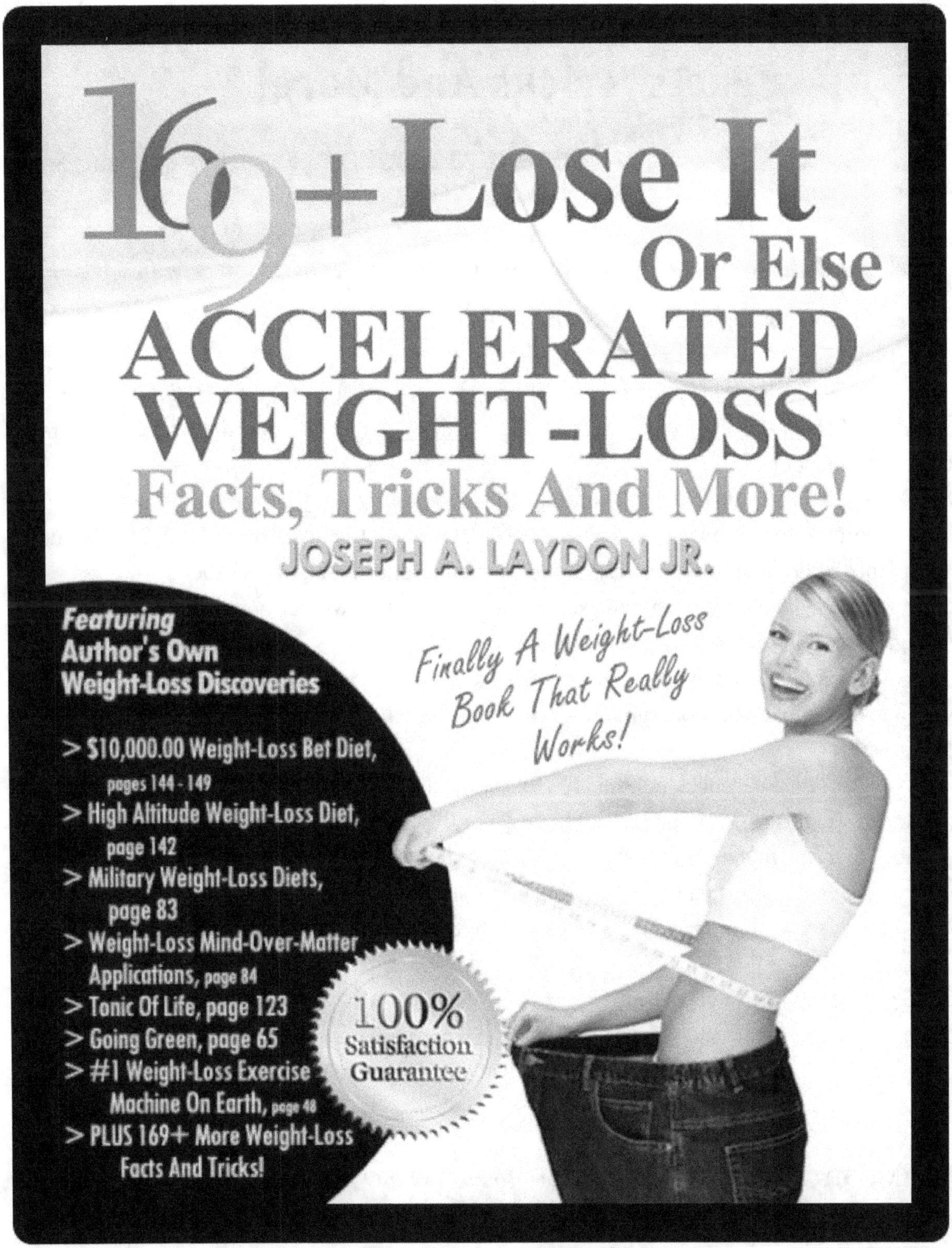

ACCELERATED WEIGHT-LOSS
Facts, Tricks And More!

JOSEPH A. LAYDON JR.

Featuring Author's Own Weight-Loss Discoveries

Finally A Weight-Loss Book That Really Works!

> $10,000.00 Weight-Loss Bet Diet, pages 144 - 149
> High Altitude Weight-Loss Diet, page 142
> Military Weight-Loss Diets, page 83
> Weight-Loss Mind-Over-Matter Applications, page 84
> Tonic Of Life, page 123
> Going Green, page 65
> #1 Weight-Loss Exercise Machine On Earth, page 48
> PLUS 169+ More Weight-Loss Facts And Tricks!

100% Satisfaction Guarantee

"169+ Lose It Or Else Accelerated Weight-Loss Facts, Tricks And More!"

UPDATED: 112203C July 2020 (Saturday)

Thank you for getting your own *169+ Lose It Or Else Accelerated Weight-Loss Facts, Tricks And More.* This weight-loss book is based on my own international weight-loss experiences and 'intensive research'.

In this weight-loss book you'll find my own diet I call the *$10,000.00 Weight-Loss Bet Diet!* This is <u>my own diet that I invented that works for me</u> as well as several others annotated in this book.

This weight-loss book is designed so you can <u>INVENT</u> your own special weight-loss diet according to your tastebuds cause TASTEBUDS RULE. And in this weight-loss book you get plenty of tasty options so to INVENT your own special weight-loss diet.

Plus, I give you unique exercise and Mind-Over-Matter options to enhance your safe weight-loss goals (as per your doctor's advice).

This may be the only weight-loss book that has you INVENT your own special tasty weight-loss diet and is complimented with unique exercises and Mind-Over-Matter applications.

OK, check out the HUGE Table Of Contents where you'll find at least a few dozen weight-loss facts and tricks I know you'll want to incorporate into your own special weight-loss diet (upon your doctor's approval). I wish you a vibrantly healthy future starting this very split second – <u>"Cause YOU BELIEVE you will lose those many unhealthy pounds starting today, tomorrow, next week,… while you read this revealing weight-loss book "</u>.

Published By Joseph A. Laydon Jr.

Website: https://www.survivalexpertblog.com
                 https://www.survivalexpertblog.com/52-survival-books/
E-Mail: wwwsurvivalexpert@yahoo.com

MOST IMPORTANT NOTE: Throughout *"169+ Lose It Or Else Accelerated Weight-Loss Facts, Tricks And More"* you will see me making references to my other documents (Newsletters, Books,…). I've kept these references in case you become a full subscriber - www.survivalexpert.com

Copyright & Disclaimer

IRISAP DISCLAIMER STATEMENT

The author of "169+ Lose It Or Else Accelerated Weight-Loss Facts, Tricks & More!" and owner of Intensive Research Information Services And Product(s)(IRISAP) is exercising his right under the First Amendment to self-publish and co-author this informational product to better educate the public with respect to alternative weight-loss diets. The author is publishing this information based upon his "intensive research" and his experiences of losing weight. Author is not a "doctor" and doesn't claim to be a doctor. Author is demonstrating through this book how to lose weight safely.

This weight-loss book is designed to help the reader become more aware of alternative ways to lose weight while under the direction of the reader's doctor. The information within this weight-loss book is for educational purposes only. Professional medical advice from "qualified doctors" is ALWAYS and HIGHLY recommended.

Advice is neither implied nor intended. IRISAP and authors\writers of resource materials are not responsible for the purchaser's and third party activities and is in no way responsible for sickness or death or successes. THE PURCHASER OF THIS WEIGHT-LOSS BOOK IS SOLELY RESPONSIBLE FOR THIRD PARTY DISCLOSURE AND RESPONSIBLE FOR THEIR ACTIONS AND ANY PRIVATE OR PROFESSIONAL ACTIONS TAKEN FROM THIS INFORMATIONAL PRODUCT. This WEIGHT-LOSS BOOK is Copyrighted and VIOLATORS WILL BE PROSECUTED! If the consumer DISAGREES with ANY portion of this DISCLAIMER STATEMENT, the consumer MUST immediately (upon receipt) return this entire informational product for a full refund.

Table Of Contents

Contents

Dedication

This is my 1st Self-Published Book and it's dedicated to my parents

Joseph and Rosana Laydon,

my big brother Joe

and my sister Linda

who are all in Heaven.

Introduction

Welcome to *169+ Lose It Or Else Accelerated Weight-Loss Facts, Tricks &*
More! This weight-loss book consolidates THOUSANDS of weight loss facts, tricks, ideas,
plans,... from the 60-pound *2012 Ultra-Advanced Anytime Anywhere Survival Program TOTAL*
Package (2012 U-AAASPTP).

It gives you more than 169+ weight-loss facts, tricks, ideas, plans,... and "related data" to support
a safe and successful weight-loss regimen. And it's complimented with more healthy
information to avoid, prevent and fight maladies from minor headaches to killer cancers.

This weight-loss book addresses many weight-loss facts & tricks so to combine one favorite with
another to <u>ACCELERATE</u> weight-loss. A healthy weight is complimented with many other
healthy benefits and at the same time avoiding many minor to serious maladies.

I highly encourage you to read this weight-loss book more than a few times so to better
understand all the related data.

If this is the only Survival Product that you have purchased from IRISAP - please go to
www.survivalexpertblog.com   for more information. Any questions, please write me a note
(see web site).

> Sincerely,
> **Joseph A. Laydon Jr.**

PS You can browse <u>www.survivalexpertblog.com</u> right now.

IMPORTANT NOTE: This Survival Book has grown to insure you get you get more than your
money's worth. The sub-headlines on the cover of this book do not match the corresponding
page numbers.

169+ Lose It Or Else Accelerated Weight-Loss Facts, Tricks And More!

You're about to read 169+ international weight-loss facts tricks and more

(**HUNDREDS** of individual healthy facts beyond weight-loss,...) - OK, let's start with Acai.

ACAI: Acai is becoming a very popular health supplement in the United States. Acai palm tree grows in the massive Brazilian Rain Forest. Acai berry fruit is smaller than a grape with a large seed complimented with super nutritious pulp. An acai branch offers 700-900 acai berries. Acai is offered just about everywhere. I talked to a General Nutrition Center (GNC) representative., he told me Acai is like a laxative. Again, that comes from a GNC representative; and we all know how laxatives affect our bodies.

ACTIVITIES THAT BURN CALORIES: Exercise is the active use of the body to build or maintain strength, endurance, to make the body healthier and it burns calories! A 170-pound person can burn 95 calories per hour just sitting (110 lbs person burns 65 calories), whereas the same 170-pound person can burn as much as 600 calories per hour running a 10-minute mile (110 lb person burns 360 calories). The following are common activities of one-hour duration and the calories burnt for a 170-pound person. Use your best judgment (or purchase a Calorie Burner Scale from any grocery store) to determine the calories burnt.

Activity	Calories Burnt
Typing	125.
Ironing	150.
Slow Dancing	235.
Mopping	285.
Shopping	285.
Fishing	290.
Volleyball (6 people)	295.
Walking	360.
Golfing	390.
Fast Dancing	475.
Tennis	505.
Mowing the lawn	515.
Swimming Slow	595.

Swimming Fast----------------------------720.
Weight Training---------------------------850.
See Exercise.

ADKINS DIET: Want to lose 10 pounds in 10 days? Dr. Robert C. Adkins, M.D., wrote an eye opening book *"Dr. Adkins' New Diet Revolution,"* on a new way to lose weight. Instead of cutting down on fat and easing up on the total calories consumed like most experts and doctors advise us to do; Dr. Adkins has a much different approach. A different way to BURN THE FAT! To burn-off the fat, Dr. Adkins states that you must first eliminate carbohydrates from your diet. Eliminate carbohydrates like bread, dairy products other than cheese, cream or butter. Eliminate fruits, grains, pasta, potatoes, processed food, starchy vegetables, sugar and white flour. Other foods\drinks that are high in carbohydrates and should be avoided are beets, candy, carrots, potato chips, chocolate, corn, crackers, fruit juice, hoagies, junk food, maple syrup, molasses, pizza, pretzels, rice, sodas and yams.

Why eliminate carbohydrates?
When you cut back on the consumption of carbohydrates, this uses up your body's glycogen, which is a starch stored in the muscles and liver. When there is no more glycogen, your body then BURNS ITS OWN FAT FOR FUEL! Burn-off the fat and lose those unwanted pounds! What foods can you eat on a carbohydrate restrictive diet? According to Dr. Adkin's book, eat low or no carbohydrate foods like cheese, and eggs. Eat fats which include butter, olive oil and mayonnaise in reasonable amounts. Eat fish, fowl, meat and shellfish. I highly advise you to read Dr. Adkins book and then consult your physician about this diet.

How would I know if this diet is working for me?
Go to your local drug store or grocery store and purchase a bottle of Ames Ketostix #2880P (50 strips). These are reagent strips for urinalysis. What you're looking for or want is ketosis. The strip will turn darker colors depending on the ketones present. The darker the color the more fat metabolism is taking place. It especially works better with a routine exercise plan in conjunction with the carbohydrate restrictive diet. The author tried this diet and lost 05 pounds within a week!

- **Ketone** -- A substance which is usually not harmful when found in small amounts in the urine. This could happen in dieting and when identified, gives you information on carbohydrate and fat metabolism.
- **Ketosis** -- A pathological accumulation of ketone bodies in the body.

WARNING: Diabetics must consult their physician. I highly advise everyone to read Dr. Adkins book prior to considering this diet.

ALFALFA SPROUTS: Alfalfa sprouts furnish only 10 calories per cup, no fat and have only a trace of sodium. Even though alfalfa sprouts are low in protein, it's one of the richest foods in mineral content. Alfalfa is an aid in weight loss. Alfalfa sprouts take up space in your stomach while providing fiber. Alfalfa is an excellent source of chlorophyll (nature's deodorant) which is thought to have antibacterial action. It may also help to heal wounds. In supplemental form alfalfa can help reduce body and breath odor. When shopping for alfalfa at the grocery store, the best tasting alfalfa sprouts are 02 to 02 1/2 inches in length. See *Gardens Alive* in the POC Section.

AMINO ACIDS: Amino acids are the "building blocks" of protein. The 22 known amino acids are vital to your health because they help build, repair, renew and provide a source of energy. If any amino acid is low or missing, the effectiveness of all the others will be reduced and must be obtained from food or supplements. Of the 22 known amino acids, eight of them are not manufactured by the body. Here are seven of them: Isoleucine, Leucine, Lysine, Phenylalanine, Theronine, Tryptophan and Valine. Here are a few amino acids and what they do for you:

Carnitine: Carnitine can help in the breakdown of fats so that they can be used as energy for the body. Carnitine is a factor in making muscles operate at their best possible strength level.

Cysteine: Cysteine is the principal source of sulfur. Sulphur helps to ***detoxify*** your body, promote improved healing and boost resistance to disease. Cysteine is important to the growth of nails, skin and hair.

Methionine: Methionine is believed to help ***cleanse*** the liver and kidneys, control cholesterol and wash out toxic waste. Methionine helps strengthen nails and improve pliability and tone of the skin.

Ornithine: Ornithine helps stimulate the immune system. Ornithine also appears to play a role in body energy.

Taurine: Taurine could possibly help retard the development of hypertension. Taurine helps strengthen brain-wave patterns. Taurine helps ***increase the white blood cells that fight infections.***

For a great source for aminos, see Health Science in the POC Section and see *Apple Cider Vinegar*.
Follow the recommended dosage and instructions from the label and as per your doctor's instructions.

AMISH WEIGHT-LOSS FOODS AND CANCER FLUSHERS: You ever known an Amish person to be overweight or get cancer? Me neither. I believe I talked in detail about all or most of these healthy foods in the 667-page Gettysburg Program. Here are the foods that help flush carcinogens (cancer-causing agents) out of your body and fight specific cancers from the get go. Plus they're also great to help you meet your weight-loss goals:

- Beans = colon cancer
- Beets = cervical cancer
- Blackberry Tea = general
- Broccoli = general
- Brussels Sprouts = general
- Cabbage = general
- Carrots = colon cancer
- Cauliflower = breast cancer & general
- Chives = stomach cancer
- Garlic = stomach & colon cancer
- Leeks = stomach cancer
- Onions = stomach cancer & general
- Pears = colon cancer
- Radishes = general
- Shallots = stomach cancer
- Spinach = lung cancer & general
- Sweet Potatoes = general
- Tomatoes = stomach, pancreatic & general
- Vitamin C = mouth, esophagus & stomach cancers

ANGSTROM MINERALS INDIUM: You'll hear me talk about *"The Missing Trace Mineral That Heals – Indium."* STOP right now and go to that segment before we go any further. OK, you ready? Let's carry-on with *Angstrom Minerals Indium*.

Indium, a very rare mineral, was originally patented in 1980 and meets the FDA's GRAS (Generally Recognized As Safe). FDA studies state it would take 20,000-times the normal dosage to hurt a human. Studies of *Indium* by Dr. Henry Schroder indicated:

a) Trace Minerals: *Indium* helps the body absorb more trace minerals. Thus, relating to a healthier mind and body.

b) Anti-Cancer: *Indium* supplementation caused lower incidence of tumors. *Indium* was found to be highly anti-carcinogenic (anti-cancer). Indium inhibited growth of MCF-7 (cervical cancer). Carcinoid and pancreatic tumors were also treated using *Indium*.

c) Weight-Loss: *Indium* helps with **weight-loss** by having beneficial effects on the thyroid which is directly linked to revving-up the metabolism.

d) Life-Span: The US ranks 17th in the world when it comes to lifespan. *Indium* could have Americans live longer, offer vibrant health, give the elderly independent lives versus sickly lives in nursing homes.

e) Glaucoma: *Indium* is used in the treatment of glaucoma. It aids to reduce the eyeball pressure by as much as 10 to 35 percent.

f) Blood Pressure: The SILENT KILLER - high blood pressure, has more than 125,000,000+ Americans in its deadly grip. And most Americans have no idea their blood pressure is dangerously high. *Indium* along with a chromium supplement is noted to lower high blood pressure (hypertension). And *Indium* is also noted to raise blood pressure for those afflicted with low blood pressure (hypotension)

g) Diabetes: This amazing healthy mineral - *Indium* has been used to drastically lower or eliminate all together, the insulin medication for Type 2 diabetic patients. And it's noted to demonstrate its healing ways in as little as the very 1st day.

h) Alzheimer's Disease: The Austrian Morbus Alzheimer's Society conducted a study and found that 35% improvement in the group taking *Indium*. Improvements in the Alzheimer's patients included better normal behavior, better short-term memory, improved stamina, and more important, some patients who were already independent, returned to self-care status.

Note: Long-term benefits of *Indium* include (but not limited to) are ADD improvement, visible signs of aging reduced, autism, lower blood pressure, remedy stress-related aid in weight-loss,...

ANTI-FAT FOODS: According to Isabelle Martin, author of *Foods That Make You Lose Weight or Negative Calories*, the following foods can be labeled as ANTI-FAT FOODS because they burn as many calories as they supply. These foods contain 75 to 95 percent water and an average of 25 calories an ounce. So what are you waiting for, eat up!!!

Anti-Fat Foods: Artichoke, Asparagus, Beets, Broccoli, Cauliflower, Celery, Chicory, Cucumber, Dandelion, Endives, Green Beans, Green peppers, Green Cabbage, Horseradish, Lettuce, Onion, Radish, Spinach, Swiss Chard, Turnip, Watercress and Zucchini.

As a matter of fact, most of the fruits and vegetables in EAT THE RIGHT STUFF (667-page *Gettysburg Program*) may be considered FAT-FIGHTING FOODS, as long as your diet is low in fat and consist of the foods that are listed above. The vegetables and fruits in this section are all very low in fat content and provide a deluge of other health benefits for you now and is a good healthy investment for your future. A healthy diet, drinking good, clean, contaminant-free water and exercise go hand-in-hand.
WARNING: SEE YOUR DOCTOR prior to any dieting or exercise plan.

ANTI-FAT SPICES: Spices stimulate the digestive juices and contribute to the to the DESTRUCTION OF FAT. Hot Mustard in particular can temporarily speed up the metabolism as much as 07 to 08 hours. Research has indicated that the metabolic rates goes up ten (10) percent after a meal. This is called the "thermic effect." The lower the fat content the higher the "thermic effect." This "thermic effect" can double if you do some light exercise one-half hour after you've eaten. A study conducted at Stanford University showed that light exercise burned 2000 calories per week, speeds up weight loss and is good for your heart.

ANTI-FAT SPICES: Basil, Clove, Fennel, Garlic, Mint, Parsley, Sage, Savory, Tarragon and Thyme.

APPLE CIDER VINEGAR (ACV): In 5,000 B.C., Babylonians fermented the fruits of the date palm. This date vinegar was credited for having superior healing qualities. Vinegar is even mentioned in the Bible (four times in the Old Testament and four times in the New Testament). Claims of curative and restorative powers of apple cider vinegar are legendary. This fabulous liquid is associated with believers who say it can lengthen life, improve hearing, mental powers and vision. Vinegar has been used thousands of years for folk medicine, hair and skin care. Vinegar comes from the French word "vinaigre" -- Vin for wine and Aigre for sour, thus wine that has gone sour. Vinegar is an acid liquid made from beer, cider and wine by a means called acetous fermentation meaning alcohol mixes with oxygen in the air. The alcohol is changed into acetic acid and water. The acetic acid gives vinegar it's unique tart taste. Vinegar contents has the basic nutrients of the original food from which it was made. Here's an example: Apple Cider Vinegar (ACV) has beta carotene, pectin, potassium... All which are very beneficial for your health as annotated in this book.

ACV is packed with amino acids, healthful enzymes and trace elements. It contains more than thirty needed nutrients, a dozen minerals and several Vitamins, essential acids and enzymes. ACV has a tart taste and a germ-killing acid and pectin for those heart healthy concerned. ACV is a great source of calcium, chlorine, fluorine, iron, magnesium, phosphorus, potassium, silicon, sodium and sulfur. The ***body requires 22 essential minerals for health and 19 of them are found in ACV!*** Potassium in ACV is known for its aid to overall circulation.

Here are some healthy benefits as a result of taking (ACV):

- **Arthritis:** ACV with water taken daily may bring arthritis relief by helping dissolve calcium deposits in the joints and eliminating them through excretion.

- **Brain Power:** ACV can boost brain power. Potassium helps oxygenate the blood as it boosts circulation and helps thin the blood resulting in clearer thinking and brain power.

- **Digestive Aid:** ACV is a natural digestive aid, helps keep the kidneys function properly, helps prevent germs from growing in the urinary tract and bladder which cause infection and inflammation. ACV destroys microorganisms, including bacteria, fungi, viruses..., as well as preventing poisons from reaching the rest of your system. Two tablespoons of ACV to a glass of water at each meal is helpful in maintaining a healthy digestive tract, which reflects your all-around health.

- **High Blood Pressure:** High Blood Pressure, the "Silent Killer," can be countered by ACV (potassium) by countering the damage done by sodium. Potassium in ACV stops excess fluid retention, and regulates the body's water balance and needed in muscle and nerve functions.

- **Infection:** Bacteria like everything else, require moisture to survive. Bacteria pulls the moisture out of your body's cells for their survival and growth. If your resistance is low and they multiply, you can become very ill and in the worst case, death. To help keep the moisture in your cells and keep the germs away is from them is a proper diet with sources of potassium. According to D.C. Jarvis, M.D., if there is sufficient potassium in each body cell, it will draw the moisture from the bacteria, thus impeding its survival and its potential to multiply.

- **Sleep Deficit:** According to a recent study at Cornell University, more than *50 million Americans suffer from sleep deficit and the fatigue from lack of sleep*. Sedatives, over-the-counter medications, narcotics, alcohol and a combination of these are widely used to overcome sleep disorders.

  Vermont folk medicine has a treatment for sleep deficit. Simply add *three teaspoons full of ACV to a cup of honey*. Take two teaspoons full of this mixture when preparing to go to bed. You should be asleep within 30 minutes. If not, take two more teaspoons full and two more every time you wake up or have trouble sleeping.

- **Weight Loss:** ACV has been noted to help *stimulate the metabolism into high gear!* ACV provides potassium which promotes proper chemical reaction in your body as well as the acid nature of vinegar enhances certain conditions of your body are just right for *fat burning!* It has been noted that the following ACV concoction also *suppresses the appetite:* Add two teaspoons of ACV to a glass of water for each meal.

Apple Cider Vinegar (ACV) promotes digestion. Add one to two tablespoons of ACV in a glass of warm water. Drink this concoction prior to each meal. It is extremely helpful in taming that appetite and **melting away excess fat**.

According to the Diet Research Center in England, better reducing and firming with ACV - mixture of 03 parts ACV to 01-part almond or olive oil - **helps the body rid excess fat**. The ACV and honey cocktail should be taken 03 times daily. (1/2 teaspoon honey plus 01 teaspoon ACV in a glass of distilled water at room temperature). Exercise and EATING THE RIGHT STUFF is also recommended.

There are other benefits of ACV. For an *authentic* ACV product see Health Science & Live Longer Products in the POC Section.

True Apple Cider Vinegar (that is alive), is a little cloudy with sediment resting at the bottom of the bottle. *DO NOT purchase* the store brand vinegar because its been deadened by pasteurization, which diminishes mineral content and many other health benefits.

100% ACV is made from apples that are grown in certified organic fashion. *INSURE* you purchase unfiltered and unpasteurized ACV. READ the label. I doubt you'll find healthy vinegar products at your local grocery store.

You can purchase very inferior ACV in your local grocery store, but if you want the good stuff see Health Science and The Family News in the POC Section. If you go to your local health food stores, *look for* Spectrum (unfiltered, natural organic) ACV. Distributed by Spectrum Naturals, Inc., 133 Copeland Street, Petaluma, CA 94952. Get ***Bragg's Apple Cider Vinegar*** at your local healthfood store.

APPLES: *"An Apple A Day Keeps The Doctor Away?"* The apple may be the King of the fruit world. Apples have been eaten by man since at least the New Stone Age, nearly 6,000 years ago. There are several thousand varieties of apples due to grafting; from the wild apple to produce strains that are less resistant to disease and apples that have particular flavors and colors. Two main groups of apples are sweet one's for eating and sharper varieties for cooking or making alcoholic drinks. Apples are rich in many needed minerals and Vitamins and may help "Keep the doctor away." Apples are rich in soluble fiber which has the ability to **lower blood cholesterol** levels and **lower your blood pressure**. Apples also **help to dampen the appetite** and the juices in apples are noted to kill infectious diseases.

According to Dr. James Anderson at the University of Kentucky School of Medicine, soluble fiber prevents hunger pangs by steadying your blood sugar level. Apples have virtually *no saturated fat, cholesterol or sodium*. A medium apple furnishes only 81 calories. Apples contain pectin for those heart healthy wannabe's. Eat an apple prior to bedtime. The pectin will keep your brain chemicals levels stable throughout the night. You'll *wake-up happy and refreshed!*

According to studies, apples even the aroma can also calm you down reducing anxiety. The juices in a fresh apple are noted to be *strong virus fighters*.

According to a study at Michigan State University, subjects who ate two apples a day had *less tension, fewer headaches and less frequent emotional upsets.*

According to a study at Yale University, researchers noted that the scent of spiced apples produced a calming effect which *aids to lower blood pressure!*

According to Italian, Irish and French researchers, apples help keep the cardiovascular system healthy. Apples put a dent in blood cholesterol. A research team headed by R. Sable-Amplis at the University of Paul Sabatier, Institute of Physiology, in Toulouse, was excited to find that *apples triggered a 28-point drop in cholesterol in normal hamsters* and a *spectacular 52-point drop in cholesterol in animals with genetically high cholesterol!* Dr. Sable-Amplis asked a group of 30 middle-aged, healthy men and women at the university not to change their diet except to eat 02 or 03 apples every day for a month.

By month's end, the apples *lowered the cholesterol in 24 of the 30 participants and HDL went up and LDL dropped!* One participant's cholesterol dived 30 percent! Dr. Sable-Amplis thinks the apple's secret is *pectin* which is a soluble fiber.

According to a French study, eating 02 apples a day may *lower your cholesterol level by at least 10 percent and by as much as 30 percent!* Why? Apples and prunes are *rich in a soluble fiber called pectin*. Studies reveal that consuming 15 grams of pectin per day for a few weeks can result in a *05 percent reduction in total serum cholesterol*. Read about *Apple Cider Vinegar*.

Note: I love Granny Smith apples. I eat them <u>nice and slow</u>. How? I take a sharp knife and slice off one small section at a time. This technique has me eating slower and enjoying the apple - thus filling me up. See *Count To 20*.

AROMA THERAPY: Chicago's Smell and Taste Treatment and Research Foundation has scientifically proven that one could lose weight by merely sniffing a fragrance before starting a meal by fooling the brain into thinking you're full. Specific odors act on the satiety center in the hypothalamus. Hypothalamus is the area of the brain that makes you feel full. Consumers can get the benefits of Aroma Therapy by using a device called a "Thin Pen." These pens come in a set of three.

ASPARAGUS: Asparagus is undoubtedly one of the *most healthiest foods on Earth!* Asparagus provides no fat, no cholesterol and hardly a trace of sodium. Four spears of asparagus provide only 13 calories. Asparagus is **so low in calories** that you would have to really eat huge amounts of it to gain weight. Asparagus is full of three food based nutrients that help in the defense of cancer. These elements are Vitamin A, Vitamin C and the mineral selenium which are excellent for its antioxidant properties.

Asparagus also contains small amounts of cholesterol-lowering fiber. Asparagus is ideal for heart-healthy menus. According to studies at the University of California and Mount Sinai School of Medicine in New York, regular asparagus consumption demonstrates lower rates of cancer and heart disease.

BAKED BEANS WEIGHT-LOSS: Now let me tell you about a man from Great Britain who lost a lot of weight by eating baked beans every day. Twenty-eight year old James Skeates from Suffolk, England lost a lot of weight by eating baked beans for 02-months. *"I was getting through two tins a day, eating them in my breaks at work, then at home with jacket potatoes, wholemeal bread or pasta. I was never hungry, but the weight kept coming off."* Skeates was reported to weigh-in at 133 kilos and 06-months later he lost 38 kilos, for a new weight of 95 kilos. By the way to convert from kilograms to pounds, multiply the kilos (kilograms) by 2.205 which will give you pounds. OK OK, I'll do it for you.

Skeates initially weighed-in at 133 kilos (kilograms) X 2.205 = 293.265 pounds. He ate 02 cans of baked beans each day for 06-months. At the end of 06-months he weighed in at 95 kilos (kilograms).

95 kilos X 2.205 = 209.475 pounds. So 293.265 - 209.475 = 83.79 pounds. He lost 83.79 pounds. And if you take 83.79 ÷ 2.205 = 38 kilos (kilograms).

Anyway, on an average, Skeates lost .4655 pound a day or 3.2 pounds a week or 13.965 pound a month. Not bad. As recommended by physicians, the weight came off real slow. Last time I checked, doctors recommend that dieters lose about 02-pounds a week to be on the very safe side.

1st Note: Kilogram means 1,000 grams. And 01 kilogram is equal to 2.205 pounds.

2nd Note: Date of news story - 26 September 2007.

BANANAS: A medium bananas furnishes only 100 calories, has hardly any sodium and is a modest source of Vitamin C. Bananas also furnish fiber for the heart healthy concerned and provides potassium which helps controlling blood pressure. Bananas are packed with Vitamin B6 which helps prevent depression. One banana provides 35% of the B6 RDA. Eating a banana *helps combat hunger pangs* and leaves you feeling satisfied and full. Bananas also help you remain alert and energetic because of the fructose sugar that is encased in fiber and carbohydrates are *slowly released* into your system.

In the 1930s, medical literature noted that bananas were a cure for ulcers. Experimenting with mice, researchers isolated a chemical in ripe and unripe bananas that suppressed acid secretion, thus blocking the development of ulcers in animals.

Modern teams of British and Indian researchers have discovered why the banana-eating rodents end up with about 1/3 fewer and less severe ulcers. Bananas work just like the most sophisticated drugs (carbenoxolone), but without the side-effects like high blood pressure. Bananas strengthen the surface cells of the stomach lining, forming a sturdier barrier against noxious juices. The British researchers' bottom line: "The role of bananas in folk medicine as an antiulcerogenic agent, at least against gastric ulcers, appears justified...."

BEAN DIET: According to Maria Simonson, Ph.D., Sc.D., Professor Emeritus and director of the Health, Weight and Stress Program at John Hopkins Medical Institutions in Baltimore, *"If you keep beans in your diet, you'll lose more weight and you'll lose it faster."* That's because beans, which are very low in fat and calories, give you a feeling of fullness that can last up to four hours longer than meals without beans.

BEANS: Beans are high in fiber, **low in fat,** low in sodium, low in cholesterol and packed with Vitamins, minerals and mother nature's way of providing protein from plants. Beans are a source of water-soluble fiber, which helps lower BAD low-density lipo-proteins (LDL), rich in B Vitamins, folic acid and the minerals copper, iron, magnesium, potassium and zinc. Beans are economical source (pennies per pound) of delicious nutrition. Beans have been shown to lower cholesterol.

According to studies at the University of Kentucky, University of Minnesota and studies in the Netherlands, beans consumed on a regular basis can lower cholesterol.

At the University of Kentucky, Dr. James Anderson, regularly prescribes dried beans - a cup of cooked pinto or navy beans a day - to lower blood cholesterol. Dr. Anderson has documented that cholesterol levels drop by an average of nineteen percent, even with men with extremely high cholesterol counts-over 260 milligrams per deciliter. One man brought his cholesterol down from 274 to 190; another participant lowered his from 218 to 167! Beans were noted to sweep the bad cholesterol LDL out of the blood and improved the critically needed good cholesterol HDL. Dr. Anderson's bean diet improved the ratio an average of 17 percent! Potentially *life-saving* numbers, uh!

Beans are also considered good bets as cancer preventers. Beans are concentrated carriers of protease inhibitors which are enzymes that can counteract the activation of cancer-causing compounds in the intestine.

Protease inhibitors can turn off oncogenies which are carriers found in every normal cell that when activated may lead to cancer. Beans are rich in compounds called lignans that are anticancer on their own and are converted by colon bacteria into hormone-like substances that according to some scientist may help fight off breast and colon cancer. According to researchers at the Nutritional Science Department, University of California, Berkeley, beans are good for your colon because they help increase "fecal output" which is noted as a sign of good health and helps alleviate symptoms or reduce chances of colon or rectal cancer, diverticular disease, hemorrhoids and bowel irregularities. *"Fecal output"* also appeared to stimulate colonic bacteria to throw off chemicals called volatile short chain fatty acids, that help lower blood cholesterol, blood pressure and may inhibit colon cancer. See *Bean Diet* and *Baked Beans Weight-Loss*. See *Arrowhead Mills* and *Akpharma* in the POC Section.

BELL PEPPERS: Bell Peppers are some of the *most nutrient-dense* foods available. One-half cup of raw bell pepper provides only 12 calories. An average bell pepper provides more Vitamin C than a cup of orange juice. Peppers are rich in Vitamin A to help resist infections. Vitamin B is provided to help absorb nutrients in food as well as helping to *improve your metabolism*. When bell peppers are mature, they become sweeter. Mature bell peppers may be orange, purple, red and yellow. Purple peppers may lose their color when cooked. According to my research, green peppers are the immature stage of the vegetable.

BERRIES: If you're *watching your weight*, try eating some berries. Berries are low calorie - low fat sweets, that have hardly any sodium, a great source of potassium and *supplies fiber that helps you absorb fewer of the calories that you do eat*. Berries are also an aid in the improvement of your blood pressure. A cup of strawberries has the lowest count of only 45 calories and a cup of blueberries has the highest count of 81 calories. The calorie count for raspberries and blackberries fall in between these two very tasty treats. Berries have natural fructose sugar to satisfy your sweet-craving, therefore an *aid to weight-loss!*

Did you know blueberries are a common Swedish folk remedy for diarrhea? In Sweden, dried blueberry soup has been used by physicians to treat childhood diarrhea. According to Finn Sandberg, professor of pharmacology at Uppsala Biomedical Center in Sweden, 05 to 10 grams (1/3 of an ounce) of dried blueberries is the dosage for diarrhea. Why do blueberries work so well against diarrhea? Blueberries contain high concentrations of compounds that KILL both bacteria and viruses! In Canadian tests, crushed blueberries destroyed nearly 100 percent of polio viruses within 24 hours, even when the blueberries were diluted 10 times!

According to Dr. Amr Abdel-Fattah Ismail, formerly a plant physiologist with the United States Department of Agriculture and now vice-president of the Maine Wild Blueberry Company, states that blueberry soup is a popular cold remedy on the European ski slopes.

BINGE EATING: According to Adam Drewnowski, Ph.D., director of the Human Nutrition Program at the University of Michigan in Ann Arbor, Michigan, there are usually two triggers to an eating binge: *"Either you're on a diet and your body needs the extra food or you overeat because you're trying to suppress some emotional-stress, loneliness, depression or anger."*

Form an *Antibinge Hotline* of at least six friends you can call when you're lonely or bored says Dr. Scher, Ph.D., director of training for the Graduate Hospital Eating Disorders Service in Philadelphia.

BLOATING FOODS: According to Dr. Elson M. Haas, author of *"The False Fat Diet,"* says that certain foods make you look fat. They bloat you up, puff you up,... You'll look larger than you really are in the chin, hips, stomach, thighs,... He calls these bloating foods the "Sensitive Seven" which are corn, dairy products, eggs, peanuts, soy, sugar and wheat. Get his book to better understand the *"Sensitive Seven."*

BODY MASS INDEX (BMI): What is Body Mass Index (BMI)? Below is the formula to measure your body fat.

ARE YOU OBESE?
BODY MASS INDEX (BMI) FORMULA

How to calculate your own BMI.

STEP ONE: Multiply your weight in pounds by 0.45 to get kilograms.
Example: 140 pounds X .45 = 63 kilograms.

STEP TWO: Multiply your height in inches by 0.025 to get meters.
Example: 67 inches X 0.025 = 1.675 meters

STEP THREE: Square the answer in STEP TWO to get your height measurement in meters.
Example: 1.675 X 1.675 = 2.805

STEP FOUR: Divide your weight in kg (STEP ONE) by your height in meters (STEP THREE).
Example: 63 divided by 2.805 = 22.45.

RESULTS AND RECOMMENDATIONS: A BMI of 19 to 25 is healthy.
A BMI of 27 to 30 means you are at risk and it is advisable to lose weight (see your doctor).

NOTE: BMI is a standard measure of body fat used to monitor obesity.

BREAD: Whole grain bread provides approximately 70 calories per slice. Bread is a natural source of fiber and complex carbohydrates and provides protein. **Bread itself isn't fattening, it's the butter, cream cheese, margarine, mayonnaise... that you put on it. Bread can be an aid to weight-loss!** According to Dr. Bjarne Jacobsen, a Norwegian scientist, people that ate less than two slices of bread on a daily basis, weighed 11 pounds more than big bread eaters. According to researchers at Michigan State University, some **breads actually reduce your appetite!** Students who ate 12 slices of dark, high-fiber bread (pumpernickel, whole wheat, mixed grain, oatmeal,...) **lost five pounds in two months** compared to students who **ate white bread** who were hungrier, ate more fattening foods and **lost no weight!**

WARNING: It is noted that one fake food is white flour. Approximately 98% of bread, pancakes, pastries, spaghetti, are made with white flour. Some of these products are caramel colored to make you think you are eating 100% whole wheat products. READ the ingredients or make your own bread, pancakes, pasta... READ the important data below!

According to a special report from Vita-Mix, compared to whole wheat, **white bread is missing**:

* 72% of chromium   * 78% of Vitamin B-6
* 78% of dietary fiber   * 96% of Vitamin E
* 50% of folic acid   * 62% of Zinc
* 72% of magnesium   * many phytochemicals

The **missing nutrients in white bread are critical** to:
- **appetite control**
- cell communication
- fetal brain development
- immune function
- preventing free radicals
- and 500 other body functions

BREATHING: Breathing helps burn calories. When you exercise not only are you revving-up your metabolism, working all your muscles, you're breathing. That oxygen is like a fuel for the fire to help burn the fat. Just like a real fire, your body needs, heat - fuel - and oxygen to burn fat - you gotta breathe. One lady (forgot her name) on TV Infomercials, offers a weight-loss program using exercise in conjunction with deep breathing exercises. See *Special Breathing Exercise* and *High Altitude Weight-Loss Diet*.

BROCCOLI: Did you know broccoli is America's favorite vegetable? One stalk of cooked broccoli furnishes only 45 calories and .2 grams of fat. According to the U.S. Department of Agriculture, broccoli is the **leading source of dietary fiber**, packed with potassium, provides Vitamin B, low in fat and even calcium (for strong bones and teeth). Broccoli is noted for its cancer-fighting properties (chemoprotectant). Broccoli may be the number one cancer-fighting vegetable. Researchers at Johns Hopkins of Medicine in Baltimore have isolated a 'chemoprotectant' substance called sulforaphane which has been identified in broccoli. Sulforaphane may be the most potent cancer protecting agent to date!

Sulforaphane actually stimulates the body's cells to produce cancer fighting enzymes. Other cancer-fighting chemicals are indoles, carotene and Vitamin C. Broccoli is noted to help **flush fat** out of your system.

BROMELAIN: Bromelain is a natural enzyme found in pineapples. This nutrient increases the body's ability to **break down fats and protein promoting body metabolism!** See Pineapples. *Follow the recommended dosage and instructions from the label and as per your doctor's instructions.*

BRUSSELS SPROUTS: One-half cup of raw Brussels sprouts provide only twenty calories while one-half cup of cooked Brussels sprouts provides 30 calories. A member of the cruciferous vegetable family (broccoli, cabbage, cauliflower), Brussels sprouts can fill you up and help you **lose weight**. A cooked cup of this tasty treat is rich in Vitamin C, provides a good share of Vitamin A, iron, potassium, riboflavin and rich in protein. Brussels sprouts are very **low in fat** and sodium and provide fiber.

Brussels sprouts are a good bet to inhibit cancer, especially colon and stomach cancer. According to Dr. Saxon Graham's 1978 study in Buffalo, New York, Brussels sprouts emerged (along with cabbage and broccoli) as **outstanding in saving lives from colon cancer!**

According to a study in Norway, eating more cruciferous vegetables, including Brussels sprouts may **suppress the precancerous growths** in the colon called polyps in which cancer initially surfaces. Brussels sprouts and other cruciferous vegetables may also **cut the risk of bladder, esophageal, lung, rectal, stomach and rectal cancer!**

BRUSSELS SPROUTS TASTY RECIPE: Here's my quick recipe for Brussels sprouts. I normally don't eat or like the taste of Brussels sprouts till I cooked em' up this way.

Ingredients: 24 Brussels sprouts, sharp knife, frying pan, coconut oil, bowl, fork, sea salt and wooden spoon.

Step 01: Take a frying pan put it on one of your burners at medium heat.

Step 02: Immediately and spoon-out 05 good oversized scoops of coconut oil (will be semi-solid at room temperature) and put them in the frying pan and wait till the coconut oil starts sizzle.

Step 03: Procure 24 Brussels sprouts and cut off the base (stalk) of each of them. Then remove 03 or 04 outer leaves (debris,…) and place them in the frying pan.

Step 04: Every couple minutes or so, gently stir the Brussels sprouts in the frying pan with your wooden spoon till they are all golden brown.

Step 05: Remove to Brussels sprouts to a bowl and sprinkle them with sea salt. Fork-in and enjoy with a cold bottle of beer.

Note: I tried cooking the Brussels sprouts with other oils but coconut oil is the tastiest and it's a Medium-Chain Triglyceride (MTC) meaning it helps you burn fat far better than other oils that aren't MTCs. See *Coconut Oil*.

CABBAGE: One cup of raw, coarsely shredded cabbage furnishes only 15 calories, while a cup of cooked cabbage is only 29 calories, .1 gram of fat and is low in sodium. Raw cabbage is high in Vitamin C and potassium. Cabbage is known to **reduce the risk of cancer** of the gastrointestinal and respiratory tracts. Cabbage **stimulates the immune system and kills bacteria and viruses**. Cabbage is also noted to help **flush fat out off your system**. Cabbage also **prevents and heals ulcers** according to studies at Stanford University School of Medicine.

This same study found that a quart of cabbage juice a day **healed ulcers 83% faster** than standard treatments producing results in three weeks or less. These same benefits of cabbage can be found in other cabbage vegetables like Brussels sprouts (miniature cabbage), cauliflower, turnips, kale, broccoli, Chinese broccoli and Chinese cabbage. Studies in Greece, Japan and the United States have indicated that people who eat the most cabbage not only have the **least colon cancer** but also have the **lowest death rates**.

According to A.M. Liebstein, M.D. *"cabbage is therapeutically effective in conditions of asthma, cancer, diseases of the eyes, gangrene, gout, pyorrhea, rheumatism, scurvy, tuberculosis... Cabbage is excellent as a vitalizing agent, blood purifier and anti-scorbutic."*

In 1931, a German scientist experimenting with deadly radiation noted that rabbits **survived a lethal dose of radiation** if they ate cabbage leaves prior to exposure. French scientist came to the same conclusion during 1950 studies. In 1959, 02 United States Armed Forces researchers fed diced raw cabbage (with broccoli & beets) to guinea pigs before and after giving them 400 rads of deadly whole body X radiation. All the guinea pigs that were not fed vegetables died within 15 days and **more than half of those guinea pigs pre-fed vegetables survived!** The guinea pigs that were fed vegetables after the radiation exposure lived longer. It was concluded that those guinea pigs fed cabbage and broccoli before and after their exposure to radiation were the **most likely to survive**. Beets proved to have no effect.

CANDIDA YEAST: Are you always **sick, tired and overweigh?** It may be an unknown problem called candida yeast or candida albicans. Candida yeast are single cell fungi that cause disease.

They live in your body like your intestines and throughout your digestive tract. When out of control, candida yeast is linked to bloating, fatigue, indigestion, joint pain, painful menstruation,... When candida yeast is permitted to multiply, they emit toxins that circulate everywhere and cause sickness even **weight gain**. When yeast grows uncontrollably your immune system is on major defense trying to protect you. But in the war between your defending immune system and the candida yeast, your immune system is weakened which may cause you to become even more sick.

What causes candida yeast to grow uncontrollably? Why are people sick, tired and overweight? Causes are:
- Standard American Diet (processed - refined foods)
- Refined foods rich in sugar and yeast
- Birth control pills
- Antibiotic drugs (kills good bacteria)
- Weakened immune system
- Pregnancy
- Hormonal changes

So what can one do to fight candida yeast infection? Yeast thrives on foods made with yeast like breads, processed foods that have sugar and flour and preserved foods like cheese (mold). So change your diet like:

- STAY AWAY from processed foods.
- EAT fresh fruits.
- EAT fresh vegetables (no mushrooms - fungi).
- EAT fish (low fat).
- EAT chicken (low fat).
- EAT eggs (no sugar).
- DO NOT ABUSE antibiotics.

See your doctor and get the book *The Yeast Connection* by William G. Crook, M.D. And yiu must see Apple Cider Vinegar, Coconut Juices & Slices and Coconut Oil.

CAN OF SARDINES: Sardines in oil are one of my favorite tasty foods and they may be a great aid to help your weight-loss goals. Here's a quote from Muscle Mag (December 2009): *"heavyweight when it comes to omega-3 fatty acids. These 'phat' fats have been found to **stimulate fat burning** so you drop more blubber, and they aid in fending off a range of diseases almost biblical in scope - cancer, diabetes, Alzheimer's and heart disease, to name a few. Best of all they're ridiculously cheap."*

I love sardines and here are the 03 brands that I eat:

- Beach Cliff Sardines (in soybean oil) (no carbohydrates & no sugars)

- Brunswick Sardines (in olive oil) (no carbohydrates & no sugars)

- King Oscar (in extra virgin olive oil) (no carbohydrates & no sugars)

Note: A can of sardines has a long shelf life of approximately 05-years, so stock-up when they go on sale.

CAPSICUM (CAYENNE): Herbal parts are taken from berries and fruits. It acts as a catalyst for herbs and provides apsaicine, capsacutin, capsaicin, capsanthine, capsico, PABA & Vitamins A, B1, B2, B3, B5, B6, B9, C (rich source), E, ascorbic acid, calcium, dihydrocapsaicin, homocapsaicin, homodihydrocapsaicin, iron, magnesium, phosphorus, potassium, selenium, sulphur and zinc. Capsicum is the source of over 100 varieties of Cayenne Pepper, from heat ranges of mild paprika to the extremely hot habanera. It's been used for **medicinal purposes for thousands of years!** Capsicum aids digestion, improves circulation and stops bleeding from ulcers.

It is noted to also be good for the kidneys, lungs, spleen, pancreas, heart and stomach. It's also noted to help remedy chronic fatigue, depression, gastric ulcers and prostration. Skin ointments that contain capsaicin have been noted to significantly **relieve the pain of arthritis, herpes zoster and diabetic neuropathy** (causes pain and tingling in the legs). Capsaicin is noted to deplete Substance-P, a neuropeptide produced by the nerves that carry pain sensation. You'll find many new pain-relieving products on the market containing capsicum-capsaicin! Most herbalist have noted that cayenne pepper **stops bleeding!**

Below is a list of capsicum and their measurements in Scoville Heat Units (SHU). Most actual cayenne pepper is rated between 30,000 to 80,000 Scoville Heat Units. Cayenne just refers to one variety of capsicum. ALL hot peppers are capsicum.
- Paprika - 0 Scoville Heat Units.
- Jalapeno - 50,000 to 80,000 Scoville Heat Units.
- Serrano - 100,000 Scoville Heat Units.
- African Bird - 200,000 Scoville Heat Units.
- Mexican Habaneras - 250,000 to 300,000 Scoville Heat Units (*HOT!!!*).

Researchers in Great Britain and Japan have found that **cayenne can cause the body to burn up to 25% more calories in a day** than it normally would!

Cayenne has the ability to deplete a chemical in the pain-transmission nerves known as Substance-P. That is why you'll see amazing products from companies in POC Section that have capsaicin as one of the ingredients.

Cayenne is being tested as an **all-around analgesic-painkiller!** According to Thomas Barks, Ph.D., head of the Department of Pharmacology at the University of Arizona Health Sciences Center in Tucson, a single injection of capsaicin **fights certain types of chronic pain** in guinea pigs for weeks! Rubbing an ointment of capsaicin on the skin, actually **numbs the pain locally!**

In his book, "**Left for Dead**," Richard Quinn the author, relates a **fascinating true story**. He was struck with a heart attack which was followed by bypass surgery. The bypass surgery was supposed to "make him as good as new." Well it didn't, and his cardiologist stated, "there is nothing more we can do." After months of moping, Richard Quinn took some advice from a friend. Richard **purchased only 69 cents of cayenne pepper (red)**, filled several capsules and swallowed them! The very next morning, Richard Quinn got up and shoveled 04 feet of wet snow off his 28-foot porch! That happened in 1980. Richard Quinn studied the medicinal values of herbs and *launched his own company* "Heart Foods Company Inc." **Read** Richard Quinn's book, "Left for Dead" at your local library, purchase it at your local bookstore or order it from R.F. Quinn Publishing Company by going to   http://www.cayennecompany.com His book is packed with information on cayenne pepper and other herbs.

The Thais (Thailand) use capsicum chili peppers as a seasoning and as an appetizer with their meals. Their blood is infused with chili pepper compounds several times a day. Thais physicians have for some time credited regular consumption of chili peppers as the reason that thromboembolism (**life-threatening blood clots**) **are** <u>rare</u> **among Thais compared to Americans!**

German researchers as early as 1965 found chili peppers beneficial for the blood as a fibrinolytic (clot-dissolving) stimulant. After more testing, Sukoon Visudhiphan, M.D. and his colleagues at the Siriraj Hospital in Bangkok suggested that the frequent stimulation of the clot-dissolving mechanism by chili peppers helps **keep the Thais immune to thromboembolism (life-threatening blood clots)!** SEE Heart Foods Company Inc., Sato Pharmaceutical, American Botanical Pharmacy, Blessed Herbs, Frontier Cooperative Herbs, Starwest Botanicals Inc., and *University of Natural Healing Inc.*, in the POC Section.

WARNING: Eating great quantities of capsaicin\cayenne is not advised for those suffering from ulcers and hemorrhoids. Eating high amounts of chili pepper by men in India was linked to a 1987 study to higher rates of cancer of the oral cavity, esophagus, larynx and pharynx.

However, according to Dr. Terry Laesione, University of Nebraska Medical Center, small doses of capsaicin actually act as antioxidants to block cell damage and may help prevent cancer. High doses and low doses of the same chemical may have the opposite effect in fighting cancer. *Follow the recommended dosage and instructions from the label and as per your doctor's instructions.*

CARBOHYDRATES VERSUS PROTEIN DIETS: The diet war between carbs and protein has been going on since the 1970s. Which is the better diet? A high protein (carbohydrate restrictive diet) or a carbohydrate diet (fruits & vegetables)? Here's my personal answer: See the *"$10,000.00 Weight-Loss Bet"* and the *"Raw Food Diet."*

CARROTS: Carrots are one of the most flavorful and lowest priced foods available. A cup of shredded raw carrots furnishes only 48 calories while a cup of sliced cooked carrots provide 70 calories. A medium sized carrot furnishes only .1 gram of fat and only 25 milligrams of sodium. A source of Vitamin A and a moderate amount of Vitamin C, carrots are a potential for **preventing cancer**. According to several dozen studies, a high carotene intake has the potential to **prevent cancers** of the lung, esophagus, stomach, intestines, mouth, throat, bladder and prostate. Carrots are a good source of potassium and high in soluble fiber.

An exciting aspect of carrots is their promise in **curtailing some of the most deadly, incurable cancers, notably of the lung and pancreas**. According to a 1986 Swedish study, carrots were designated as one of two prominent dietary barriers to pancreatic cancer and the other was citrus fruits. It was noted that eating carrots "almost daily" substantially **cut the chances of cancer of the pancreas**.

According to a study, by a team of researchers at State University of Buffalo, New York, noted that men eating the most high carotene foods, including carrots, were about **half as likely to develop squamous cell lung cancer**. They concluded the difference between high risk and low risk is only one carrot! According to Dr. Menkes, eating just one carrot a day might **prevent 15,000 to 20,000 lung cancer deaths each year** in the United States! Even after years of smoking, **carrots may ease the cancer threat** by simply retarding the disease progression.

According to a study in New Jersey by National Cancer Institute epidemiologist Dr. Regina G. Ziegler, three vegetables surfaced in preventing lung cancer - carrots, sweet potatoes and dark-yellow winter squash. Dr. Regina G. Ziegler discovered that men who ate a half a cup of carrots or sweet potatoes or winter squash a day, were **half as likely to develop lung cancer** compared to those who hardly ate any of the vegetables.

She also found that **non-smoking women exposed to cigarette smoke could slash their risk of lung cancer by eating more carrots!** See Smoker's Body Starts Healing Itself and other Smoking POCs in the POC Section.

WARNING: Carrots are very good for you, but if you've been snacking on these tasty treats to lose weight, then read this: Eating carrots may **raise the blood sugar too high**, raising the insulin level so you want to eat more and more! So take it easy on the orange rabbit food!

CAULIFLOWER: Cauliflower is a bit more costly but worth it when it comes to your health. One cup of raw cauliflower furnishes only 31 calories, provides a good source of Vitamin C (one cup equals 100% of RDA) low in sodium and low in fat. Cauliflower is noted to help **flush fat** out of your system. Cauliflower is one of the vegetables **recognized by the Committee on Diet, Nutrition and Cancer of the National Academy of Sciences** as one of the **best bets for preventing cancer!** Cauliflower has established itself as being high on the list of anticancer vegetables. A close cousin to cabbage, broccoli and Brussels sprouts - all of these vegetables are linked to lower cancer rates, especially of the colon, rectum, stomach and possibly the bladder and prostate. Norwegians who eat their fair share of cauliflower (along with broccoli, Brussels sprouts & cabbage), have fewer and smaller precancerous polyps of the colon.

According to a study by Dr. Lee Wattenberg, laboratory animals were fed cauliflower and then given powerful carcinogens like nitrosamines. The animals that ate cauliflower did not readily develop cancers as those animals that didn't eat cauliflower.

CELLULAR HEALING: The cell is the basic unit of all living things. Many **HEALING ASPECTS** that you read throughout this book **BEGAN AT THE CELLULAR LEVEL!** Through proper nutrition, exercise, supplements, your thoughts and other treatments (alternative and conventional), **YOUR BODY HAS THE ABILITY TO HEAL ITSELF!** Read this statement 25 more times right now - you must BELIEVE **your magnificent body has the ability to heal itself** for **weight-loss** and many other healings throughout your body. OK. ready that statement 25 more times before we move on.

We'll take a closer look at this remarkable working miracle! This single unit of life has its own organization and function.

* The nucleus of the cell is the command headquarters for the entire unit. Imagine this if you can - messages encoded within the nucleus of each cell would require 3,000 volumes of books, with each book having 1,000 pages, with each page having 1,000 words!

- Each cell can replicate itself to an exact likeness. When a cell is worn-out or aged, it will self-destruct.

- Each cell has an energy factory called the mitochondria. The mitochondria manufacture all the energy it needs to live and do its work.

- Each cell also has a protein manufacturing plant called the endothelial reticulum.

- Each cell has a storage warehouse called the golgi body. The golgi body stores the manufactured product until it is needed.

- Each cell has a sentry or security force. The security force allows only that substance that is needed to enter the cell interior and lets waste material exit the cell.

Now do you understand the importance of proper nutrition, exercise, and an overall healthy lifestyle. One more time, **YOUR BODY HAS THE ABILITY TO HEAL ITSELF!**

Now let's get back to your shallow breathing. Notice your breathing right now as you read this. YOU'RE A SHALLOW BREATHER! You're taking in only 20% of the oxygen you could take in if you weren't a shallow breather! And think of what all that EXTRA GOOD OXYGEN will do for YOU at the cellular level!

Remember you have 100,000,000,000,000 cells in your body right now and all are aching for that precious fuel- oxygen! And they're all trying so hard to keep you healthy. With the proper nutrition, supplements, exercise, OXYGEN, and thoughts, your body has the inherent ability to heal itself!

When you take in extra oxygen and hold it in your lungs for 15 - 20 seconds or more, that vital nutritious oxygen goes to your lungs and the oxygen is passed on to the blood running throughout your lungs. But now that blood has more nutritious oxygen than it's had in a long time. The cells throughout your body are dilated and hungry waiting for more of the same precious fuel - oxygen. That vital fuel fires-up every cell in your body which reflects INCREASED ENERGY and may have a beneficial side-effect of weight loss and other healing benefits!

Another healing fact you have to know about deep breathing is that it's aerobic breathing. Aerobic meaning an injection of more oxygen into your body to stimulate blood circulation. Most folks know the word aerobic from vigorous exercise. Vigorous exercise noted to **speed up the metabolism to lose weight.** But with deep breathing you get the same aerobic injection of oxygen without the vigorous sweating exercise of running 03 miles, jazzercise, calisthenics, stair-stepping... So do your aerobics while watching TV! See *Special Breathing Exercise.*

CHERRIES: A cup of sweet red cherries furnishes only 82 calories, whereas a cup of sour red cherries furnishes only 52 calories. Cherries may be a <u>**great diet aid**</u>. If you enjoy sweets, substitute that 300 calorie candy bar with cherries that will not only satisfy your sweet tooth but fill you up. Cherries are a good source of Vitamin A, low in sodium, a modest fiber content for your heart and no fat.

According to a 1950 writing by Ludwig Blau, Ph.D., in the Texas Reports on Biology and Medicine, claimed he **cured his crippling gout that confined him to a wheelchair by eating 06 to 08 cherries each day!** He noted that as long as he ate cherries, the **gout stayed away!** He also annotated that **12 others who suffered from gout** also ate or drank cherry juice and they **were also completely free of gout!**

Prevention magazine printed Ludwig Blaus's advice and **testimonials started to pour in** to *Prevention* magazine! Many wrote and said initially consuming 15 to 20 red or black cherries a day then 10 a day after that worked to remedy their affliction with gout!

According to a study at Forsyth Dental Center, cherry juice to be **a potent antibacterial agent against tooth decay!** They noted that black cherry juice blocked 80 percent of the enzyme activity leading to plaque formation which is the groundwork to tooth decay.

Note: I was raised eating cherries straight of the cherry trees in our yard - Mmmmmmmm!!!!

CHICKEN: Eat chicken instead of high fat and high cholesterol red meat. 04 ounces of cooked white meat provide only 245 calories, while dark meat provides 285 calories. Chicken has **far less fat and cholesterol than a T-bone steak**, but is equal in protein. Cook with the skin on the chicken but DO NOT EAT THE SKIN (too much fat).

WARNING: Chickens are a great money-maker. To insure those pecking chickens grow as fast as possible, some chicken farms may introduce chemicals to the chickens so they weigh the most in the least amount of time. These chemicals are passed on to the consumer - YOU! Before you purchase that poultry, investigate where and how it was raised. You might be better off buying your chicken meat from a small poultry farmer who has no need to pump his chickens up with hormones and chemicals! You'll probably save some money too!

CHINESE DIET: Chinese consume 300 more calories per day than Americans, yet they have **lower rates of obesity**, heart disease and cancer. What's their secret? The Chinese diet consist of high fiber, non-fat, antioxidant-rich fruits and vegetables which is only 15% of calories from fat. This diet reflects their **low rates** of cancer, heart disease and **obesity**. The Chinese also exercise a great deal more than Americans. While Americans are driving or riding everywhere they go, even very short distances, Chinese are bicycling everywhere they go!

WARNING: Don't be fooled by the Chinese restaurants in the United States. Many do not serve the healthy, authentic Chinese foods found in China. Ask for nutritional facts of each meal before you order! See Chinese Restaurant Syndrome in Doctor Words.

CHITOSAN: Chitosan comes from the shells of crabs, shrimp,... and is noted to attract fat molecules. Chitosan can attract up to 04-times its own weight in fat which prevents the fat from the food you eat from being digested by your body. Chitosan acts like a magnet to absorb fat. If you consider chitosan (non-prescription) as a supplement, insure you get an authentic product and insure you see your doctor. See *Chromium Picolinate* and *Conjugated Linoleic Acid*.

CHROMIUM PICOLINATE: Chromium picolinate is an essential trace mineral which facilitates the action of insulin, glucose and protein and fat metabolism. Chromium picolinate is noted to enhance the body's sensitivity to insulin and may reduce blood glucose levels thus reducing complications from diabetes. **This micronutrient may help ameliorate a diabetic condition!**

Chromium enhances the body's sensitivity to insulin (a hormone that helps metabolize sugar). Chromium has been noted to reduce complications from diabetes by lowering blood glucose levels by 18% and glycosylated hemoglobin by 10%.

Chromium has been noted to **stimulate fat loss!** Chromium may do this by having an effect on the satiety center of the hypothalamus which is part of the brain that signals that you're full and no longer need to eat anything else. Chromium also seems to enhance the thermogenic effects of carbohydrate foods. Chromium also tends to **build muscle mass at the expense of fat!**

Chromium may enhance thermogenic reactions by activating the sympathetic nervous system, which **increases caloric burning**.
Follow the recommended dosage and instructions from the label and as per your doctor's instructions.

CITRUS AURANTIUM: Do you like Seville oranges? Well those small tasty oranges have an ingredient in them that may support your weight-loss plan. The unique ingredient is called citrus aurantium. Citrus aurantium tells the fat cells to speed-up their release from fat storage. Citrus aurantium also helps boost the metabolism and the growth of muscle cells. Remember the more muscle you have the more calories you'll burn. See Muscles.

COCONUT JUICE & SLICES: According to **Cookycoconuts.com**, nutritional values change as the coconut matures. Move aside Gatoraide - for the liquid inside the coconut is coconut water or called coconut juice and is one of the **HIGHEST sources of electrolytes on Earth**. Electrolytes are ionized salts in blood, tissue fluids and cells including salts of sodium and potassium. A substance that can conduct electricity when it is in solution. So? So what? We need electrolytes because our entire body is an electrical system and we need those electrolytes to keep us performing at our best whether we're running in a marathon or sitting behind a desk.

And the coconut juice is consumed to prevent dehydration, and is used in some areas of the world to hydrate casualties via intravenous tubes and needles.

The fresh white coconut meat is protein rich and loaded with coconut oil. Coconut oil is rich in what is called lauric acid which is found in Mother's milk. Lauric acid has anti-bacteria, anti-fungal, and anti-viral agents.

The super healthy fresh coconut oil and fresh white meat have a laundry list of super healthy benefits like:

- Anti-Bacteria
- Anti-Fungal
- Anti-Viral
- Candida Albicans
- Chronic Fatigue
- Chron's Disease
- Diabetes
- Digestive Disorders
- Energy Booster
- Heart Disease
- IBS (Irritable Bowel Syndrome
- Immune System Booster
- Lowers Cholesterol
- Metabolism Booster
- Rejuvenate Skin
- Thyroid Function
- Weight-Loss
- Wrinkles

Bottom line, now you know plenty of good reasons to mix plenty of fresh coconut slices in your trial-mix.

Note: *Cookycoconuts.com* recommends the best brand coconut oil is Tropical Traditions. See Tropical Traditions in the POC Section. See Coconut Oil below.

COCONUT OIL: Coconut oil got a bad rap years ago. Sixty-five percent of coconut oil's saturated fat is mostly made up of medium-chain triglycerides (MCTs). Populations like Polynesian Puka Puka and Tokelau islanders that consume most of their fat from coconut oil have **low rates of heart disease!** See MCT in Doctor Words.

Coconut oil (MCT), unlike other oils, is less likely to attribute to obesity. Why? Your body easily converts coconut oil into energy rather than depositing calories as body fat.

Coconut oil also *kills germs!* It contains anti-microbial components like mother's milk. The Polynesian Puku Puku and Tokelau islanders live in an environment ideal for parasites. There protected from parasites by the coconut oil in their diet.

It may be wise to avoid processed products like margarine, chips, cookies... that have trans-fatty acids. According to a study Dr. Walter Willett, of Harvard University, **trans-fatty acids double the risk of heart attack**. Trans-fatty acids may also contribute to **cancer, diabetes and obesity**. Read the contents before you purchase the product. Look for **"partially hydrogenated oils." If you read this, AVOID IT!** See Omega Nutrition.

COENZYME Q10 (COQ10): If you're tired of feeling sick & tired all the time, may be something as simple as a single supplement may be the answer - it's called Coenzyme Q10 (CoQ10). As you age, your Q10 levels diminish. If you had no Q10 in your body, you'd be dead real quick. The point in this segment is to make you aware of this very special supplement so you can get your vibrant energy back so you can achieve your weight-loss goals. OK, let me tell you about CoQ10.

CoQ10 was discovered in 1957 by Fred Crane, M.D., from the University of Wisconsin. He isolated CoQ10 from beef hearts. CoQ10 is a Vitamin-like substance that resembles Vitamin E which may be more powerful as an antioxidant. Of the 10 common coenzyme Qs, only CoQ10 is found in human tissue. CoQ10 declines with age and should be supplemented in the diet. CoQ10 plays a crucial role in the **effectiveness of the immune system and the aging process!**

The New England Institute reports that *CoQ10* alone is effective in **reducing mortality** in experimental animals afflicted with tumors and leukemia. It's noted that *CoQ10* may be helpful in the **complete remission** of many cancers!

In Japan, *CoQ10* is being used in the **treatment of heart disease, high blood pressure and enhance the immune system!**

Research has revealed that **CoQ10 benefits** allergies, asthma, and respiratory disease as well as treating the brain for anomalies of mental function associated with Alzheimer's Disease and schizophrenia. The amazing *CoQ10* is also beneficial in **aging, candidiasis, diabetes, multiple sclerosis, periodontal disease and obesity**. **AIDS** is a primary target for research on CoQ10 because of its **immense benefits to the immune system**. The use of *CoQ10* is a major step forward in the **prevention and control of cancer**.

Use caution when purchasing CoQ10 because not all products are offered in its purest form. CoQ10's **natural color is bright yellow\orange** and has very little taste in the powdered form. CoQ10 should be kept away from heat and light since pure CoQ10 will deteriorate in temperatures above 115 degrees Fahrenheit. Sources of CoQ10 are mackerel, salmon and those tasty sardines. **Sardines contain the largest amounts of CoQ10.** See *Can Of Sardines*.

One study published in the American Journal of Cardiology (1985), 150mg of CoQ10 taken daily by heart patients for 04 weeks **reduced the incidence of angina attacks** from 5.3 to 2.5 per day. The researchers concluded that CoQ10 actually **strengthened the diseased heart**, which allowed it to reach higher levels of energy before pain or oxygen deprivation occurs.

In another study published in the American Journal of Cardiology 1990, a long-term study of 126 patients with severe cardiomyopathy that took supplements of CoQ10 **prolonged their lives by years**, not weeks or months - YEARS! In some patients the **disease was eliminated entirely!**

Other published studies have noted that *CoQ10* helps a wide variety of illnesses, including AIDS, cancer, chronic fatigue, periodontal disease... See *Institute For Vibrant Living* in POC Section.

WARNING: To date, no side-affects have been documented. Insure you purchase **authentic CoQ10**. Some companies put dyes in their **fake** CoQ10 to achieve the orange color that is found naturally in pure CoQ10!
Follow the recommended dosage and instructions from the label and as per your doctor's instructions.

COLD WATER CURES: If there is one thing I hate more than 08-legged spiders, it's cold frigid water. I can still hold my own when it comes to cold weather to include being soaking wet with cold water (surface or submerged) but I just have a lot of *"Art Of Suffering"* memories when it comes to cold water. Anyway, did you know plain ol' cold water has some very beneficial effects?

According to Gurudev Khar Khalsa, a noted Sat Nam Rasayan Healer and Kundalini Yoga Teacher from Los Angeles, California: *"Cold Water Massage Therapy is one of the healthiest and most inexpensive of therapies. Simply massage the body with almond oil before taking a shower. Shower in cold water until your body temperature rises and no longer feels cold, but toasty and warm. Make sure the bathroom is heated. Never get out of a cold shower into a cold room."*

And here's list maladies remedied by cold water and complimentary benefits of taking cold showers - Brrrrr:

- Acne
- Allergies
- Anxiety Attacks
- Asthma
- Awake
- Blood Cholesterol Lower
- Blood Circulation
- Blood Pressure Reduced
- Blood Sugar Lowered
- Body Feels Warmer
- Body Odor Eliminated
- Calming Effect
- Cleanses Circulatory System
- Clearer Mind
- Complexion
- Concentration Improvement
- Depression Eliminated
- Dry Skin
- Eliminates Poisons & Toxins
- Energy
- Feelings Of Euphoria
- Five Senses Improved
- Flushes Organs
- Focus Improvement
- Hair Improvement
- Headaches Eliminated
- Heart Problems
- Heightened Awareness
- Immune System Booster
- Learning Improvement
- Less\No Colds
- Less\No Flu
- Leg Bloating\Pain,...
- Libido Improvement
- Mental Faculties Improved

- Migraines Eliminated
- Mood Improvement
- Muscle Cramps
- Pain
- Panic Attacks
- Positive Thoughts
- Pulse Rate Lower
- Rashes
- Refreshed
- Skin Improvement
- Sinusitis
- Sleep Improvement
- Strengthens Nervous System
- Strengthens Mucous Membranes
- Stress Buster (see *Stress Busters*)
- Sweating Reduced
- Utility Bill Reduced
- Zest For Life

I've told you before that the **BLOOD RULES!** It's apparent to me that cold showers get the blood moving thus the many benefits of plain ol' Cold Water Cures!

CONJUGATED LINOLEIC ACID (CLA): CLA is a fatty acid that's opening eyes in the medical field. CLA helps you to a healthier body in different ways. CLA helps reduce the risk of cancer, heart disease and asthma. CLA is an antioxidant. CLA helps boost the immune system. CLA not only **helps burn fat** it also helps build muscle. And the best news is CLA can be found at your local drug store as an over-the counter supplement.

COTTAGE CHEESE: One-half cup of cottage cheese provides approximately 84 to 120 calories depending on the brand you purchase. Insure that you purchase cottage cheese that is 01 to 02 percent milk fat. Cottage cheese provides a healthy source of calcium, Vitamin B, and riboflavin and is a great **weight-loss food**. Try whipping cottage cheese instead of using cream cheese. Use cottage cheese for all sorts of recipes instead of fat-laden sour cream or cream cheese.

Note: If you want a sweet rewarding treat, try adding a few tablespoons of pure maple syrup to a cup of cottage cheese. I've ate this sweet treat since I was a kid. The great taste will SURPRISE you.

COUGH DROPS: Here's a neat trick to cut calories, fat and unnecessary carbohydrates when you get that strong craving to eat. Drop a cough drop in your mouth. But not any cough drop. Cough drops that have menthol - eucalyptus have been noted to **stop that craving** to eat those snacks you really shouldn't be eating.

COUNT TO 20: 20 minutes that is! Why? Next time you get a food craving, make yourself wait 20 minutes. Most food cravings that **aren't due to hunger** will subside in 20 minutes. If after 20 minutes, you still feel hungry, drink plenty of clean water and EAT THE RIGHT STUFF! Walking and other vigorous exercise has been noted to kill food cravings.

CUTTING FAT & CALORIES IN COOKING:
- Trim fat before cooking.
- Roast or broil meat on a rack.
- Brown meat, then drain fat before continuing to cook in pan.
- Remove fat (skim from top) from stews or soups after chilling.
- Use low fat cooking methods such as bake, broil, microwave, roast, stir-fry or braise.

DETOXIFICATION THERAPY: Detoxification Therapy aids to **rid the body of chemicals and pollutants and can expedite a return to health**. Forms of Detoxification Therapy include, Colon Therapy, Hydrotherapy, Hyperthermia, Fasting, Juice Therapy, Massage... See Fasting.

DHEA (DEHYDEROEPIANDROSTERONE): DHEA has been seen on **"CNN" and even CBS' 60 Minutes!** Researchers at the University of Wisconsin wrote, *"The role DHEA plays in aging and disease is perhaps the greatest discovery of this century!"* It is probably the **best all-purpose anti-aging** therapy in the world! DHEA is noted to be the most abundant hormone in the blood stream.

Its concentrations drastically increase during puberty and then sharply decrease after age 25. Scientific research validates its many benefits in **treating obesity**, acting **against tumors**, **cardiovascular disease** and many other catastrophic illnesses. There have been over 4,000 published articles involving the use of DHEA.

Miraculously your body converts DHEA into whatever hormone is needed to maintain balance such as estrogen, testosterone, progesterone and cortisone. **Thousands of senior citizens** have reported a return to **youthful vigor** after DHEA for only a few months. Many reports suggest strongly that Alzheimer's Disease is reversible with DHEA! Maintaining DHEA levels in the body has been shown to be important in improving memory, preventing Alzheimer's disease and osteoporosis in post-menopausal women.

According to a 12 year study published in the New England Journal of Medicine in 1986 (315,1519-24), reported that of the 242 men aged 50 to 79 studied: "A 100 microgram per deciliter increase in DHEA sulfate concentration corresponded with a **48% reduction in mortality** due to cardiovascular disease and a 36% reduction in mortality for any reason. The natural level of DHEA sulfate was measured and those individuals with higher levels **lived longer and had much lower risk of heart disease.**"

Research by Dr. A. Schwartz, a researcher at Temple University, has proven beyond question, DHEA is **effective in weight control** because of its ability to block an enzyme named G6PD (glucose-6-phosphate-dehydrogenase) which is essential for fat tissue production and also promotes cancer cell growth. **No matter what you eat, DHEA still has benefits of weight loss!**

DHEA can now be obtained without a prescription from many health food stores or thru mail-order.

However, a **natural source of DHEA comes from the plant Dioscorea villisa L., commonly called Dioscorea, also known as the Mexican Yam**. The Wild Yam is best explained in an article in a 1992 National Geographic article titled *"Under the Spell of the Trobriand Islands."* The most prized commodity in their culture is the miraculous yam! These are the **MOST YOUTHFUL PEOPLE ON EARTH!!!!** Catastrophic disease there is virtually unknown... The Mexican Yam product is available to you in just a couple of days and it's called Endogen and its available to you right now!

It is recommended that you have a blood test to find out your level of DHEA at this time. Once you consume this amazing supplement your dosage should put you at a DHEA level that you were at in your twenties! Remember what I annotated on the prior page - your level of DHEA takes a nose-dive after the age of 25! DHEA levels for women should be approximately 200-400 mcg/dl and 500-700 mcg/dl for men. SEE your doctor concerning a blood test for DHEA and consumption of this amazing supplement.

WARNING: Insure the DHEA you purchase is *U.S. pharmaceutical-grade DHEA!* *Follow the recommended dosage and instructions from the label and as per your doctor's instructions.*

DIATOMACEOUS EARTH (FOOD GRADE): Diatomaceous Earth (DE) - is a safe product from Mother Nature Herself. DE is the fossilized remains of microscopic shells created by one celled plants called DIATOMS. DE is a fine white powder resembling baby powder. Magnified 7,000-times a single DE particle looks like a Rice Chex cereal. It's tubular, hollow with many holes throughout the structure and it's many super razor sharp edges and almost as hard as a diamond. DE has been used for centuries to safely kill all sorts of parasites - insects. Once the insect comes in contact with it, it cuts into the critter and dries it up. It's used to kill all sorts of pest insects like fleas, ticks, ants, bedbugs, flies, scorpions, box elder bugs, silverfish, aphids, mites, beetles, cockroaches, centipedes, spiders,... Simply by rubbing DE on your pet's fur, within 48-hours it will have killed most or all the fleas, ticks, mites,...

I know what you're asking: *"Why the heck do I need to know about DE?"* As I stated before DE is a food grade product. It's safely consumable for pets and us humans too. Remember when I said DE is *"used for centuries to safely kill all sorts of parasites - insects."* DE within the body goes after parasites. It's used to safely de-worm your critters from horses to them 9-life critters or even small like pet mice.

Now let me concentrate DE for us humans. As I stated before - imagine this - *"Magnified 7,000-times a single DE particle looks like a Rice Chex cereal. It's tubular, hollow with many holes throughout the structure and it's many super razor sharp edges and almost as hard as a diamond."* As you consume DE (me, I put a teaspoon in a 16-ounce plastic bottle, fill it with V-8 Juice - Spicy Hot, I shake it real good for 30-seconds and pour it all in a glass) it's like a DETOX!

DE by the MILLIONS have a strong negative charges. These MILLIONS of DE travel throughout your digestive tract ATTRACTING and ABSORBING:

- Bacteria
- drug residue
- E-Coli
- Endotoxins
- Fungi
- Heavy metals (mercury, lead,...)
- Pesticides
- Protozoa
- viruses

DE also scrubs away at the small and large walls of your entire digestive tract, even the long tract of your colon. Testimonials from using DE are common. Testimonials like:

- better health - 15 trace minerals
- clearer skin (acne, age spots, psoriasis)
- colon cleanser
- fights against polyps (cancer)
- fights against cancers
- fights against ulcers
- gums stronger
- hair grows stronger & faster
- healthier colon
- healthier respiratory tract
- healthier urinary tract
- increased energy
- joint pain
- ligament pain
- lower blood pressure
- lower cholesterol
- Menopause - less symptoms
- nails grows stronger & faster
- regular bowel movements
- teeth stronger

Yes, there's more. But don't believe a word I'm saying. Go to *Diatomaceous Earth (food grade)* in the POC Section and go to those websites and you decide if DE is for YOU and your critters.

WARNING: There are 02 types of DE. One type is used for swimming pool filters. <u>**NEVER NEVER NEVER**</u> use this type of DE for inhalation of this type of DE can cause a lung disease called silicosis. See DE in the POC Section for all natural and safe DEs.

DIET FAILURES: If you don't know it by now, dieting is a mega big bucks business. Most of those companies that promote their weight-loss programs do not keep accurate information on their results. Informal surveys have demonstrated that **VERY FEW** dieters will have maintained their weight-loss 12 months later. Who benefits from these diets? Probably the person selling those diet programs.

- Most of these diets are not only boring, but they are unnatural, especially if they involve special diet foods and eating schedules. Permanent and healthy eating habits aren't part of the program.
- Dieting more often than not lowers the body's metabolism. Believe it or not, your body shifts into the survival or starvation mode and cuts back its calorie needs in order to survive. Why does your body do this? According to my research, it dates back to prehistoric times. Your **body is simply trying to survive like it instinctively did during the winter months when food was lacking back during those cave man days!**
- Dieting changes the percentage of fat in the body. Quick weight loss (not recommended) removes both fat and muscle tissue from your body.

When your weight is regained (another fad diet failure), it comes back in the form of fat and you're probably weighing more! Frequent dieting and weight gain is called *"yo-yo dieting."* Yo-yo dieting may put strain on your heart and was considered very unhealthy. On nationwide television in August and September of 1995, researchers were noted to say that yo-yo dieting isn't as dangerous as previously thought.

However, you get nowhere with yo-yo dieting. You're simply wasting your hard-earned money. Your morale and motivation aren't at their peak level either. So see your physician. , EAT THE RIGHT STUFF and EXERCISE regularly meaning at least 03 times a week for at least 20 to 30 minutes per workout.

Many studies have noted that healthy eating habits, meaning EAT THE RIGHT STUFF, **STARTING AND MAINTAINING AN EXERCISE PROGRAM** and losing weight gradually are the most effective ways of reducing your weight **PERMANENTLY!** Replace fat with complex carbohydrates and protein. Supplements of Vitamins and minerals are also recommended.

WARNING: You must see your physician prior to starting any diet or exercise program. See my *$10,000 Weight-Loss Bet Diet*.

EGGS: While serving in the U.S. Army at Fort Davis, Panama, we would often have height & weight check-ups to insure we were not overweight which is against military regulations. One soldier often told me he had a friend that always **lost a lot of weight** to meet military height & weight standards. What did he do? He ate nothing but eggs. Why? Eating eggs has you on an all protein diet - meaning a carbohydrate restrictive diet. No carbs in the body, then the body has no other fuel to burn than fat. The combination of daily physical training and eggs insured extra fat was burned-up real quick.

ENZYMES: Enzymes are **SO IMPORTANT** for your health. Enzymes are **ESSENTIAL** for all chemical changes in your body. There are three types of enzymes:

- Metabolic enzymes which keeps your body functioning to its peak performance.

- Digestive enzymes in order to **properly digest food**.

- Food enzymes which are found in **RAW FOOD!** These enzymes also aid in proper food digestion. Enzymes are destroyed when food is cooked or heated above temperatures of 118 degrees.

Enzymes make minerals, proteins, Vitamins and other components of our body work. Enzymes are vital to life and your performance. Every physical act from blinking, breathing to walking can not take place without enzymes. Each year new enzymes are discovered and their amazing responsibilities they have with respect to your health.

To date, thousands of enzymes have been discovered. For example, one very important enzyme is called Superoxide Dismutase (SOD). It's a super antioxidant and it working right now as you read this book! Without this enzyme, you would age very quickly! A 10-year old without SOD would look like a 70-year old person! Amazing uh! See *Raw Food Diet* and *Juice Therapy*.

ENZYME THERAPY: Enzyme Therapy uses a variety of enzymes to assist the digestion and assimilation of vital nutrients derived from foods and nutritional supplementation. Certain forms of Enzyme Therapy may be used to reverse disease states and return the body to homeostasis (balance). Take a re-look at *Enzymes* above.

EXERCISE: Exercise is the bodily exertion for the sake of restoring the organs and functions of the body to a healthy state. Benefits from regular exercise are improved self-confidence, increased capacity for physical work, increased endurance, increased muscle tone, reduced risk of heart attack, induces weight-loss,...

Also, according to researchers at Scripps College, exercise keeps your brain in shape. Research indicates that there is a 20% difference in the ability to reason & remember and physical reaction times between people who exercise and couch potatoes.

In this Survival Book, I give you different exercise that will no doubt help you lose weight. Put your own exercise routine together and start losing that unwanted and unhealthy weight so you can be the most healthy and attractive YOU!

Here's my **#01 pick for exercise machines**. It's the *Nordic Track Cross Country Ski Machine*. I've owned 02. Back in 2005, I LUCKILY found my second machine at the *Twice Is Nice Shop* in Belleville, IL. This machine probably cost about $1,000.00 bucks brand new. Anyway, I got on it and tried it out and it worked fine. Guess what I paid for it? Only $25 bucks - best purchase I have ever made in my life! I still have it.

Anyway, being in the military (Infantry, Special Forces {Green Berets}, I've had plenty plenty plenty and plenty of physical training butt whoopins handed to me. I gotta tell you, Nordic Track Cross Country Ski Machine will give you that butt whoopin you need and WILL DEFINITELY help you lose that unwanted and unhealthy weight REAL QUICK!!!!

If you can get one, get it for your health for your future!!! For more butt whoopins, see U.S. Army Rifle Drills, Exercise Mind-Over-Matter Trick, Activities That Burn Calories, Exercise Videos, Military Weight-Loss Exercises And Diets, Rucksacking, Run-Swim-Ruck-Shoot, SERE Weight-Loss Plan, Swimming Fat Burners, Tantric Toning, Walking and Water Polo.

EXERCISE MIND-OVER-MATTER TRICK: Here's a neat Mind-Over-Matter application. As you know I strongly believe in Mind-Over-Matter applications and you can read about em' throughout this Survival Program. And like I've always said, *"If you don't believe ain't nuthin' gonna happen!"* Here's a Mind-Over-Matter application that's backed-up by a wise researcher and scientific proof!

First of all, your conscious mind knows the difference between what is real life and what is fantasy. But your subconscious doesn't know the difference. That's why many Mind-Over-Matter applications tap into the subconscious so the user does the impossible.

According to Dave Smith, Ph.D,. a sports psychologist at Chester College, England *"We found that the parts of the brain that control movement are stimulated by thinking about movement."* And muscle increases the metabolism which burns calories - fat even when you sleep.

"To a certain extent, the mind (subconscious mind) can't tell the difference between really doing something and imagining it. You need to imagine that you are actually doing something athletic."

Dave Smith, Ph.D., says you don't have to sweat you need to CONCENTRATE. *"Close your eyes and imagine how you'd move your body, what it would feel like."* Dr. Smith states **just 05 concentrated minutes a day should do the trick.** That 05-minutes a day translates into 22-pounds a year! Want proof?

Dr. Smith did a study at Manchester Metropolitan University using 03 groups of people. The 1st group concentrated on muscle contractions 20-times a day for a whole month. The 2nd group actually did the real exercise. Dr. Smith found that the 2nd group that did the actual exercise, increased their strength by 33%. The 1st group that imagined the muscle contractions increased their strength by 16%! The 3rd group that did nothing increased their strength by 0%.

Now who can use this Mind-Over-Matter application? YOU can! And YOU can do it just about anywhere (except driving or activities that endanger your life or other lives). Try doing it before you go to sleep at night. So try it, **BELIEVE IT**, YOU HAVE TO BELIEVE IT WORKS! Your mind is an AMAZING MACHINE no computer can match! See *Vision Therapy* and *Vision Boards*.

EXERCISE VIDEOS: Exercise videos may definitely get you to lose that unwanted weight. Besides helping you lose weight, you can exercise in the privacy of your home and exercise according to your schedule. **DO NOT** purchase any exercise videos. Why? Cause there are plenty of em' at your local library. Below is a list of exercise videos I found at one of the libraries I go to (Scott Air Force Base, IL) and I didn't list the ones that are already checked out. OK, let's start with All Day Yoga (alphabetical order).

- All Day Yoga
- AM And PM Workout
- Anyone Can Dance Hip Hop
- Biggest Loser Workout
- Biggest Loser Workout 2
- Body Target Abs
- Buff Moms To Be
- Burn & Firm Circuit Training
- Cardio Pilates
- Dance For Weight-Loss
- Dance It Off
- Dance To Fitness
- Dance Yourself Thin
- Easy Pilates
- Evening Stress Release Yoga
- Everybody Steps
- Fat Burning Walk II
- Fat Burning Yoga
- FIRM, The - Body Sculpture System
- Get Moving - Walking For Weight-Loss
- Hula Workout – Beginners

- Hula Workout - Weight-Loss
- Lift Weight To Lose Weight 2
- More Yoga For The Rest Of Us
- New Ballet Workout, The
- Pilates Abs & Waist
- Pilates Advanced Workout
- Pilates Abs & Butt
- Pilates Butt & Hips
- Pilates Complete For Inflexible People
- Pilates Complete For Weight-Loss
- Pilates For Every Body
- Pilates On The Go
- Pilates Principles
- Pilates Weight-Loss Workout For Beginners
- Pilates Workout For Dummies
- Power Yoga
- Shrink Your Female Fat Zone
- Stay Ball Core Workout
- Tae Bo
- Tae Bo - Foundation Energy
- Tae Bo - Strength & Power
- Tai Chi For Beginners
- Total Body Sculpt W/Gilad
- Total Body Yoga
- Ultimate Step Circuit
- Urban Hip Hop
- Walk Away The Pounds
- Weight-Loss Walk - 4 Miles
- Yoga Conditioning For Weight-Loss
- Yoga Fit Kids
- Yoga For Beginners
- Yoga For The Rest Of Us
- Yoga For Weight-Loss
- Yoga Zone - Fat Burning
- Zumba – Advanced

- Zumba – Beginners
- Zone Pilates Mat & Ball Workout

See *Wheat Germ Oil For After-Burner Performance.*

C'mon, go to the library and get a few videos and START MOVING. C'mon STOP READING THIS Survival Book and WALK to your local library and get them exercise videos NOW! I can still see you sitting there. You're still reading this aren't you? OK, let's carry-on with *Fasting.*

FASTING: Fasting is an economical, effective therapy for a wide range of conditions like allergies, arthritis, headaches, hypertension,... By relieving the body of the task of digesting foods (NO FOOD), fasting allows the system to purge itself of toxins thus expediting the healing process. During the fast, the liver converts stored sugar into glucose for fuel. When stored sugars are depleted, fat is burned for fuel.

Most fasts only last a few days (02 - 04 days). Some medical experts have their patients go on a fast but also have them drinking plenty of fresh fruit juice, fresh vegetable juice, pure water, or a combination of these drinks. The fast would last a few days, time enough for the body to purge itself of toxins. Some medical experts consider fruit & vegetable juice as food and have their fasting patients drinking only pure water. See Juice Therapy and Detoxification Therapy.

FEELING FULL FOODS: Here's a real quick list of nutritious foods that make you feel FULL, but aren't high in calories. These foods will help you lose that extra unhealthy weight. Use these foods as part of your healthy meals to start losing weight today. Are you ready? Here they are:
- Apples
- Apricots
- Broccoli
- Cantaloupe
- Carrots

- Celery
- Cucumbers
- Eggplant
- Grapefruit
- Honeydew
- Lettuce
- Mushrooms
- Oranges
- Papaya
- Peaches
- Pears
- Pineapples
- Raspberries
- Spinach
- Squash
- Strawberries
- Tomatoes
- Watermelon.

See other nutritious foods in this Survival Book and see Enzymes, Tonic of Life and Water.

FIBER: Fiber comes from plant foods. There is no fiber in foods like eggs, beef, cheese, chicken, pork... Fiber is not digested; it provides no calories. Fiber speeds up the elimination of waste and combats constipation. Fiber helps remove cholesterol (**lowers cholesterol**) and **cancer-causing chemicals** out of your bodies system.

Nutritionists recommend at least 35 grams and up to 70 grams of daily fiber. Fiber helps food pass through the intestines faster and **lowers the absorption of fat!**

So if you eat any fatty foods insure that fiber is consumed during your meal. A diet high in fiber can be a factor in lowering cholesterol levels. Remember, fiber comes from plant foods. Read the Nutritional Facts on all food products that you purchase. Stay away from the foods that are high in saturated fats, sodium and cholesterol. Choose foods that are have little or no fats, sodium and cholesterol but have ample protein, carbohydrates, fiber, Vitamins...

According to Dr. Elaine Fox, (Chief Nutritionist and the Executive Director of the North Nassau Health Center, New York -- The Guide to a Healthier Diet – "Eat Well Be Well" VIDEO), fiber is the indigestible portion of food (fruits, vegetables & whole grains). Fiber draws water to it thus increasing the health of the gastrointestinal system. If food stays in the lower bowel (colon) for too long, bacteria breaks down residues of fat that cause cancer producing chemicals.

Fiber increases the transit time (time between when the food is consumed to when it is eliminated), so that the residue of food doesn't stay in the lower bowel too long which may cause bacteria that could break down residues of fat causing cancer producing chemicals. Transit time should be between 24 to 36 hours. Good nutrition balances the transit time. If transit time is beyond 36 hours, gradually increase your fiber.

Fiber also helps to bind cholesterol. Consuming fiber seems to lower cholesterol as well as being nutritious. Any whole grain has fiber as well brown rice (verses white rice), oat bran, wheat bran, fruits and vegetables (especially carrots).

FISH: Heart-health experts have found the benefits of eating fish are even greater than previously realized. In 1985 the New England Journal of Medicine found that **"the consumption of as little as one or two fish dishes per week may be of preventive importance in relation to coronary heart disease."** *Omega-3 fats* in fish benefits the heart by making the blood less prone to the abnormal clotting process that can lead to a heart attack. See Capsicum – Cayenne Pepper now!

Fresh fish rates high for keeping blood pressure in a healthy range. Jichi Medical School in Japan have shown that levels of **"good" HDL cholesterol were high among Japanese who eat the most fish!** Fish may also help those who suffer from arthritis.

According to Dr. Joel Kremer of Albany Medical College in New York, daily supplements of EPA (eicosapentaenoic acid) fish oil brought dramatic **relief to inflammation and stiff joints** caused by rheumatoid arthritis. Fish is **less fattening** and more digestible than beef. Fish is high in mineral selenium which has proven to chase away the blues.

There are about twenty varieties of fish that can be purchased at your local supermarket. Four ounces of fish furnishes anywhere from 89 calories to 236 calories, with raw haddock having the lowest calorie count of 89 and four ounces of canned herring rates the highest calorie count of 236.

- Salmon is low in saturated fat and high in **Omega-3 fatty acids**. Salmon provides only 233 calories per 4.5-ounce steak and only 06 grams of fat per 03-ounces.

According to researchers at the University of Cincinnati, Ohio, researchers have successfully **blocked both migraine headaches and kidney disease with Omega-3 fish oils**. Migraines generally **eased up in about 60 percent** of those who took fish oil capsules for six weeks. The number of migraine attacks **dropped from 02 per week to 02 every 02 weeks and they were less severe!**

Those patients diagnosed early of kidney disease, showed a retardation of kidney deterioration by switching from animal fat to Omega-3 fish oils. According to Dr. Uno Barcelli, assistant professor of medicine at the University of Cincinnati, "It seems fish oil must be used relatively early in the disease process." Fish oil therapy had no effect on patients with advanced kidney disease.

Is fish a brain food? It sure is! Fish is noted to be food for thought! According to Dr. Judith Wurtman, principal investigator at MIT, the high protein in fish, namely the amino acid tyrosine, may be a **boost to the brain** neurotransmitters norepinephrine and dopamine, which **energizes your mind and making you feel more alert**. Three or four ounces of fish (broiled or grilled) is sufficient.

WARNING: Fast food fish is noted to have 1/10 of Omega-3 fish oil compared to a can of Chinook salmon. Fast food fish is mostly made from whitefish already low in fat and Omega-3's. Too much Omega-3 may block normal blood clotting and lead to excessive bleeding. Researchers have discovered that Omega-3 fish oil capsules can actually aggravate diabetes by producing a steep rise in blood sugar and a drop in insulin secretion.

FIVE DEADLY WHITES, THE: I'm here to tell you that it's very important to not only "Eat The Right Stuff" (healthy foods throughout this Survival Book) but it's very important to AVOID *"The Five Deadly Whites."* <u>THIS SUBJECT IS VERY IMPORTANT</u> so here it goes:

What are the Five Deadly Whites (FDWs)?
The five deadly whites are (listed in order as the most dangerous threat to your health): Meat, Dairy, Salt, Sugar and White Flour.

- **Meat** - Meat contains fat and fat is already linked to many cancers, heart disease, stroke, diabetes... Meat eaters consume over 50 pounds of fat (cholesterol) each year!

- **Dairy** - Pasteurized milk changes the calcium to an inorganic form which can not be assimilated by your body. Animal products are noted to be sources of LDL (bad cholesterol).

- **Salt** - Your body needs sodium but the sodium chloride (table salt) may be toxic to your body! For more information and a far superior sodium product see Whole Salt.

- **Sugar** - Sugar is linked to a wide variety of health problems and noted to hinder your immune system. For an alternative to aspartame see Super Sweet Stevia.

- **White Flour** - White flour is missing most of the good ingredients prior to its processing. It's bleached, synthetic Vitamins added and it's called "enriched." Remember the saying concerning bread "The whiter the bread, the sooner you're dead!" See Bread and Whole Salt.

Now let's look at each one of these **FIVE DEADLY WHITES** and see what they are and WHY they're a serious health threat to you and possibly others around you. We'll start with meat.

FIRST DEADLY WHITE: MEAT

What is the definition of meat?

Meat is defined as the edible flesh (soft tissue of the body - animal) of mammals as distinguished from that of fish or poultry. Edible flesh including poultry and some fish and shellfish.

Sounds harmless to me. How can meat be harmful to my health?

Meat contains fat and fat is ALREADY LINKED to heart disease, many cancers, many degenerative diseases too numerous to annotate and DON'T forget about obesity - FAT makes you fat. Americans consume HUGE AMOUNTS of fat each year.

As of 2014, the average American consumes approximately 85 pounds of fat and oil each year!

You already read the multitudes of deaths caused by heart disease and cancer in the previous sections! Fat and cholesterol go hand in hand and where you find a high cholesterol count, odds are you'll find THE SILENT KILLER - hypertension - high blood pressure!

If meat is so dangerous, people should be dropping dead all around me!

They are! As I stated in the introduction, more than 1,400,000 Americans die each year from Heart Disease, Cancer, and Stroke. Imagine that many people in front of you! Each year the death toll starts all over again! 01, 02, 03, 500, 20,000, 500,000, 1,000,000, and 1,400,000 plus!!!

I need to eat meat. What about all the protein and other nutrients I'd be missing if I didn't eat meat?

Yes you do need those vital essentials and nutrients. However, when any food is heated and cooked, the heat causes a chemical reaction. Protein and those very important enzymes aren't the same beneficial nutrients anymore! They're practically worthless to your body. So now you're consuming meat that has fat that is harmful and DEADLY in more ways than one and the nutritional value is just about worthless!

I thought meat was really good for you. Is it really that bad for your health?

If you think the beef you purchase at your local grocery store comes from cattle grazing on chemical-free and toxin-free grassy hillsides, well you better think again. Nowadays, it's difficult to find fresh organically raised meat. A large percentage of cattle are raised in the quickest, cheapest and most unnatural manner possible.

Why? **Money is the motivation** in the meat producing business. The use of drugs are common in raising cattle. Cattle are loaded with antibiotics, drugs, pesticides and synthetic Vitamins. Prior to being led to slaughter, cattle are loaded with tranquilizers and meat tenderizers. Other animals like chickens, lambs, pigs, veal calves are also raised in very unnatural manners. The tainted meat is passed-on to the consumer.

Why are so many Americans afflicted with heart disease, cancer and dozens of other diseases? Depending what and where you buy it, meat is loaded with saturated fat. Saturated fat is linked to heart disease, cancer and many degenerative diseases.

In other words, **saturated fat is linked to suffering and death!** If you must eat meat, purchase the **leanest** meat you could find. To make it juicier, put some Extra Virgin Olive Oil on it and make sure there are PLENTY of fruits, vegetables and good clean water! If you like a salty flavor without the salt, try Bragg Liquid Aminos. It contains 15 healthy amino acids! See Health Science, Olive Oil, Whole Salt, and **$10,000.00 WEIGHT-LOSS BET Diet**.

SECOND DEADLY WHITE: DAIRY PRODUCTS

Dairy products are harmful to my health? You're joking?

First we'll talk about milk. I'd like to see evidence where milk-producing cows are absolutely free of drugs, toxins, antibiotics... which may be passed on to the consumer.

Second, when milk is pasteurized meaning it is heated to temperatures of 160 degrees or more, that heat causes a chemical reaction that changes calcium to an inorganic form which cannot be assimilated or used by your body as previously thought.

Third, dairy products - animal products are a source of low-density lipo-protein (LDL) BAD CHOLESTEROL! **High cholesterol leads to heart attacks, heart disease, stroke and other cardiovascular diseases!** Americans have on average cholesterol of 212 because of the unhealthy Standard American Diet and poor eating habits.

Heart disease is the number one killer of Americans. More Americans die of heart disease than all cancer deaths combined. Approximately 1,500,000 heart attacks take place each year with approximately 250,000 which are fatal within fifteen minutes.

THIRD DEADLY WHITE: SALT

Did you know the word "salary" comes from the Latin word *"sal,"* which means salt. The Roman soldiers were said to be "worth their salt." They were often paid in salt rather than money. Salt also known as sodium chloride is composed of 40 percent sodium and 60 percent chloride. It's essential to life and is a very important mineral to your body. Without it, you would die. This mineral helps maintain fluid levels between the cells and the blood system and also acts as an electrolyte to help chemical and electrical reactions in your body.

However, if you're consuming too much salt, high blood pressure may surface. Salt related health problems are caused by diets consisting of high quantities of REFINED sodium compounds and a couch-potato life style. Table salt (the stuff you but at the grocery store) is an inorganic (not usable by your body) compound of sodium and chlorine.

It's toxic! Table salt lacks more than 80 minerals which protect your body from the toxic effects of pure sodium chloride! Table salt, which is almost pure sodium chloride is heated in an oven and **stripped of its vital buffer minerals** and may contribute to cardiovascular disease.

If you like a salty flavor without the salt, try Bragg Liquid Aminos. It contains **15 healthy amino acids!** See Health Science and Olive Oil and Whole Salt for a different and **healthier alternative** to sodium chloride. If you must have your salt, SEE *The Grain and Salt Society*.

FOURTH DEADLY WHITE: SUGAR

Sugar is a sweet crystalline carbohydrate, sucrose. During the American Revolution, Americans consumed about 20 pounds of sugar per year. Today it's about **140 pounds of sugar & sweetners per year!** The average American consumes 100 grams of cane and beet sugar daily. Of the refined foods that Americans eat, none is so damaging as sugar. **Sugar has been linked to degenerative disorders such as aging, cataracts, diabetes, hypoglycemia, tooth decay and stomach problems**.

Sugar has also been linked to impairing the immune functioning system. Studies have shown that sugar can distort the chemistry of antibodies or reduce lymphocyte cells which are important to the immune response. To compound matters, a diet high in cholesterol, saturated fats and sugar only increases the risk factors associated with heart disease. The **more processed foods that you eat the more processed sugar you consume**.

Consumable products like cake, canned vegetables, cookies, medications like cough syrup - cough drops, ketchup, frozen vegetables, salad dressing, soft drinks, soups, TV dinners and even tobacco products like cigars, cigarettes and pipe tobacco. Try replacing raw honey for that refined unhealthy sugar and read about stevia.

An unknown sweet health threat is called aspartame; a synthetic sweetener (brand names NutraSweet & Equal) has been **linked to many health problems**.

What is aspartame?

More than 30 years ago, a chemist in search for a medicine to relieve ulcers came across a new discovery we now know and use as Aspartame. Aspartame, a synthetic sweetener (brand names NutraSweet & Equal) has been **linked to many health problems**.

Aspartame is linked to many health problems?

Yes, aspartame is noted to generate methanol in the intestinal tract, which small amounts of this toxin could cause significant eye problems. Methanol is a **colorless, poisonous liquid used chiefly as a solvent, fuel...**

Aspartame is noted to cause brain tumors in rats. **An <u>increase of the incidence of brain tumors in the U.S. has been noted since aspartame was added to our food supply!</u>** According to the National Cancer Institute, the incidence of common primary malignant brain tumors is on the rise coinciding with the licensing of aspartame for use in beverages in July 1983.

Are there other health problems associated with Aspartame?

You bet! It's also suspected of causing seizures. H. R. Roberts, M.D., F.A.C.P., **testified before Congress and the FDA**. He feels aspartame may be responsible for the increasing number of eye problems. He advises patients afflicted with vision problems like black spots, blurred vision, bright flashes, decreased vision, tunnel vision and other eye problems, **eliminate aspartame** from their diet for a month prior to any aggressive treatment. In many cases, restricting aspartame may alleviate many of these vision symptoms.

Aspartame is also linked to the following symptoms\afflictions:
- aches & pains
- anxiety attacks
- blindness
- confusion
- depression
- difficulty breathing
- edema
- fatigue
- headaches
- hearing loss

- heart palpitations
- hyperactivity
- memory loss
- menstrual problems
- muscle aches
- nausea
- numb arms
- ringing in the ears
- skin lesions
- sleeplessness...
- many more!!!

I don't consume any synthetic sweeteners like NutraSweet & Equal, so I'm OK, right?

You're a long way from being OK! A long way! In 1991 there were 1,500 products sweetened with aspartame. One year later there were 4,000 products sweetened with aspartame. By 1996 there may be **more than 15,000 products containing aspartame!**

Many products containing aspartame are probably in your kitchen right now and you've been consuming them for months or years! If you've suffered or are currently suffering from any of the symptoms or afflictions annotated on the previous page, first look at the least intrusive treatment - YOUR DIET and look into the your consumption of Aspartame! **An alternative to aspartame is called stevia!**

What is stevia?

The Japanese developed a method of refining the sweet glycosides out of the stevia leaf creating a new product called Stevioside which is **300 times sweeter than sugar!** At the time of this writing the FDA allows stevia to be used as nutritional\dietary supplement and not as a food additive (food manufacturing companies cannot use it). Stevia is noted to be superior to aspartame (brand names NutraSweet & Equal) which has been linked to health problems. Stevia may be purchased at health food stores or from Body Ecology (1-800-4STEVIA) and Consumer Direct (1-800-947-6417).

WARNING: If you must use any sugar product, use it sparingly.

What about saccharin, is it safe?

Saccharin is a white crystalline powder, having a taste about 500 times sweeter than cane sugar, used as a calorie-free sweetener. Let me give you a quote from Sweet'N Low's pink sugar packet that contains saccharin and is sold everywhere: **"Use of this product may be hazardous to your health. This product contains saccharin which has been determined to cause cancer in laboratory animals."** Sweet'N Low is a granulated sugar substitute. If you use this product, read and reread the **"WARNING"** till it sinks in!

FIFTH DEADLY WHITE: WHITE FLOUR

White flour is missing most of the good ingredients (bran and germ) prior to its final processing. It's bleached, synthetic Vitamins added (coal-tar-derived--**carcinogenic**) and it's called *"enriched."* Go figure! Remember the saying I gave you concerning bread - "The whiter the bread, the sooner you're dead!"

Even when bread is baked, the chemical reaction with heat used to bake the bread actually destroys many of the nutrients that were there prior to baking!

FLAX SEED: In 1909, the average U.S. person consumed approximately 125 grams of fat per day. Today (data from 1998) the average person in the U.S. **consumes approximately 175 grams of fat, an increase of 40 percent or about 50 extra pounds per year and increasing!** Of the total increase in the consumption of fats and oils, shortening, margarine, refined salad oil and cooking oils account for fifty percent. This increase in fat over the years is undoubtedly **linked to the increase in degenerative diseases**.

In order to extend the shelf life of many products, **essential fatty acids (good fat) have been purposely processed out of most foods**. This is profitable for the manufacturer, but **UNHEALTHY** to the American consumer - YOU! Approximately **80% of Americans are deficient** in essential fatty acids. Flax seed has a high content of essential fatty acids.

Flax seed supplies the body with needed essential fatty acids and richer in Omega-3's than fish oil and packs more fiber ounce for ounce than oat bran!

Listed below are some observed benefits of flax seed:

- Seriously ill cancer patients were treated with flax seed oil and low-fat cottage cheese by Dr. Johanna Budwig. Over a period of approximately 90 days, **tumors gradually receded. Symptoms of anemia, cancer, diabetes and liver dysfunction were completely alleviated!**

- According to a study in Great Britain by Dr. Sinclair, a relative **deficiency of the essential fatty acids** plays an important part in the **causes of arteriosclerosis, coronary thrombosis, diabetes mellitus, hypertension, multiple sclerosis and certain forms of malignant diseases!**

- Dr. J.R. Vane shared the 1982 Nobel Prize for Medicine for his work proving how the metabolism of Omega-3 fatty acids helped prevent heart problems.

- A U.S. physician, Dr. Donald Rudin discovered that Omega-3 fatty acid deficiency is the basic cause of major mental illness, because fatty acids provide the substance upon which niacin and other B Vitamins act to form the prostaglandin-3 series tissue hormones which are special mission fatty acids that regulate neurocircuits through the whole body.

The **Food and Drug Administration (FDA) has recently entered into a 03-year, $2 million contract with the National Cancer Institute (NCI) to research the effect of flax seed on various health concerns**. The FDA will conduct experiments confirming flaxseed's role in fat and cholesterol metabolism, bone mineralization and the immune system. This research will make flaxseed one of the most intensively-studied nutrients used in any food product.

Flax seeds are a **great source of healthy soluble and insoluble fiber** as well as protein. Just 1/4 cup (50 grams) of flax seed provides 20 grams of fiber. Remember fiber is noted to ameliorate, heal, prevent:

- Colon cancer.
- Constipation.
- Diverticulosis.
- Hemorrhoids.
- Improves blood sugar metabolism.
- Lowers blood pressure.

- Lowers cholesterol.
- Protects against other cancers.
- Rectal cancer.
- **Weight loss**.
- Much more...

FORCED HYDRATION: This is a term used in the military that directs the soldier to drink water according to a preplanned schedule that insured the soldier is adequately hydrated at all times. Forced Hydration is implemented to AVOID heat casualties. But you can use Forced Hydration to **help you lose weight**. Experts state to drink 08 08-ounce glasses of water per day.

Water is a **natural appetite suppressant** and has NO FAT, NO CARBOHYDRATES, NO CALORIES. Set a *Forced Hydration* schedule and stick to it. Don't drink tap water - drink purified water. I gotta tell you, **many an ex-chubby folks have attributed their weight-loss to drinking plenty of pure water**. So drink up.

GARCINIA CAMBOGIA: A weight-loss herb from India. This herb has an ingredient that blocks excess glucose from turning into fat. One over-the-counter product that has a garcinia cambogia extract is called Citrimax. Garcinia cambogia ia a metabolic enhancer. It revs-up your fat-burning engine and is a natural appetite suppressant. **HOLD THE PHONE!!!**

As of this update (23 March 2014) – Garcinia Cambogia has been touted as a real option to helping you lose all that unhealthy weight that's been holding you down for years. You know the famous health professional Dr. Oz? I'm gonna give you a quote from a website and give you the website itself:

According to Dr Oz - *"this is in my opinion, the biggest breakthrough in weight loss supplements to date. Not only is it super effective but very affordable"*.
http://celebeautymag.com/diet/burn-fat.html   NO, I ain't making a dime on this referral!

GARLIC CLOVE APPETITE SUPPRESSANT: If you have an urge to eat just for the heck of it (depression, stress,...) and not related to being hungry, try this appetite suppressant. Rub a clove of fresh garlic on your upper lip. This should suppress your appetite even if you do eat anything. See Healing Garlic.

GERSON DIET: In 1919, Dr. Max Gerson developed a diet to eliminate his own migraine headaches. The Gerson Diet consist of foods that are low in fat, grain & protein products while utilizing large amounts of fresh, raw vegetable juices and other raw foods. Dr. Gerson found that through his research, he discovered not only did this diet eliminate his migraine headaches, but most other health problems like arthritis, diabetes and even **terminal cancer!**

GLYCEMIC FOOD INDEX (GFI): Folks across the world are using the following GFI as part as their weight loss goals. You've even seen TV commercials offering meals using the GFI. Glycemic Food Index (GFI) means the way your body responds to different foods that increases the sugar levels in your body. The higher the sugar levels the harder it is for your body to maintain a healthy weight. Some foods with high GFI ratings flood your body with sugars while other don't and the sugars they do release are slowly released for energy, metabolism and minimum or no weight gain.

Each food is given a rating between 0 - 100 with a top rating of 100 for high glycemic foods and a rating toward 0 rating being low glycemic foods. Bottom line, the foods with a **low *GFI* rating** give you the better results for weight loss. Let's start with fruits:

Fruit GFI Ratings:
Cherries---------------------------22
Grapefruit---------------------------25
Prunes-----------------------------29
Apricots (dried)--------------------30
Apple------------------------------38
Peach (canned in juice)-----------38
Pear (fresh)------------------------38

Plum--------------------------------39
Strawberries-------------------------40
Orange, Navel------------------------42
Peach (fresh)------------------------42
Pear (canned)------------------------43
Grapes------------------------------46
Mango------------------------------51
Banana-----------------------------52
Fruit Cocktail-----------------------55
Papaya-----------------------------56
Raisins-----------------------------56
Apricots (fresh)----------------------57
Kiwi--------------------------------58
Figs (dried)-------------------------61
Apricots (canned)--------------------64
Cantaloupe--------------------------65
Pineapple (fresh)---------------------66
Watermelon--------------------------72
Dates-------------------------------103

Vegetable GFI Ratings:

Broccoli----------------------------10
Cabbage----------------------------10
Lettuce-----------------------------10
Mushrooms--------------------------10
Onions-----------------------------10
Red Peppers-------------------------10
Carrots-----------------------------49
Green Peas--------------------------48
Corn (fresh)-------------------------60
Beets-------------------------------64
Pumpkin----------------------------75
Parsnips----------------------------97

Bread GFI Ratings:

Pumpernickel----------------------41
Sourdough------------------------53
Stone Ground Whole Wheat----53
Pita Whole Wheat-----------------57
Whole Meal Rye------------------58
Hamburger Bun--------------------61
Croissant--------------------------67
Taco Shell-------------------------68
White------------------------------70
Bagel------------------------------72
Kaiser Roll------------------------73
Bread Sufiing----------------------74
Whole Wheat 100%---------------77
French Baguette--------------------95

Bean & Pea GFI Ratings:

Chana Dal---------------------------08
Chickpeas, Dry----------------------28
Kidney Beans, Dry------------------28
Lentils------------------------------29
Lima Beans (frozen)-----------------32
Yellow Split Peas--------------------32
Chickpeas (Canned)-----------------42
Blackeyed Peas (Canned)----------42
Baked Beans------------------------48
Kidney Beans (Canned)------------52
Note: See *Baked Beans Weight-Loss*.

Soup GFI Ratings:

Tomato------------------------------38
Minestrone---------------------------39
Lentil--------------------------------44

Follow the recommended instructions from the label and as per your doctor's instructions.

GOING GREEN: I will talk about the super healthy wonders of juicing and to INSURE you get the super health benefits of juicing you might want to compliment it with Going Green. In other words, add a super healthy green powder to your glass of juice. Why?

Cause most or all of the green powder products that I've ever seen are LOADED with green foods, fiber, vegetables, fruits, minerals, vitamins,... Your best bet to *Going Green* is of course a health food store. Any questions, ask the employee. They're supposed to be knowledgeable in that area. WAIT - I've listed 02 different 'green powder' products that I use:

a) Essential Greens: Essential Greens (17.6 oz) offers a great healthy supplement. Essential Greens is a 'super concentrated greens drink mix' and some of the healthy ingredients include Aloe Vera Gel, Barley Greens, Carrots, Chlorella, Green Tea, Hawaiian Blue-Green Algae, Kale, Plant Based Enzymes, Prebiotic Fibers, Spinach, Tomato, Wheat Grass,... and much more. Essential Greens can be found in just about any health food store.

b) All Day Energy Greens: *All Day Energy Greens* (11.36 oz.) is ABSOLUTELY LOADED with all kinds of nutrients like Acerola (fruit) Extract, Alfalfa (leaf) Powder, Aloe Vera (leaf) Powder, Apple Fiber Powder, Apple Pectin Cellulose Powder, Carrot Juice Powder, Chlorella (cracked cell), Ginger (root) Powder, Horsetail (herb) Powder, Organic Barley Green (ariel) Juice Powder, Parsley (leaf) Juice Powder, Red Raspberry (leaf) Powder, Rose Hips (fruit) Powder, Stevia (see Super Sweet Stevia), Watercress Powder, Yucca (root) Juice Powder,... OK enough - I'm tired of writing down all the healthy ingredients. You must see *Institute For Vibrant Living* in the POC Section. Call them NOW and they'll send you healthy info on all they're great products. At the time of this writing (October 2009), they sent me a very informative, all-color, 36-page booklet solely dedicated to one of their products - All Day Energy Greens. Insure you ask for this booklet.

Important Note: Even if you don't juice (extract juices from vegetables, fruits,... using a juicer machine) and you drink store-bought juice, still consider adding a super healthy green powdered product to your juice.

If I don't have time to juice, I simply add a few spoonfuls of *All Day Energy Greens*, a few pinches of cayenne pepper and a good squirt of Braggs apple cider vinegar to a big bottle (14 fluid ounce) of *V8 Spicy Hot* and I'm set for the whole day (keep cold). I could literally live off this super healthy concoction. YES, I'm drinking some right now as I write this Important Note. OK, let's carry-on with *Goji*.

GOJI: Gogi is another supplement that is very popular in the United States. Gogi berries grow in China and Mongolia. Gogi berries have been used in Chinese, Tibet and India medicine for thousands of years. It's used to avoid and fight cancer, help eyesight, boost the immune system, protect the liver, reduce blood glucose, lower cholesterol levels, improve memory,... Now here's what makes Gogi work. Goji is loaded with a bounty of antioxidants and complimented with vitamins and minerals. Goji is being touted as a **DETOXIFIER** which aids to clean the body of toxins thus **losing weight**.
Follow the recommended dosage and instructions from the label and as per your doctor's instructions.

GRAPEFRUIT: A grapefruit furnishes only 80 calories, is rich in Vitamin C, calcium, potassium, pectin, high in delicious fiber and free of fat and sodium. Grapefruit can economically fit into most budgets. According to Dr. James Cerda of the University of Florida, grapefruit is noted to **dissolve fat and cholesterol!**

It's made up of long-chain molecules for fuel and it fills you up! It's great for helping you lose weight. Consumed before bedtime, grapefruit can help promote sound sleep. When consumed in the morning, grapefruit is noted to help prevent constipation. Drink 06 ounces of grapefruit juice prior to each meal. Grapefruit juice contains the enzyme amylase and suppresses the appetite.

GRAPEFRUIT JUICE: Drink 06 ounces of grapefruit juice prior to each meal. Grapefruit juice contains the enzyme amylase and **suppresses the appetite**. According to Dr. James Cerda of the University of Florida, grapefruit is noted to **dissolve fat and cholesterol**. It's made up of long-chain molecules for fuel and it **feels you up!** It's great for helping you **lose weight!**

GREEN TEA: The tea that we drink is approximately 80% *"black tea"* and approximately 20% *"green tea."* Here's the secret behind green tea: Approximately 30% of the tea leaf is made up of an ingredient called polyphenols. Polyphenols are noted to have both **antioxidant and anticancer properties!** Here's the difference in the preparation between black tea and the remarkable qualities of green tea. When black tea is prepared, the tea leaf is crushed. When the leaf is crushed, the polyphenols are oxidized by the enzymes within the leaf, thus neutralizing their antioxidant and anticancer properties. The actual oxidation turns the leaf black!

In preparation of the green tea, the leaf is first dried and heated, which blocks this enzymatic destruction of the polyphenols. Green Tea contains the antioxidant and anticancer properties while containing less caffeine. The green tea extracts actually remain stable after brewing the tea leaves in hot water. Green Tea has twice the concentration of powerful catechins as black tea leaves.

Instant Green Tea has approximately 03 times more catechin than black tea. The stronger the cup of Green Tea, the greater the anticipated health benefits. **Green Tea** has joined the ranks of broccoli, garlic, oats,... and other foods and supplements that **may protect people from cancer!**

Benefits of drinking Green Tea:

- **Antioxidant Protection** -- Antioxidants are very important in **protecting you against cancer, heart disease and aging!** Polyphenols extracted from the green tea have **more scavenging effect on oxygen free radicals** than even Vitamin C and E (known antioxidants).

- **Antitumor\antimetagenesis activity** -- According to a study published in the Journal of the National Cancer Institute, 902 Chinese with esophageal cancer and 1,552 healthy Chinese in Shanghai, China discovered that **consuming green tea reduced esophageal cancer risk by 57% in men and 60% in women!**

In other studies, animals consuming green tea and green tea extract were noted to be significantly **protected against ALL forms of cancer!** Green tea has a antimutagenic effect (blocks the development of carcinogens in the intestinal tract and the blood).

According to Dr. Fung-Lung Chung of the American Health Foundation in Valhalla, N.Y. stated that Green Tea consumption may explain **Japan's lower death rate for lung cancer**. Dr. Chung stated that **Japanese men smoke more than Americans, but have a lower risk of lung cancer!**

- **Cholesterol lowering** -- The polyphenols in green tea as well as catechins are noted to lower blood fat levels. In a 02-year study of 1,306 males in Japan, it was noted that **green tea consumption was instrumental in cholesterol reduction**. Nine cups or more of green tea per day resulted in a 08 mg\dl reduction. The participants <u>did not change</u> their dietary habits or any other variable.

In another study involving 6,000 nondrinking, nonsmoking, women of 40 years or older, consumed at least five cups of green tea per day. The study found a **50% reduction in stroke rate!** See Smoker's Body Starts Healing Itself and other Smoking POCs in the POC Section.

- **Antibacterial properties** -- Green tea is also noted for its antibacterial properties. According to Japanese studies, green tea extract **inhibited the growth of many bacteria that cause cancer!** Green tea is noted to inhibit growth of all 24 bacterial strains isolated from infected root canals. For more information on Green Tea see *Natures Distributors, Inc.*

Follow the recommended dosage and instructions from the label and as per your doctor's instructions.

GUINNESS WORLD RECORD WEIGHT-LOSS FACTS: If you think you can't go without your hamburgers or lose any weight then read these 03 Guinness World Record Facts:

a) Longest Survival Without Food & Water: On 01 April 1979, Andreas Mihavecz was arrested and put in a holding cell in Hochst, Austria. The police forgot about Mihavecz for 19 days. On 18 April 1979 he was discovered in his cell close to death!

b) Most Male Weight-Loss: The most weight-loss for a man was Jon Monnoch of the USA. His heaviest weight was 1,400 pounds. In a 16-month period, he dropped his weight down to 476 pounds, a reduction of 924 pounds!

c) Most Female Weight-Loss: The most weight-loss for a woman was Rosalie Bradford of the USA. Her heaviest weight was 1,199 pounds. From January 1987 to February 1994, she dropped her weight down to 282 pounds, a reduction of 917 pounds!

GYMNEMA SYLVESTRE: This climbing plant is native to the forest of Central and South India. Gymnema Sylvestre has been used since the sixth century B.C. This amazing herb is noted to **lower blood sugar and could repair damage to the cells in the pancreas!**

According to 1990 animal studies on diabetic rats, fasting **blood glucose levels returned to NORMAL** after 20 to 60 days of treatment. Autopsies on these rats demonstrated that the islet and beta cells of the pancreas (produces insulin) had doubled in number compared to the control group! Destruction of beta cells **was thought to be irreversible!**

Human studies demonstrated that 05 of 22 diabetic patients taking 400mg of Gymnema Sylvestre per day for 18 to 20 months as a supplement to oral drugs could **discontinue their drugs and the remaining reduced their doses!** Researchers concluded that "the beta cells may be **REGENERATED** in Type II diabetic patients on GS4 (Gymnema Sylvestre) supplementation." *Follow the recommended dosage and instructions from the label and as per your doctor's instructions.*

HEALING BLACK DIRT (HSOS): Find some rich black dirt and you may find some healing dirt that may remedy several maladies. And now there's evidence that rich black dirt may contain a specific healing bacterial ingredient. There's good bacteria and bad bacteria and rich black dirt may contain good bacteria called **homeostatic soil organisms (HSOs)**.

HSOs when in the human body, destroy dangerous organisms that are bad for our health like molds, parasites, yeast, and other microorganisms that interfere with proper digestion and absorption of food.

Millions and millions of North Americans are sickly because their HSOs intake is deficient. According to Jordan Rubin, N.D. *"...soils have been depleted of HSOs, and out intake has dropped."*

Research indicates that as many as 92% of people suffering from many gastrointestinal problems from indigestion to irritable bowel syndrome could find relief in 04-months from taking HSOs. According to Paul Goldberg, D.C. *"HSOs help crowd out the bad organisms that prevent proper digestion and trigger pain."*

And HSOs may offer some fighting help when it comes to preventing arthritis. According to gastroenterologist Joseph Brasco, M.D., co-author of *"Restoring Your Digestive Health"* - Research shows that the more HSOs people eat, the lower their risk of ever developing arthritis. And HSOs may offer some help to remedy asthma and allergies. According to the National Institute of Allergy and Infectious Diseases, 35 million Americans are afflicted with allergies or asthma.

According to Paul Goldberg, *"...when patients take 04 to 18 HSO caplets daily for 04 months, their asthma and allergy symptoms are reduced by 70%. When immune cells are regularly exposed to healthy HSOs, they learn to stop overreacting to dust, animal dander, pollen and other harmless particles in the environment. That means less lung, airway and sinus inflammation."*

HSOs are known to help prevent and or remedy:
- Asthma
- Constipation
- Food Allergies
- Heartburn
- Indigestion
- Irritable Bowel Syndrome
- Joint Stiffness
- Pain
- Rheumatoid Arthritis

No you don't have to go look for and eat rich black dirt to get your intake of healthy HSOs. HSOs can be found at local healthfood stores. And see the Vitamin Shoppe in the POC Section. And see *Indium*.
Follow the recommended dosage and instructions from the label and as per your doctor's instructions.

HEALING GARLIC: As early as 1500 B.C., it is noted that Egyptians listed 22 garlic prescriptions for a variety of ailments including heart problems, headaches and physical weakness. Hippocrates, a Greek physician, recommended garlic as a remedy. Chinese Herbal Code indicates that aged garlic has been used for heart problems for over 1,000 years. Garlic was used by folk healers to fight infection, cleanse the system of harmful substances, reduce high blood pressure and stimulate the immune system.

Recently, the medical field has rediscovered the value and benefits of natural medicines from the plant world. One herb from the plant field noted for its wide range of therapeutic qualities is GARLIC. Garlic research has focused on many areas including:

- Anti-bacterial effects.
- Anti-viral effects.
- Antioxidant.
- Blood pressure.
- Cancer prevention and care.
- Cardio vascular care.
- Cholesterol.
- Memory improvement.

Garlic contains Vitamins A, B1, C, E, calcium, germanium, iron, potassium, selenium, sulfur, zinc and a score of trace elements (see additional mineral and Vitamins information below). According to Dr. Gerhard Schrauzer of the University of California at San Diego, selenium, one of the important trace elements from garlic, offers protection against cancer and atherosclerosis and helps normalize blood pressure!

Germanium, another important trace element found in garlic, stimulates oxygen circulation throughout your body. The United States produces approximately 250 million pounds of fresh garlic each year which is an increase of 100 million pounds over the last decade!

European, Oriental and American doctors have recognized the powers of garlic. Doctors and scientist say that garlic has a wide range of detoxifying and microbe fighting properties. Sulfur compounds and allicin are attributed to the wonder healing of garlic. Allicin, one of the sulfur compounds in garlic is one of the most active.

It is activated when whole fresh garlic is cut or crushed. It is responsible for garlic's odor, but more important, allicin is what gives garlic its *medicinal power*. Allicin is effective against bacteria which causes dysentery, strep throat, staph infections, typhoid along with treating diabetes, hypertension, high cholesterol, vaginitis and the list goes on.

Garlic has both antifungal and antibacterial actions. Garlic's allicin was tested against staphylococcus aureus and found to be equivalent to 15 penicillin units/mg! Garlic has been shown to interfere with the growth of influenza viruses, reduce levels of coliform bacteria in the large intestines and **inhibit tumor growth!**

Garlic has a potent substance called ajoene. Formed with allicin, it is responsible for garlic's heart-saving, anti-thrombotic reaction. Tests have indicated that ajoene is at least as potent as aspirin in preventing aggregation of blood platelets and keeping blood from clotting. Garlic is also one of the few foods that contain an adaptogen called germanium.

Garlic is one of the very few foods that contain an adaptogen called germanium. This substance promotes the healing by alerting the immune system, reducing harmful deposits and destroying free radicals, dangerous byproducts that float throughout the body and cause a decline in health.

Garlic contains over 70 sulfur compounds that work together to initiate biological activities such as antibacterial, antibiotic, antiviral, antifungal, cancer fighter, cardiovascular helper, heart nutrient, high blood pressure medicine, immune booster and a skin cancer fighter.

According to an analysis conducted by the Department of Agriculture, a single clove of garlic contains minerals and Vitamins along with its unique high concentration of sulfur compounds:

- 7 calories
- .01 mg B1
- .004 MG B2
- 1.4 mg calcium
- 1.5 gm carbohydrate
- .01 grams of fat
- .07 mg iron
- .02 mg niacin
- 10 mg phosphorus
- 26 mg potassium
- .31 grams of protein
- .9 mg sodium
- .7 mg Vitamin C

In the former Soviet Union, garlic is used to kill bacteria and fight infections. Garlic has been tested to be **more effective than antibiotics** for specific types of bacterial infection called 'gram negative.' Throughout Europe garlic has earned the name *'Russian Penicillin.'* During World War II, garlic (Russian Penicillin) was widely used on the Eastern Front.

According to the United States Department of Agriculture, California, the largest producing state of garlic, produced approximately 500 million pounds of garlic in 1994.

According to many studies conducted around the world, aged garlic extract **reduced total cholesterol levels by up to 30 percent!** Garlic also **raised HDL** (good cholesterol) and reduced hardening of the arteries while lowering LDL (bad cholesterol).

According to Tufts University Diet and Nutrition Letter, two cloves of garlic per day may be **as potent** as some cholesterol-lowering drugs. Garlic may also prevent blood clots that could block arteries and lead to stroke.

Reduce heart disease risk by adding garlic to your diet (see your doctor)! Another report notes that garlic helps prevent heart attacks and strokes by controlling atherosclerosis (plaque and fat formations inside the arteries which leads to blockages in the circulatory system), high blood pressure, high cholesterol and high triglycerides.

According to 1970's studies from German physician, Dr. Hans Reuter, of Cologne, Germany, the effectiveness of garlic against heart disease is based on three fronts -- controlling cholesterol, blood pressure and fatty deposits in the arteries. Dr. Hans recommended consuming just one to three cloves of garlic per day.

The British medical Journal, The Lancet, published a study by two Indian cardiologists. The study showed that raw garlic protects you from heart disease. EAT THE RIGHT STUFF and insure garlic is part of your diet.

Dr. Bordia and Dr. Bansal of the Department of Medicine at R.N.T. Medical College in Udaiipur, India, found that **garlic demonstrates to control cholesterol so effectively that it overcomes the cardiotoxic effects of butter fat!** In controlled experiments, subjects were given a meal that included a 1/4 pound serving of butter.

As expected, blood cholesterol levels soared. The experiment was repeated, but this time 50 grams of raw garlic (two cloves) were added to the butter. Results were astonishing! The **garlic lowered blood cholesterol by more than 25 percent** from the pre-meal fasting level.

According to Dr. David Kritchevsky, associate director of the Wistar Institute in Philadelphia, *"I was doing postdoctoral work in Switzerland, when I discovered that my landlady, a **66-year-old woman who looked 44 and acted 22,** attributed her good health to the fact that she ate a clove of garlic chopped up in her salad every single night."* This discovery motivated him to begin a serious investigation into garlic's possible impact on heart disease.

The National Library of Medicine, in Bethesda, MD, contains over 125 scientific papers (from 1983 to the present) written about the medicinal value of garlic.

HIGH ALTITUDE WEIGHT-LOSS DIET: Here's another true weight-loss story. How would you like to lose weight and lose it quickly? And get this – you can eat 03 fat-rich restaurant type meals a day and you don't have to do any exercises - none!!! Sounds crazy uh?

Well I actually lived what I call the *"High Altitude Weight-Loss Diet."* Back 1987 while serving with the US Army Special Forces, our A-Team (Green Berets) deployed to Ecuador. We were at a location that was so high up (near Cotopaxi) that we were unable to do any physical training – we couldn't breathe normally to do any running, any exercise at all.

Every day I ate restaurant meals, had a brewski now & then when off duty and still lost weight very fast. I distinctly remember laying in bed in that hotel room and I was laboring trying to breathe. My body was working extra hard every second - 24-hours a day trying to get the vital oxygen it needed.

Again, we were so high up our bodies weren't use to the lack of oxygen so our bodies were trying extra extra hard to breathe every second 24-hours a day. I remember having some time off and asked one of the Ecuadorian soldiers we were training to help me shop for some new clothes that would fit me. I wasn't familiar with the small towns nearby.

As it turned out, I was not only skinny, I turned even skinny skinny!!! I lived in that environment for about a month or so and lost may be a pound of weight a day and remember I ate fat-laden and sugar-laden foods and did absolutely no exercise – no exercise!!

What I call the *High Altitude Weight-Loss Diet* really and truly works! I would ASK YOUR DOCTOR BEFORE YOU CONSIDER THIS DIET. And NO, Denver, Colorado (Mile High city) isn't high enough (5,680-feet). We were located near Cotopaxi (7,884 feet to 19,344-feet) at an approximate elevation of 9,226-feet.

That's real high and nearly dangerous cause altitude sickness and dangerous epoxy starts at 10,000 feet – if my memory serves me correctly.

MOST IMPORTANT NOTE: In my humble opinion (I ain't no bariatric physician) I sincerely believe the *"High Altitude Weight-Loss Diet"* could GREATLY REDUCE OR BANISH the USA and the world's OBESITY PEOBLEM once and for all. Think of what this diet could do if you ate super healthy food instead of fat-rich food like I did. I have my own documented PROOF of this unique diet and I CHALLENGE ANYONE TO PROVE ME WRONG!!!! Yes, that includes YOU! SEE $10,000.00 Weight-Loss Bet Diet at the end of this book.

WAIT! Here's why I think the *"High Altitude Weight-Loss Diet"* works. I already told you my body was working overtime to try to breathe even just laying in bed. You ever see folks who stop smoking and they immediately start gaining weight? Well their body is already trying to heal itself from all the years of smoking. Let me interrupt real quick and let me give you my researched data from the Gettysburg Program (full version) – **at www.amazon.com**. Here's my own "intensive research" for how your body starts healing itself once you STOP SMOKING:

Smoker's Body Starts Healing Itself: OK, if I quit smoking today, will my health improve? It sure will! It will also save you a great deal of money too, depending on the severity of your smoking habit. The following are some compiled facts of what happens when you quit smoking, from the American Cancer Society and the Center for Disease Control:

- **Within 20 Minutes** -- Your blood pressure and pulse rate drop to their normal levels and the temperature in your hands and feet will increase to your normal levels.

- **Within 08 Hours** - The carbon monoxide in your bloodstream will have decreased to its normal level and the oxygen in your bloodstream will have increased to its normal levels.

- **Within 24 Hours** -- Your chances of a heart attack decrease!

- **Within 48 Hours** -- Your nerve endings will start re-growing and your smell and taste will be enhanced.

- **Within 02 Weeks To 03 Months** -- Your circulation will improve, walking will improve, walking will become easier and lung function will increase by up to 30%!

- **Within 01 To 09 Months** -- Your coughing, sinus, congestion, fatigue and shortness of breath will decrease; cilia will regrow in your lungs, increasing their ability to handle mucous, clean the lungs and reduce the possibility of infection; your body's overall energy will increase.

- **Within 01 Year** -- Your increased risk of heart disease due to smoking will be cut in half!

- **Within 05 Years** -- Your risk for lung cancer from smoking will have been cut in half, your risk of stroke will be on the way to being reduced to that of a nonsmoker; your risk of cancer of the mouth, throat and esophagus will be half what it was when you smoked!

- **Within 10 Years** -- Your lung cancer risk will be that of a nonsmoker and precancerous cells will have been replaced with normal cells.

- **Within 15 Years** -- Your risk of coronary heart disease will be that of a nonsmoker!

See Smokenders and other Smoking Cessation *POCs* in POC Section.
Follow the recommended instructions only as per your doctor's approval.

OK, here's my point, the High Altitude Weight-Loss Diet really and the body of a smoker have something in common – both bodies are **struggling to survive** (entire body) which burns calories, burns fat - 60-seconds every minute, 24-hours a day, 07-days a week, 30-days a month, 365-days a year.

HOODIA: Hoodia is another very popular weight-loss supplement in the United States. Hoodia is so popular that there are dozens of Hoodia products out there and they all advertise their product is the authentic Hoodia containing Hoodia gordonii also known as P57.

At this time, I found no credible medical evidence that even Hoodia gordonii works for weight-loss much less any Hoodia-type product. My humble advice is to save your money ($20 - $50 per bottle – 01-month supply) and simply read this entire Survival Book and you decide what is best for you and your healthy future. You Must See *Garcinia Cambogia.*
Follow the recommended dosage and instructions from the label and as per your doctor's instructions.

HOT WEIGHT-LOSS: When the urge to eat is overwhelming try a HOTTTTT Indian, Mexican, or other spicy cuisine. According to Maria Simonson, Ph.D., Sc.D., professor emeritus and director of the Health, Weight and Stress Program at the John Hopkins Medical Institutions in Baltimore, *"The flavor is so intense that you'll find yourself **eating much smaller portions** than you would of bland or sweet foods."* An additional **bonus** of **HOTTTT spicy foods, spices and herbs** is that they heat your entire body which **speeds up your metabolism!** Read about Cayenne Pepper. See *Kalahari Appetite Suppressant*.

HYPNOTHERAPY: Hypnotherapy was used and noted to effective back in ancient times! Once it was endorsed by the American Medical Association (AMA) in 1958, hypnotherapy grew in its applications, methods and especially its credibility.

Hypnotherapy is a technique whereby the practitioner can speak directly to the unconscious mind and can therefore communicate with that part of the mind that controls everything from perception to memory, as well as monitoring all the physical functions of the body.

Hypnotherapy can be effective in treating a wide variety of conditions from anorexia nervosa, asthma, depression... Hypnotherapy is the quality of interaction between the expert and the patient using hypnosis or not. The process of **discovery and recovery from psychoemotional traumas** that affect the productive living of life. Hypnotherapy is used in treating or addressing many common psychosomatic problems such as addictions, pain, phobias, stress, **weight control**...

Indian Gator Aid: Here's the 1st Gator Aid made by Indians hundreds of years earlier. Equal parts of chia seeds (mint-tasting) and prickly pear juice with water was a known endurance drink for the Pima and Tohono O'odham Indian tribes.

INDIUM: Indium is a trace mineral meaning it's needed by the body in very very small amounts as compared to sodium and dozens of other minerals. Indium is Element #49 on the Periodic Table of Elements. It's a soft mineral, which does not dissolve in water unless compounded (other elements added). It's 99.99% pure, and is the 10th most scarce element of all available elements. Indium was discovered in 1883.

So, what's the big deal about Indium?

Indium is a natural trace mineral and in recent years, is proving to be a leading mineral to fight aging, reverse aging, fight and ameliorate diseases of all kinds. For centuries, thousands of years, ancient cultures have used minerals to fight ill health and stay healthy, like the Chinese and other cultures have used mineral-rich seaweed. Greeks used iron enriched water. Pioneers drank rusty water for their iron. Indium is called *"the missing trace mineral."* Until recently has its supplementation to the daily diet been linked to helping the body heal itself and according to the manufacturers, all it takes is 01 single drop a day.

What's the healing secret behind Indium?

Indium, a rare trace mineral through its unique ingredients helps the body improve its own health in many ways (keep reading). And it somehow gets the body to absorb MORE of other trace minerals as well as recycle them through the body again thus helping the body perform at peak performance. Like I said before, your body is mostly made-up of water and minerals (74+).

Indium levels in the soil and human bodies were found so low, that even special recording equipment was unable to record any traces of indium. That may indicate indium may not be needed to sustain life, but aid in vibrant health. Just 01 single drop of indium per day, has recorded many many healing testimonials across the globe.

Can you give me some healing accounts of Indium?

Sure, there are many, but here's an <u>abbreviated</u> listing:

- Alzheimer's Disease
- Acne
- Allergies
- Anti-Aging
- Anti-Depressant
- Backache
- Blood Sugar Normalization
- Bruises, Cuts, Scratches,... Healed Faster
- Cancer (reduced tumors)
- Circulation
- Diabetes (Type Two)
- Dizziness
- Energy Level Increase

- Exercise (longer workouts)
- Glaucomic Eye Pressure
- Hair (restores original color & enhances re-growth)
- High Blood Pressure
- Immune System Enhancement
- Inflammation
- Intestinal & Bowel Maladies
- Lethargic Appetite
- Libido
- Lifespan Increase
- Memory Improvement
- Menopause
- Menstruation
- Mental Clarity
- Migraine Headaches (decrease)
- Morbus Parkinson's Disease
- Nausea
- Pain (general)
- Prostate (PSA)
- Red Blood Cells Live Longer
- Sense of Smell Improvement
- Sense of Taste Improvement
- Sinus Pressure
- Sleep Improvement
- Trembling Hands
- Ulcers (mouth, stomach,...)
- Urinary Maladies
- Vision Improvement
- **Weight-Loss**

Is Indium safe to take?

Yes. According to tests on animals, the current Indium supplement offered by East Park Research, Inc., it would have to be 1,000 times stronger just to make a mouse sick!

Oh, before I forget, Indium has been given to race horses to improve their performance.

This sounds too good to be true but I'm still very interested in Indium. Where can I get more FREE information before I make my buying decision?
Good question. See East Park Research, Inc. in the POC Section.

JELLO: While serving in the U.S. Army at Fort Davis, Panama, I was told one diet aid used under the care of a physician is Jello! Yes, Jello. Overweight GIs would **eat Jello to lose weight!** Why does it work? Jello is mostly water and water has NO FAT, NO CARBOHYDRATES, - it's water. The overweight GIs could eat as much Jello as they wanted but were not allowed regular meals. Try NO SUGAR Jello to help you lose weight.

JUICER MACHINES: There are basically two types of juicer machines. There are centrifugal juicers that have a spinning basket and there are mastication type juicers. These juicers separate the juice from the pulp & fiber and you end up with pure juice. That's the goal of using a juicer machine, to get the pure juice, consume it so that the benefitting nutrients go right into the bloodstream almost immediately. Which juicer is best?

The Gerson Clinic in Mexico City, Mexico is having great results with **curing the "incurable!"** One reason is they use a mastication type juicer because they feel the centrifugal type juicers leave most of the nutrients in the pulp whereas the mastication type juicer machines removed three to four times more nutrients!

However, you don't have to go to Mexico, read this entire book and **USE MANY OPTIONS TO REGAIN YOUR VIBRANT HEALTH** under your doctor's approval!

While I'm on the subject of juicer machines, what about all that left-over pulp? Making your own compost is a good idea! If you want something done right, then do it yourself! Use compost to _**grow your own fresh fruits and vegetables and don't forget those Amazing Herbs**_.

To insure you have the best soil, read about earthworms on the internet and protect your crops by growing garlic around the perimeter of your garden and throughout it! Don't believe me, read about that amazing powers of Healing Garlic and see *Gerson Diet*.

JUICE THERAPY: Juice Therapy utilizes the fresh, raw juice of vegetables and fruits to nourish and replenish the body during periods of stress and illness. Juice Therapy may be used as nutritional support or as part as a health maintenance plan. Juicing delivers those needed and healthy nutrients (Vitamins, minerals, phytochemicals...).

I have read PLENTY of testimonials of regular folks that juiced and seen healing results from arthritis to cancer to **weight-loss**. And when it comes to a juicing machine, what you pay for is what you get so shop wisely. See Detoxification Therapy and see Going Green.

KALAHARI APPETITE SUPPRESSANT: Now to tie-in with Zulu Super Food, I want to tell you about the Kalahari Appetite Suppressant. The Kalahari Desert was unmerciful even to the savvy Kalahari bushmen. Food was precious and water priceless.

At times there was no food nor water. But the savvy bushmen and women had a trick to suppress their want for water and food. Throughout the Kalahari Desert are patches of tiny bushes that offer a bitter bean that resembles a lima bean. These beans are eaten by the natives to suppress the urge for water and food.

The only problem is the beans burns the tongue, throat, and stomach. The point to all this is that <u>hot</u> (I mean real hot) spicy tasting food may suppress the appetite. According to my research, the Kalahari Appetite *Suppressant* is not Hoodia. See Hoodia.

KIMCHEE: The 1st time I ate Kimchee, I said "How can people eat this?" Well, after the 2nd & 3rd try "I love it!" Kimchee is a very popular Korean food. I believe it originated in Korea. Kimchee is a combination of cabbage, other vegetables, spices,... I was told that Kimchee is made by storing its **raw contents** in closed containers in underground buried holes where it is allowed to age and ferment. The end result is a very spicy and tasty vegetable meal that still has those much needed **weight-loss enzymes!** Now here's the good part why Kimchee is a potential **great weight-loss meal!** Kimchee's:

- **total fat content - <u>ZERO</u>**
- **saturated fat – <u>ZERO</u>**
- **cholesterol content – <u>ZERO</u>**
- **calories per serving - <u>only 05,</u>...**

Kimchee also contains hot spices that will fire-up your metabolism. Now you don't have to bury cabbage in your backyard, you can buy Kimchee at most grocery stores. Let me ask you something and this is not a joke. Have you ever seen an overweight Korean? Well, there you go.

LATE EATING: Experts can't agree on exact times but they do agree that when you eat late, you're asking for it - you're inviting extra pounds of weight. Why? Cause your body - metabolism slows down, especially while you're sleeping so that food turns into fat since there is no need to burn it. What's worse is if you're eating sweets, fat-laden foods,...

Turn off your eating machine as early as 3pm and no later than 7pm. Some experts state **NO CARBOHYDRATE FOODS AFTER 3PM** and **NO EATING AFTER 7PM**.

LOSE FAT BY EATING FAT: Replace those saturated fats with Medium Chain Triglycerides (MCTs)! MCTs have been used in medicine for almost 40 years for patients who have difficulty digesting or absorbing nutrients or who need a rapidly available source of energy.

MCTs are 1/3 to 1/2 the size of long chain triglycerides (LCTs) which are found in virtually all oils in the foods we eat like butter, margarine, animal fats and vegetable oils. MCTs are much more water-soluble than LCTs meaning there are **rapidly burned for energy**.

LCTs (fat) on the other hand, may be stored in the body and utilized at a later time. MCTs may be a **great diet replacement for LCTs**. See Sound Nutrition in the POC Section for additional information or go to your local health food store and look for MCT FUEL by TwinLab.

MAGNESIUM: Magnesium relaxes the nerves and muscles. This mineral is known as the *"anti-stress" mineral*. Magnesium converts blood sugar into energy. This mineral helps keep teeth healthy and provides temporary relief from indigestion.

This mineral is necessary so that our body can use Vitamin C, calcium, phosphorus, sodium and potassium effectively. Magnesium is essential in over 300 enzyme activities, especially the production of ATP (helps supply energy to every part of your body).

Magnesium is a **must for healthy hearts!** As a matter of fact, research has indicated multitudes of **heart disease related deaths are linked to magnesium deficiency!**
Follow the recommended dosage and instructions from the label and as per your doctor's instructions.

MCBARROON DIET: According to Jan McBarroon, M.D., a specialist in weight control, *"Maintenance is what matters. It **took me years to figure out the secret**. I had to **start eating and stop dieting**." "I lost 50 pounds - five times!"* Here are some basics for her weight-loss program:

- Limit calories to 1,200 daily. For maintenance (after reaching your weight goal) limit yourself to 1,500 to 1,800 calories per day.

- 60 to 70 percent of your calories should come from carbohydrates like bread, fruits, lentils, pasta, rice, vegetables...

- No more than 20 calories of protein per day.

- Reduce fat intake to 10 to 20 percent of total calories. Three grams of fat for every 100 calories.

- Drink 64 ounces or eight 08-ounce glasses of water per day.

IMPORTANT: Most Americans **gain weight because they eat so much so late at night!** Your body has two sets of enzymes. One burns food as energy and is activated in the morning. The other enzyme stores food as fat and is activated in the afternoon and evening.

- King, Queen And Pauper - Eat like a king at breakfast, a queen at lunch and a pauper at night! Exercise daily and supplement your diet with these nutrients!

- **Chromium Picolinate** - Regulates blood sugar levels and keeps a lid on insulin, which is an appetite stimulant and fat-making hormone!

- **Super Blue Green Algae (SBGA)** - A pure plant protein and an excellent, non-stimulating appetite suppressant. Cuts hunger! See Super Blue Green Algae.

- **Garcinia Cambogia Extract** - A metabolic enhancer. It revs-up your fat-burning engine and is a natural appetite suppressant. See Garcinia Cambogia.

MEDITERRANEAN DIET: People in the Mediterranean have been noted to **develop far less heart disease than Americans**, even though they drink, smoke and even consumed as much or more saturated fat than Americans! What are they doing different?

Their diet consists of an oil they use on their vegetables, grain-rich dishes and meats. They even dip their bread in it!

It's olive oil! Yes, olive oil. One added bonus of monounsaturated fats, they maintain HDL (high density lipoprotein) that helps prevent heart disease. Olive, peanut and canola oils are noted to be highest in monounsaturated fats. Insure you read the Nutrition Facts label on any cooking oil. Look for the word *"monounsaturated."* Look for the least amount of saturated fats and the most monounsaturated fats.

WARNING: INSURE you use **"cold pressed"** olive oil! Use all cooking oils sparingly! See Olive Oil.

Why are people who live by the Mediterranean Diet, healthier than Americans despite their high tobacco consumption, low exercise level and modest health-care system?
The Mediterranean Diet is a diet low in meat, but high in cereal, fruit, grain, legumes, monounsaturated fats-nuts and vegetables. Recent French Study found that the Mediterranean Diet after a heart attack was 70 percent more life-saving than the Standard American Diet (low-fat diet-less than 30 percent fat calories). Some Harvard Researchers favor the Mediterranean Diet over the Standard American Diet.

A research effort called the Seven Countries Study, examined 12,763 men ages 40 through 59 in the Netherlands, Finland, Italy, Greece, Croatia and Serbia, Japan and the United States. Ten years after their initial screening, the study reported several important results:

- Mediterranean groups had **lower death rates** from all causes than the northern European and American groups.

- **Lower mortality from coronary heart disease** in the Mediterranean countries.

- Men at the peak of their lives (45 years) have **longer life expectancies** in Greece than in any other European or North American country despite their high tobacco consumption, low exercise level and modest health-care system.

The Mediterranean Diet is based on traditional eating patterns evolving over centuries in Greece, Italy, North Africa, Southern France, Spain and several Middle Eastern nations. All share a general pattern of cooking and ingredients.

The diet is rich in fruits, vegetables, legumes and grains. The **principal fat is olive oil!** Lean red meat is eaten only a few times a month and in small portions. Eating foods from animal sources - namely dairy products, fish and poultry is low to moderate. Wine is drunk with meals.

Plenty of crusty country-style bread is enjoyed with each meal. The major fat used in the Mediterranean Diet is olive oil! Olive oil is primarily a monounsaturated fat, which is noted to lower harmful low-density lipoprotein (LDL) blood cholesterol and may increase good high-density lipoprotein (HDL) blood cholesterol. Olive oil isn't the only key to a healthy diet.

Here are some **Mediterranean eating tips**:
- Switch to olive oil (extra virgin).
- Avoid butter and margarine. There is nothing wrong with putting olive oil on toast or whole grain bread.
- Cut meat consumption. If you do eat meat, insure it's lean. Try small portions of poultry or fish with plenty of vegetables.
- **INCREASE** fruit and vegetable consumption.
- Eat plenty of whole grain bread. The darker the better (ingredients not burnt).
- Eat a salad at the beginning and end of each meal.
- Wine at each dinner meal. It's been noted that a couple glasses of wine each day may protect against coronary heart disease.

MELATONIN: Melatonin is a natural hormone which is used as an organic **alternative to sleeping aids and as a treatment for jet-lag**. There have been **4,000 articles published on melatonin**. Melatonin is inexpensive. It is a nonprescription supplement. According to my research, it has no toxic properties.

Research indicates the following values of melatonin: a transducer, an overall governor of all energy functions, anti-aging, anti-arteriosclerotic, anti-infectious, anti-stress, anticarcinogenic, antitoxic, regulates endogenous opioid system, regulates hormone system, regulates immune system, regulates mineral metabolism, regulates oxidation reduction, regulates respiration...

Swedish researchers Walter Pierpaoli and Georges Maestroni of the Institute of Integrative Bio-Medical Research in Locarno, Switzerland, noted that when 10 healthy aging mice were given melatonin, their **lifespan increased** to 931 days, compared to 755 days for the control group.

Not only did **melatonin prolong their lifespan** but they also noted **positive action on their performance and reversed or delayed symptoms of age-related debility, disease and cosmetic decline!**

- **Cancer** - Many research studies have noted that melatonin enhances the ability of experimental animals to withstand stress by **enhancing and maintaining efficient immune function**. Melatonin may **inhibit** the growth of a variety of **tumor cells**. In one study melatonin was injected during the afternoon **influenced the regression of mammary tumors** in rats and counteracted the development of breast cancer.

- **Depression** - Depression, at one time or another, affects everyone. It may be a pronounced in the elderly during the winter months. This is called Seasonal Affective Disorder (SAD). SAD is directly related to the reduction of daylight hours during the winter months. SAD may be affectively treated with high-intensity light. Increasing the brightness of the light cycle has been noted to increase the level of melatonin released during the dark cycle. One researcher (J. Beck-Friis) noted that one syndrome of **severe depression is related to low melatonin levels** and abnormal melatonin\serotonin cycling.

- **Insomnia** - The majority of insomniacs are the elderly. In a double-blind placebo trial, Austrian researchers noted the effects of 20 young healthy volunteers that were exposed to artificial insomnia. The benefits of melatonin were exceptional. Their **overall sleep improved, including a reduced number of awakenings** during their sleep and a **reduction in time they were awake before they fell asleep**.

Follow the recommended dosage and instructions from the label and as per your doctor's instructions.

MELONS: Melons on an average provide approximately 55 calories per cup. Melons provide one of the **highest fiber content** of any food, while providing generous amounts of Vitamin A, Vitamin C, more than 800 milligrams of much needed potassium (1/2 cantaloupe). Melons are a great source of 'pure' water (grown organically).

MILITARY WEIGHT-LOSS EXERCISES AND DIETS: Here is a complied list of all the Military Weight-Loss Exercises And Diets in this book. These **really work** in helping you meet your weight-loss goals. Let's start with Eggs.

- Eggs
- Forced Hydration
- High Altitude Weight-Loss Diet
- Jello
- Rucksacking
- Run-Swim-Ruck-Shoot
- SERE Weight-Loss Plan
- Swimming Fat Burners
- U.S. Army Rifle Drill Exercises (07)
- Water Polo

And don't forget the other weight-loss applications I used with great success - see $10,000.00 Weight-Loss Bet Diet, Apple Cider Vinegar (APC), Apples, Cabbage, Carrots, Coenzyme Q10 (CoQ10), The Five Deadly Whites, Healing Garlic, Hot Weight-Loss, Juice Therapy, Mind-Over-Matter and Raw Food Diet. OK, let's carry-on with Mind-Over-Matter.

MIND-OVER-MATTER: Folks, call it what you like (Biofeedback Training, Guided Imagery, Meditation, Prayer, Vision Therapy...), there is something happening here! **YOU HAVE NO IDEA OF THE POTENTIAL OF YOUR MIND AND WHAT IT CAN DO TO ENHANCE YOUR LIFE!** In this Survival Book, I've tried to reveal several Mind-Over-Matter Therapies that work!

INSURE you read this Survival Book at least a few times and consider (with your doctor's approval) using these Mind-Over-Matter Therapies in conjunction with other conventional and alternative therapies and treatment. See *Exercise Mind-Over-Matter Trick, Vision Therapy, Your Picture, Mutt And Jeff Mind-Over-Matter*, and more throughout this Survival Book.

OK OK, here are a couple of my own Mind-Over-Matter applications that have happened to me. So I BELIEVE in Mind-Over-Matter Applications. OK, Let's start with Soda Drink:

a) Soda Drink:
Time-------1973
Location---High School
Subject----Faked-Out My Taste Buds

It was my senior year in high school and I was talking to a friend by the soda machine. Back then I'd always always drink grape sodas. Well I put my money in the machine while talking to my friend. I just "brailed" my way through the motions of inserting the money, selecting the soda, grabbing the grape soda, opening it and began drinking without looking at the grape soda - all while talking to my friend.

Well I drank at least half the grape soda. While in the process of swallowing a gulp of the grape soda, I looked at the can to realize it wasn't a grape soda but a cola!!!!

As I looked at the can the tastebuds in my mouth went from tasting grape to tasting cola!!! I fooled myself - I was so sure I was drinking grape soda - the cola didn't register on my tastebuds!!!!

This is absolutely a true story and ever since then, I've been interested in Mind-Over-Matter applications.

Why Mind-Over-Matter applications? Cause if there is one untapped power - it's your mind and you can use various Mind-Over-Matter applications to IMPROVE your life! There is ALWAYS room for improvement for everybody and that means YOU!

b) 01 In 52 Card Pick:
Time-------Spring 1985
Location---Fort Bragg, North Carolina
Subject----Author's Own Dowsing Technique

One day while working at the U.S. Army Special Forces Weapons Branch, I was sitting in the weapons bay - classroom where we taught Phase II Weapons to Special Forces Candidates (potential Green Berets). Sitting around during our lunch break, one of the cadre broke out a deck of cards. They played a bit and then I said something like 'let me show you all something.'

I told one cadre to shuffle the cards and pick out a single card and show all the cadre but not to let me see the card that was picked. I told him to place the card in the deck and shuffle the deck. He shuffled the cards and I told him to pass the cards over and let another cadre member shuffle the cards. About a half a dozen cadre got their turn to shuffle the cards. I then told them to take the deck and cut it and place the two sections of the deck side-by-side.

I then took my right-hand - palm down and placed it or hovered it over each deck. I did this back and forth 02 or 03 times to confirm my choice. You see when I placed my hand over the deck that had the card they picked, my hand - namely the fingers would tingle! And sure enough the fingers tingled. I said *"the card is in that deck"* pointing to the deck. They looked at me like I was crazy. I told them to discard the other deck and deal the remaining cards into 06 - 07 decks with 05 or so cards per deck. They did what I told them.

With several smaller decks of cards in front of me, I again hovered my right-hand - palm down and hovered it over all the decks and once or twice more to confirm. I stated *"the card is in that deck"* pointing to the deck of only several cards.

Looking at me strangely, I told them to get rid of all the other cards and place the remaining several cards side-by-side. They did as I requested and again, I hovered my right-hand - palm down over the remaining several cards. I confidently stated *"that's the card"* pointing to it. They looked at me like I was nuts and flipped over the card I picked and the room busted in shouts!

They asked me how I did it - they thought it was a trick so I did the same "dowsing for cards" again (02 - 03 times) to prove myself and again I picked the correct card! Once I proved myself, one cadre member wanted to take me to Las Vegas and others wanted to take me to some local poker games in Fayetteville. I declined stating *"it doesn't work that way."*

How does this hand dowsing work? I'm not sure, all I know is that my hand - fingers tingle! It's a form of dowsing and most important - **I BELIEVED** in my ability to dowse with my hands. I have never tried to do this with other applications to find things like water, oil, minerals, precious metals. This is a true story - I'm sure those former weapons cadre that were present may not remember me as a weapons instructor but they will always remember me decades later for that special magic-like application to pick out 01 specific card from an entire deck of 52 cards.

c) Author's Own Mind-Over-Matter Application To IGNORE Cold Weather - Thinking Of The Past:

"Aren't you cold?" they would ask. When I worked at the post office in St. Louis (1996), I'd be on the roof taking a break with nothing on but shirt and pants. It was cold hovering around freezing temperatures. People would ask me "Aren't you cold?" I would say "no." Sometimes I would say "I don't feel it like you do." What am I doing to overcome the cold-weather temperatures?

Being in the military, one thing they (leadership) almost NEVER NEVER do is stop the training for bad weather, no matter how bad it got. As a matter of fact, they were more than a few times when as a young private, I thought I was going to freeze to death. I thought if I even dozed-off I'd be dead. I agree with this policy, just because the weather gets bad, the war doesn't stop. Besides you can use the bad weather to your advantage in offensive operations especially at night.

Anyway, through the years of training and multitude of times of being exposed to bad, miserable, weather (thousands of hours); I became immune to it. How? Whenever bad & miserable weather was around me, I simply thought of when it was really bad. I had the past and 20-years of miserable weather to draw from - I'd think of when it was really bad and when I did, the present miserable weather was nothing more than a refreshing crisp awareness that I was still alive and I just carried-on! So when faced with freezing temperatures, I knew it was nothing compared to what I survived before. Besides I knew it wasn't going to last like the long hours and days of continuous miserable near-death weather I faced many times before.

When I moved into my present house in 2007, I adopted a water garden with 06 koi fish. Today I have approximately 60 koi fish. During the winter months, I'd get in that super cold water with NO COLD WEATHER PROTECTION and clean the filters. It took about 90-minutes of being submerged in that cold water. A few years back I started wearing protective waders. My point is I tolerated that cold water cause I used my special Mind-Over-Matter Application.

NOTE: Insure you properly prepare for all cold weather environments. You don't have to go in there and *"Rambo"* it like I did!

Insure you read about other Mind-Over-Matter related applications throughout this Survival Book.

MIRACLE II PRODUCTS: Dr. LaMar also offers *Miracle II Products*. I had to bring these products to your attention because of the many Testimonials linked to using Miracle II Products. And some of Miracle II Products are:

- Miracle II Soap
- Miracle II Neutralizer
- Miracle II Neutralizer Gel
- Miracle II Skin Moisturizer
- Miracle II Moisturizer Soap

Miracle II *Products* are linked to reported Testimonials like: Acid problems (stomach), acne, AIDS, age spots, allergies, Alzheimer's Disease, athlete's foot, arthritis, bed sores, body odor, bronchitis, bruises, burns, cancer, candida albicans, cataracts, cellulite, chicken pox, cholesterol, colic, common cold, constipation, contact lens cleaner, Chron's Disease, cracked skin (hands & feet), cuts, dandruff, denture hot spots, dermatitis, diabetes, diaper rash, discolored skin, douche replacement, dry skin, ear ache, elbows, enema, energy, eye wash & lubrication, fever blisters, gingivitis, gout, Gulf War Illness, foot odor, finger nail fungus, gallbladder, hair, head lice, heels, hemorrhoids, herpes, high blood pressure, hives, hyperactivity, indigestion, insect bites, insect repellent, jock itch, kidney cleanser, knees, liver cleanser, lubricating gel, Lupus, Lyme Disease, Lymphoma-Follicular cancer, scalp, nerves, nose bleeding, odors, pancreatic, parasites, pink eye, poison ivy, poison oak, prostate, psoriasis, rash, Ryder's Syndrome, scars, scratches, sensitive mouth problems, shoe odors, shingles, sinus, skin cancer, snake bite, spider bite, spotted skin, stomach ulcers, stop smoking, stretch marks, styes, sunburn, tag warts (skin), teeth, T-Cell booster (immune system), thyroid problems, tired feet, toxemia, tumors, ulcers, ulcers (mouth) underarm deodorant, varicose veins, **weight-loss**, wrinkles, yeast infection,...

Yes Yes Yes, folks all over the world are using Miracle II Products on their pet critters and the bigger "don't let in the house" critters like horses, cows, pigs,...

While researching for this small segment, I tried to reason why these Miracle II Products work so good. It may start out with **what THEY DON'T HAVE IN THEM**. Did you know most bath and shower soaps are made and comprised of 80% animal fat!!! These ingredients (fat) in regular soap BLOCK TOXINS from leaving your body.

And it turns out these *Miracle II Products* may have a **"detoxifying" a "cleansing" process on the body** while they're used (let the body rid itself of toxins) - thus giving your body the innate ability of your body to heal itself - thus the many healing Testimonials.

This is just 01 more reason why you have to call and get your own healthy info packet from Dr. Lamar. I believe the lady at Dr. LaMar's company told me the packet cost $2.50. See Dr. LaMar's Products Inc. in the POC Section. I believe the lady at Dr. LaMar's company told me the packet cost $2.50.

MUSCLES: Recent research indicates that the more muscle you have, the higher your metabolism rate. The extra muscle makes your **metabolism go up even when you're at rest**. **Lift weights to lower your weight!** See Weight Training and Exercise Mind-Over-Matter Trick.

MUSHROOM: At this time few medicinal benefits from the popular and common mushroom in the United States, have been researched and proved. However, four Oriental mushrooms (shiitake, oyster, enoki and tree) contain compounds that can stimulate the immune system, inhibit blood clotting and retard the development of cancer.

Japanese scientists have analyzed the medicinal qualities of mushrooms, especially the shiitake mushroom which is popular in the United States. Scientists note that some mushrooms possess properties that may **strengthen the immune system against a variety of infections, cancer and possibly, autoimmune diseases like rheumatoid arthritis, polyarthritis and multiple sclerosis**.

The most common and best-studied mushroom with the **greatest therapeutic qualities** is the shiitake, also known as *"golden oaks"* in the United States. In 1960 Dr. Kenneth Cochran of the University of Michigan, launched a study of the shiitake mushroom. He discovered this mushroom contained a compound called lentinan, a long-chained sugar called a polysaccharide, which has a **strong antiviral potential that stimulates the immune system functions!**

Shiitake stimulates the immune system to produce more interferon, which is a natural defense agent against viruses and fighting cancers. The shiitake compound, lentinan, has proved itself in fighting cancers. It has been tested in leukemia patients in China and on breast cancer patients in Japan.

In follow-up Japanese test, lentinan was found to be **far more effective against influenza viruses than a powerful antiviral drug called amantadine hydrochloride**. More tests found that lentinan is a broad-spectrum killer of various viruses.

Consuming shiitake could **help lower blood cholesterol and even block the bad effects of highly saturated fats**. In one study, a group of thirty healthy young women **drove their blood cholesterol down by an average of 12 percent** by simply eating 03-ounces of shiitake each day for a week.

Could shiitake counter the effect of fat in the diet?
In another study, one group ate two ounces of butter every day for a week; their cholesterol went up 14 percent. Another group ate the same amount of butter every day for a week, but added three ounces of shiitake. **Guess what happened?** Their blood cholesterol **dropped 04 percent** instead of rising 14 percent (non-eaters of shiitake)!

MUSIC & SOUND THERAPY: Sound Therapy is based on the idea that sound and music can influence our health through both its calming and energizing effects on the brain hypothalamus and central nervous system. Sound Therapy is **used in hospitals, schools and psychological treatment programs to alleviate pain, improve movement and balance, lower blood pressure, overcome various learning disabilities, promote endurance and strength and reduce stress!**

And here's the other take on Music & Sound Therapy. Listen to your most favorite music and start working out. Before you know it you'll have gone through several songs and you're just getting started. Your favorite music will take your mind off your *"boring"* workout.

MUTT AND JEFF MIND-OVER-MATTER: Before you read this segment, read Your Picture. Read it? OK, here's another take on it. Mutt And Jeff is a term used by the British during World War II. British interrogators used Mutt And Jeff (good interrogator and bad interrogator) to get information out of German, Italian,... prisoners of war (POWs). The "bad interrogator" would start by abusing the prisoner. Then the "good interrogator" would come in and treat the prisoner with humane respect thus getting the cooperation and most important, the needed information from the prisoner. Where am I going with this?

Do the Mutt And Jeff with pictures of yourself. Put a picture of yourself at the fridge (motivates you to stop snacking,...) of you being overweight (bad picture). Put a thin picture of yourself (good picture) next to your exercise machine (motivates you to workout). You get the idea. If you don't have current overweight or past thin pictures, just paste your face to a thin body from a magazine. Your SUBCONSCIOUS doesn't know the truth.

Your subconscious will start doing its work when it sees all your Mutt And Jeff pictures throughout your home, car wallet,... Thus, you have Mutt And Jeff Mind-Over-Matter working for YOU 24-hours a day! And remember what I told you about Mind-Over-Matter applications, you have to <u>BELIEVE</u> for them to work.

NONI: Noni (Morinda citrifolia) is such a popular and bragged about health supplement that MLM (multi-level marketing) and non-MLM companies used it to boost their sales.

Forget about MLM (it only works for people at the very top - 01%), *Noni* may show some promise as a healthy supplement in support of your healthy weight-loss goals. It was first reported by Captain James Cook who between 1773 to 1775 he made many a discoveries to include recording the healthy Noni plant.

Noni (fruit, leaves, stem, seed, flowers, bark,...) has been noted to be used for: abdominal swelling, abscesses, appetite stimulant, arthritis, boils, brain stimulant, bruises, carbuncles, colic, constipation, cough, cuts, diabetes, fever, fractures, gum infections, hernia, hypertension, insecticide, jaundice, laxative, menstrual regulation, mouth infections, nausea, rheumatism, scabs, scalp insecticide, skin cracking, sores, sore throat, sprains, sties, stomach ache, stomach ulcers, toothaches, tuberculosis, urinary tract, wound poultice, wounds,... Visit your local health food store and ask about Noni to supplement your healthy diet.

NUTS TO OBESITY, CANCER AND HEART DISEASE: Nuts (almonds, macadamians, pecans, soy) may help you lose a lot a weight! Why? Well you actually need fat in your body to process food nutrients through your bloodstream. Nuts contain one of the best fats - monounsaturated fats. Studies have shown that nuts with these "good fats" actually suppressed the appetite and participants actually lost weight. Why? The body got the signal it was full because of the nutty omega fatty acids. So nuts to obesity,...

OATS\OAT BRAN: Approximately one ounce of uncooked oat bran provides 110 calories. A recent published study lasting over 12 years at the University of Kentucky with hundreds of volunteers showed that oat bran as well as wheat bran **effectively lowered cholesterol** by 20 percent, which reflects on the protection against heart disease. Oats may have an anti-inflammatory effect on contact eczema and psoriasis.

OLIVE OIL: Olive oil varies in quality. The term "virgin" is loosely applied. Originally it meant that the oil was from the first pressing of the fruit, as opposed to the second or third pressing. Olive oil when unrefined has a **greenish tinge and a pungent flavor**. It is preferred to refined oils because the health qualities are intact. I've found that Extra Virgin Italian Olive Oil (cold pressed), is one of the best bets for a quality oil.

Many studies have shown that populations using large amounts of olive oil like Italy and Greece have **lower heart disease and stroke**. Olive oil is rich in Vitamin E and a known antioxidant. Olive oil is linked to longevity, olive trees have been known to live as long as 3,000 years!

Olive oil may be one of the best choices when cooking with oils. Olive oil IS NOT saturated fat but is a monounsaturated fatty acid, which is stable at high temperatures and less prone to oxidation than other vegetable oils. Extra Virgin Oil is probably your best choice of oil. However, see Coconut Oil and see Mediterranean Diet.

ONIONS: A 1/2 cup of raw onions provide only 27 calories and are inexpensive. Onions are used in just about every dish imaginable, from appetizers to main courses to soups to even jellies. Onions can be eaten raw, they can be pickled, sautéed, deep fried, boiled, steamed... Onions help **boost the good cholesterol** which is HDL (High Density Lipo-proteins), lower total blood cholesterol, slow down blood clotting, thin the blood, kill bacteria and may even counteract against some allergic reactions.

Dr. Victor Gurewich, professor of medicine at Tufts University, prescribes and tells his patients to **"Eat onions."** Dr. Gurewich notes that raw, strong onions elevate critical HDL-type blood cholesterol. The typical therapeutic dose is only 1/2 a medium-size raw onion - or equivalent juice - each day.

Dr. Gurewich says that is usually enough to **"dramatically raise"** HDLs (good cholesterol) an **average of 30 percent in about 03 out of 04 heart disease patients!** In a few cases, **HDL levels have doubled or tripled** on the onion regimen! He says that **raw onions work best** because cooking lessons or destroys the onion's power to raise HDLs.

Raw or cooked onion works as a natural anticoagulant to **help prevent life-threatening blood clots that may cause heart attacks and strokes!**

According to a study in India, test participants were purposely fed fat-intensive meals that raised their cholesterol to dangerous levels, thus increasing the risk of blood clots. The participants were then given **only two ounces of onion**, which was added to their diet and their cholesterol levels were **quickly brought within safe limits!**

Onions may be a potential source of **possible cancer antidotes** because of their concentrated sulfur compounds that are able to turn off cell changes preceding cancer growth. Researchers at the M.D. Anderson Hospital and Tumor Institute have isolated propylsulfide in onions that in tests **blocked enzymes needed to activate a potent cancer-causing substance**.

Researchers at Harvard School of Dental Medicine discovered that putting onion extract on cultures of oral cancer cells from animals significantly inhibited proliferation of the cancer cells and destroyed some. As a matter of fact, the National Cancer Institute has funded much research on sulfides in onions and garlic, naming them promising agents in fending off cancer!

PAPAYA: Mexican Indians say that papaya has *healing powers*. A regular size papaya provides only 160 calories, Vitamin C, a significant source of folic acid, fiber and very low in sodium. It is best to pick a papaya when it is just turning yellow. Papayas provide **healthy digestive properties** (enzyme called papain) that have a direct tonic effect on the stomach.

PASTA: Pasta is found in many cuisines throughout the world like Italian lasagna, Chinese lo mein, Greek pistachio, Jewish lokshen kugel... Did you know pasta isn't fattening? Pasta itself provides approximately 110 calories per ounce, but the fattening stuff is what you add to the pasta (butter, cheese, oil, tomato sauce, ground beef...)! Pasta is rich in copper, iron, magnesium, manganese, niacin, phosphorus, protein, riboflavin, thiamin and zinc. Pasta is easily digestible, **low in fat and low in sodium**. Eat some pasta but <u>watch what you put on it</u>! Some pasta boxes will tell you their product is a *"low glycemic"* food. See Glycemic Food Index.

PAST LIFE THERAPY: Past Life Therapy (PLT) accesses information or images from possible former lifetimes, usually through hypnotic regression or some form of altered state of consciousness, for therapeutic purposes.

PLT searches emotionally or physically traumatic life memories such as promoting cathartic release (release of emotions), reframing attitudes, **changing old habits or behavior problems** and gaining conscious insight into the lessons of that life memory for therapeutic purposes; to help **patients resolve their present problems.** Also known as Regression Therapy or Transformational Therapy. Past Life Therapy may reveal why you're over weight thus having you finally losing all that extra unwanted unhealthy weight.

PEACHES: A regular size peach has only 37 calories and provides Vitamins C and A. The skin of a peach can be removed very easily by boiling it just a minute or so and then dropping it in very cold water for about a minute. Peaches are easily digestible, provide a **high fiber** content while **promoting regularity.**

PEANUT BUTTER: Nutritious peanut butter helps with weight-loss. According to Richard Mattes Ph.D., R.D. and other researchers, people who ate peanut butter felt satisfied longer than other snacks. They not only felt more satisfied but lost **15-times as much weight** as those that passed on food. A great snack is peanut butter on celery sticks - MMMMMmmmmm!

And here are some more Peanut Butter Facts to back-up this claim:

Fact 01: American consume approximately 700,000,000 pounds of peanut butter each year! That's about a katrillion zillion peanuts!

Fact 02: 02 tablespoons of peanut butter contain 16 grams of fat - the GOOD fat!

Fact 03: 02 tablespoons of peanut butter contain 190 calories!

Fact 04: 02 tablespoons of peanut butter contain sufficient amounts of folate as 05 raw carrots or 01 1/2 cups of raspberries.

Fact 05: 02 tablespoons of peanut butter contain sufficient amounts of Vitamin E as in 20 apricots or 20 bananas or 20 slices of whole wheat bread!

Fact 06: 02 tablespoons of peanut butter contain sufficient amounts of zinc as in 03 cups of cooked broccoli or 40 dried plums.

Fact 07: 02 tablespoons of peanut butter contain sufficient amounts of magnesium as 04 cups of cooked pasta or 20 cooked eggs.

Fact 08: 02 tablespoons of peanut butter contain sufficient amounts of potassium as in 02 cups of cottage cheese or 01 1/2 cups of blackberries.

Fact 09: 02 tablespoons of peanut butter contain sufficient amounts of copper as in 03 cups of cooked white rice or 06 cups of apple juice.

Fact 10: 02 tablespoons of peanut butter contain sufficient amounts of fiber, vitamins, and minerals.

Fact 11: Experts state women can have 04 tablespoons of peanut butter a day while men can go crazy and eat 06 tablespoons of peanut butter a day to cover the RDA (Recommended Daily Allowance)! Look at all that food you have to eat to get the nutrients your body needs whereas all it takes is 04 to 06 tablespoons of peanut butter a day. Plus - MMMmmmmmmm!

PEARS: Worldwide, pears are the second most important fruit crop after apples, but in the United States they rank third after apples and peaches. With 3,000 varieties in the Unites States, only a handful are commercially consumed. 06 ounces of raw pears provide only 101 calories and 46 calories per half (dried). Pears provide a fair amount of Vitamin C and iron while aiding in digestion. Pears are an **excellent source of roughage** while being an aid in regularity.

PINEAPPLES: Two slices of pineapple provide only 90 calories, Vitamin C and very little sodium. When picking fresh pineapples at the supermarket, insure the leaves are dark green. A natural enzyme found in pineapples called **bromelain is a nutrient that increases the body's ability to break down fats and protein promoting body metabolism!** Pineapple is rich in manganese and helps **satisfy your sweet tooth!**

POPCORN: Eaten as a healthy snack, plain popcorn (no butter and salt) compared to beef provides 67% as much protein, 100% as much iron and an equal amount of calcium. One and a half ounces of plain popcorn supplies as much energy as two eggs without the fat and cholesterol.

Plain fiber packed popcorn is **great for snacking** versus those potato chips, cheese crackers and other snacks that are high in saturated fat, cholesterol, sodium and sugar. Try hot air cooked plain popcorn instead of oil cooked or prepackaged microwave popcorn.

When you go to the movie theater or the stadium to watch baseball, football, soccer or any other sport, ask the vendor what kind of oil the kernels are popped in. Coconut oil is the preferred and healthy cooking oil for popcorn. See *Coconut Oil* and *Sound Nutrition*.

PORK: According to the American Heart Association, fresh pork cuts contain an average of *31% less fat* than reported in the early 1980's. Besides being lower in fat, pork is 17% **lower in calories and 10% lower in cholesterol** than in 1983. Pork offers **more nutrient value for fewer calories** as previously thought.

POSITIVE AFFIRMATIONS: First and foremost, you have to believe your mind is more powerful that you can imagine. Planting positive thoughts in your mind works if you apply it! Positive affirmations negate negative beliefs and start you to believe in yourself so you're a success and closer to your goals! Let's start with *Target Nutrition*.

Target Nutrition: You can use this affirmation / visualization to improve your eating habits from sickly fast-food to nutritious eating. Listen, there isn't a person walking this Earth that can say that fast-food restaurants help cure their maladies. Did you know most people in the United States and hundreds of millions more across the globe are overweight and have tried a diet or two - at least a diet or two? Why are so many overweight? There are a lot of factors but the main one is a hormone called insulin which has the dieter overeating and over-eating the wrong foods.

Some of you may already have the (U-AAASPTP or PAWS Program) and have the Gettysburg Program (107-page) version and some of you have the 667-page version. The 1st section gives you some of the best foods to eat to lose weight and fire-up your amazing body to heal itself. You'll notice there aren't any cheeseburgers anywhere in either version.

But the point is, you're eating habits could make all the difference in the world. Remember I told you more than a few times before, your own body has the incredible innate ability to heal itself - all you gotta do is kick-start it with 01 or 02... of 60+ alternative therapies and one of them is target nutrition.

Target Nutrition Affirmations / Visualization: As I lay in bed, just prior to sleep, **I consciously & verbally** command my subconscious to: "Compel me to eat more nutritious fruits & vegetables, drink more pure cool water and stay away from all fast-food restaurants because I want to look better, I want to feel better, I want to perform better and I want to be more healthy." Say this 05-times, go to sleep and don't worry about it. I let my POWERFUL subconscious mind work on it. Do this verbal command every night.

In the morning **just after you wake-up** do the following Visualizations and Positive Affirmations.

Today I start a new and healthier life. The 75 trillion cells in my body will be fed more nutritious food from this day forward.

I see myself eating my first healthy breakfast meal of delicious oatmeal and red succulent nutritious strawberries, a filling banana and a glass of orange juice. I am no longer eating any of the 05 deadly whites like sugar, salt, flour, fat, and dairy products. If I want to sweeten my meal, I'll use honey. If I use any fat for cooking, I'll use extra virgin olive oil. And for salt, I'll use fresh nutritious sea salt instead of processed cooked store salt.

For lunch, I see myself eating some hot vegetable soup that's low in salt. For a side dish, I'll eat a hefty but leafy salad with a tasty low fat dressing and at least 02 glasses of pure cold water.

For dinner, I'll start off with another leafy delicious salad with a low-fat dressing. For the entre I'll have a filling potato with no-fat sour cream, 03 slices of cooked turkey, peas and 02 glasses of pure, cold water.

After this meal, I will not eat after 7pm - I will not eat after 7pm. If I feel hungry, I'll slowly eat a delicious apple with a full glass of pure, cold water.

I will plan & prepare ALL my healthy meals ahead of time so to AVOID unhealthy meals. After 03-weeks, I can see I'm looking better and losing that unwanted, unhealthy weight.

HEY, while you're laying there, how about doing some Mind-Over-Matter warm-up exercises and a short run! See Exercise Mind-Over-Matter Trick right now.

POTATO: The potato originated in South America. Botanically, the potato is related to the eggplant. The potato is a tuber, according to Dr. Mike Samuels the author of *Heart Disease*. A medium potato provides only 110 calories, Vitamin C & B6, significant niacin, more potassium (don't peel, 60% is close to the skin) than a large banana and is low in sodium. A processed potato chip has **six times the calories, 400 times the fat and 250 times the salt** of the same amount of a natural unprocessed potato chip.

Do you think these saturated fat, sodium and cholesterol packed potato chips might hinder you from the healthy body and longer life you deserve? If you must have your potato chips, try making your own without the great amount of saturated fat, sodium and cholesterol. Shop around for a product that can turn potato slices into fat-free, sodium-free, low-calorie potato chips.

According to Dr. John McDougall, director of the nutritional medicine clinic at St. Helena Hospital, in Deer Park, California, potatoes are an **excellent food for rapid weight loss.** (DO NOT put the fat tasty stuff on potatoes like butter, margarine, sour cream...). Potatoes are a great source of fiber and other nutrients mentioned above, help lower cholesterol while protecting against strokes and heart disease!

White raw potatoes have high concentrations of protease inhibitors, which are compounds known to void-out certain viruses and carcinogens. Of several foods, inhibitors found in the potato were found to have the strongest antiviral powers! Potato chemicals stopped viruses better than soybean inhibitors which are considered one of the fiercest antiviral agents. Potatoes, especially the skins, are rich in chlorogenic acid, a polyphenol which prevents cell mutations leading to cancer.

Potato skins were found to have antioxidant activity - neutralizing "free radicals" that damage cells leading to many disorders including cancer.

It's a crying shame! According to the Agriculture Department and National Cancer Institute, the closest many children get to a vegetable is eating French fries!

PRAYER: Prayer predates the Bible and may be the **oldest mind power of all!** Prayer means something different to each individual. According to Dr. Herbert Benson, author of *The Relaxation Response* and *Beyond The Relaxation Response, "faith does make a difference in enhancing the power of the mind over health and disease."*

Dr. Benson states that patients who chose a prayer word or prayer to those who used a neutral word to evoke relaxation received far superior results!

Dr. Kenneth Pelltier, a Stanford University Psychologist and author of several books, including the international best seller *"Mind As Healer Mind As Slayer,"* studied people who made remarkable recoveries from life-threatening illnesses. Dr. Pelltier found they shared common characteristics, especially:

- Profound changes in their lives through meditation, prayer and other spiritual practices.

- A deep sense of the spiritual side of their human nature. Prayer is more than words. Prayer is also faith, hope and forgiveness.

See *The National Centre for Padre Pio, Inc.* in the POC Section.

PRICKLY PEAR: The following are some documented healthy wonders of the cactus called prickly pear. Let's start with *Nutrition*.

a) Nutrition: According to herbal researcher, Hall Newbegin from Berkeley, California, prickly pears cactus are loaded with amino acids, antioxidants, vitamins,...

b) Energy: According to a biochemist at Vista, California, *"Prickly pear is loaded with vitamins and amino acids that keep our bodies functioning at their peak, and thousands of regular people who take it report increased energy."* Athletes are taking prickly pear extracts and they can work out longer & harder before they become fatigued. And they recover faster from fatigue and sore muscles.

c) Pain Remedy: Researchers state prickly pear cactus contains an ingredient called betasitosterol which is a natural anti-inflammatory. And this ingredient can help reduce inflammation by as much as 65%! It may help remedy pain from achy muscles, arthritis, back pain, knee pain,...

d) Cholesterol Reduction: High cholesterol raises the risk of heart attack by 30%. Researchers have discovered that a prickly pear cactus extract can slash the bad artery-clogging - LDL cholesterol, by 34%! How does it do it? Cause prickly pears like apples, are loaded with pectin which is a soluble fiber that grabs cholesterol and evacuates it out of the body before it can get into the bloodstream.

e) Weight-Loss: Research demonstrates that prickly pear cactus helps reduce water weight - bloating. It purges the tissue of excess water. And prickly pear cactus has an added weight-loss bonus, it can reduce blood sugar by 21%. Reducing blood sugar destroys food cravings for snacking and worse yet, food binges.

Now we know one reason why Indian tribes in desert environments that had access to prickly pear fruit were so vibrantly athletic. And as far as where you can find prickly pear cacti, most folks think they're exclusive to the far southwestern parts of the United States. You can find them all over desert type regions. Heck, they're growing right now in my backyard where I was a kid in Colorado. OK, I know what you're thinking - where can I find prickly pear cactus products? See *Prickly Pear Cactus Products* in the POC Section. See *Coconut Juice & Slices* and *Indian Gator Aid*.

PRITIKIN DIET: In the 1970's, Nathan Pritikin made news with his Pritikin Program that could detour high blood pressure and high cholesterol from reaching dangerous and deadly levels. The Pritikin Program included low-fat, low-calorie, low-salt diet with a moderate daily exercise program. 893 Pritikin Program participants were studied by a team from Loma Linda University.

The 26-day Pritikin Longevity Center program demonstrated there was something to this unique program.
- 83% were able to terminate their prescription of high blood pressure medicine!
- Overweight participant lost an average of 13 pounds!
- Cholesterol levels dropped an average of 25%!
- 50% of diabetics were able to stop taking insulin!
- Participants performed better on mental ability test!
- Many people were alleviated of their tiredness and required less sleep!

PROANTHOCYANIDINS: In the 1950's, Professor Jacques Masquelier of the University of Bordeaux, France, isolated active components of the pine bark; they were found along the St. Lawrence River and other parts of the world.

There are 20,000 different types of and combinations of bioflavonoids. One particular group is **vastly superior** because it is **water-soluble** and **highly bioavailable**. This group of bioflavonoids is called **proanthocyanidins!**

The most powerful and health-enhancing and beneficial proanthocyanidins come from the bark of the maritime pine, Pinus maritima, growing along the southern coast of France from Bordeaux to the Spanish border. This bark contains the **LARGEST AMOUNTS** of the **ACTIVE INGREDIENTS!** Also called of Pycnogenol (PROANTHOCYANIDINS), these special compounds allow the Bordeaux pine to **withstand the harsh winds of winter, the blinding sun and intense heat of summer and the salty winds of the Atlantic Ocean!**

Proanthocyanidins are non-toxic and are **powerful heavyweights when it comes to antioxidants!** Dubbed OPCs for short, these OPCs can be extracted from a few certain species of pine trees... OPCs have been extensively tested throughout the world for toxicity and have been concluded as being **completely safe and non-toxic!** For superior antioxidants, you must read about *Pycnogenol* (registered trademark).

PRUNES: If you don't know it by now, prunes are well known as an excellent laxative. During the 1950s and 1960s, the United States Department of Agriculture's Western Regional Research Center devoted considerable manpower and money to find the laxative power in the prune. The USDA gave up the studies in the late '60s. Scientific evidence of exactly how and why prunes work as a great laxative are unknown at the time of this writing. However, prunes have proven their worth as a laxative.

At Essex County Geriatric Center in Belleville, New Jersey, the center's head dietician, physician and nutritionist decided to take 300 elderly patients off laxatives; many of which were constipated and dependent on their daily laxative pills. The staff began by adding two-thirds of an ounce of high-fiber bran to the morning oatmeal.

This worked 60 percent of the cases. The remaining difficult cases, the staff added up to a half a cup of prune juice a day. One year later, **90 percent of the residents were off laxatives**, preferring dietary-imposed regularity. The patients stated they felt better and the **pharmacy bills for laxatives fell by $44,000 the first year!**

PYCNOGENOL THE ANTIOXIDANT OF CHOICE: Every second of every day, our **body cells are exposed to alcohol, exhaust fumes, pesticides, pollution, processed foods, preservatives, poor nutrition, stress, tobacco smoke, toxins, x-rays...**

These environmental hazards and your own lifestyle choices cause arthritis, bruising, cancer, clogged arteries, heart disease, lack of energy, liver damage, mental deterioration, poor circulation, premature aging, susceptibility to sports injuries...

One way our bodies protects itself against pollutants, is by forming antioxidants in the form of super oxide dismutase (SOD). The most common antioxidants found in foods are Vitamins A, C, E and selenium. However, the continual bombardment of stress, environmental pollution, and food processing destroy antioxidants allowing the body to be more susceptible to disease and ill health. Your body already has a difficult time producing enough antioxidants to combat the multitude of contaminants it's exposed to every second!

Antioxidants can help ALZHEIMER'S DISEASE, ARTHRITIS, CANCER, HEART DISEASE, JET LAG, PROSTATE, STROKE...

There are 60 chronic degenerative diseases that science knows of that are caused by free radicals.

Professor Jacques Masquelier of the University of Bordeaux, France was granted a U.S. patent for Pycnogenol (*a registered trademark of Horphag Overseas Limited*). Pycnogenol is a natural plant product made from the bark of the European coastal pine, Pinus Maritima. Pycnogenol is the **most POWERFUL antioxidant today and acts as a protector against environmental toxins!** Research has demonstrated that Pycnogenol is **50 times more effective than Vitamin E and 20 times more powerful than Vitamin C!**

Studies show that Pycnogenol is rapidly absorbed and distributed throughout the body within 20 minutes. Pycnogenol helps activate Vitamin C and has it working before it leaves your body. Pycnogenol is being used in France, Finland, Holland, Germany, Switzerland and now the United States.

Pycnogenol is a perfect weapon to prevent ill health and premature aging. Using supplements to increase the intake of antioxidants can build the body's defenses and may slow down the aging process. Pycnogenol is an effective antioxidant that is possibly one of the **MOST POWERFUL FREE RADICAL SCAVENGERS AVAILABLE!**

The following are <u>only 40%</u> of some of the documented health benefits from the research of Dr. Richard Passwater, Dr. Jacques Masquelier, Dr. Morton Walker, Pasteur & Huntington Institutes and seven other leading Universities in Europe.

- Decreases Allergies\Hay fever
- Enhance Immune Resistance
- Helps Alzheimer's
- Helps Asthma\Bronchitis
- Helps Diabetes
- Improves Circulation
- Improves Joint Flexibility
- Improves Skin Smoothness
- Increases Energy, Less Fatigue
- Lowers Cholesterol
- Prevents Ulcer Formation
- Prevents Fat Formation\Cellulitis
- Prevents Wrinkling of the Skin
- Reduces Arthritis Pain
- Reduces Blood Pressure
- Reduces Infection\Flu\Cold
- Reduces Menopause\PMS\Cramps
- Reduces Risk of Cancer
- Reduces Risk of Phlebitis
- Reduces Risk of Stroke
- Reduces Stress\Depression
- Reduces Varicose Veins
- Repairs Atherosclerosis
- Resists Mutagen Attacks
- Resists Oxidized LDL
- Retards Aging
- Strengthens Capillaries

What is Pycnogenol and what can it do for me?

Pycnogenol is an extract from the maritime pine consisting of proanthocyanidins and water-soluble nutrients. Pycnogenol, a specific blend of bioflavonoids (patented), a **"super protector nutrient"** is a made up of powerful antioxidant nutrients for use to scavenge free radicals.

The mixture of nutrients can help you live better longer, stay healthier and appear more youthful. Pycnogenol is noted to **protect you from approximately 80 diseases, including arthritis, cancer, heart disease** and most non-germ diseases which are linked to the deleterious chemical action of free radicals.

It is **well known and documented** that antioxidant nutrients protect the body's cells from the attack free radicals. Free radicals form during normal metabolism and are multiplied by environmental pollutants and radiation.

Pycnogenol slows the damage associated with aging, restores elasticity and smoothness to skin because of its influence on skin protein, nourishes blood cells and blood vessels.

This amazing antioxidant alleviates hay fever, other allergies, strengthens capillaries to reduce edema, bruising and varicose veins... If Pycnogenol was not safe, it would not have been allowed to be sold in so many countries for so many years. As long as Pycnogenol is sold without drug-like claims, it is available as a nutrient-rich food supplement. Read other health benefits noted in the previous pages.

Is Pycnogenol safe to use?

Pycnogenol has been extensively tested for decades. Studies include acute and gross toxicity, mutagenicity, carcinogenic and teratogenic studies.

Can Pycnogenol help with Allergies?

It has been noted for some time that bioflavonoids can control allergies. Allergies are usually treated with antihistamines. Antihistamines work by interfering with the binding of histamine to cells after its release. Pycnogenol and other bioflavonoids act to prevent histamine release in the first place. Many physicians in Europe reported that Pycnogenol was their first recommendation for hay fever and related allergies. In their opinion, **Pycnogenol is extremely effective, safe and available at a lower cost** than synthetic drugs.

How about varicose veins?

According to a German study, 77% of 110 people (84) with varicose veins **showed a clear improvement** in the size of their varicosities.

How about Diabetic Retinopathy?

Pycnogenol has been licensed in France for years to treat diabetic retinopathy. In one clinical study where 40 patients were given 80mg to 120mg of Pycnogenol daily for a week followed by 40mg to 80mg daily for up to four months, **ninety percent** of the recipients had a reduction in micro capillary bleeding and their **eyesight improved!**

QIGONG: Until 1980, this 5,000 year old practice (QiGong), was kept as a secret within families and religious temples. QiGong is an ancient oriental technique which uses movement and breathing to stimulate the natural healing energies within the body. Practiced regularly, it has been shown to enhance overall vitality, reduce the effects of stress and assist in the resistance to disease.

The world's largest medicineless hospital, the Huaxia Zhineng Qigong Clinic & Training Center is located in Qinhuangdao, China practices QiGong. Its founder is Dr. Pang Ming, a Qigong Grandmaster who is trained in both Western and Chinese traditional medicine. Since its initial practice in 1988, the clinic has treated more than **180 different diseases (100,000 patients+) with a 95% success rate!** Beat that success rate *"conventional medicine!"* The center avoids medicines and special diets and favors exercise, love and life energy which is known as chi!

How can you look into this alternative practice? Luke Chan, the first Chi-Lei Master to be certified outside China by the Zhineng Qigong Center, has practiced Qigong and Tai Chi for 28 years. He now practices in the United States! He'll send you free information concerning his practice! See *Luke Chan* and *A Beginners Guide To Healthy Breathing* the POC Section.

RAW FOOD DIET: Probably the **BEST DIET** I've come across is the Raw Food Diet. This diet consist of raw fruits & vegetables and juicing. This diet is similar to the Gerson Diet, with the exception of consuming large amounts of grain. This diet has literally solved a wide variety of health problems where **conventional medicine has FAILED!** Yes, even **terminal cases!**

REFLEXOLOGY BLUES KILLER: Feeling blue may bring on a feeding binge. If you got the blues and you're feeling down and out, don't go kick the dog or that 9-life critter. Here's a super simple Reflexology application you can do to yourself or a fellow weight-watcher Anytime Anywhere.

The pituitary gland helps raise endorphin levels which results in making you happy. The reflex points that stimulate the pituitary gland are located center on the fleshy parts of each thumb.

With the index finger of the same hand apply firm kneading massage for a couple minutes and repeat till you're happier than 9-life critter with human servants insuring a bowl of fresh vittles, a warm bed, toys, and a clean litter box are always available 24-hours a day. And don't forget the 02 more pituitary reflex points located in the center bottom of both big toes.

REFLEXOLOGY WEIGHT-LOSS POINTS: Reflexology is a specific bodywork technique of stroking or applying pressure to one part of the body in order to effect changes in another part of the body, relax muscles and stimulate the body's own natural ability to heal itself. There are several techniques under the generic term Reflexology: Hand Reflexology, Foot Reflexology, Zone Reflexology and Body Reflexology. The Reflexologist uses a map of the body on the soles of the feet and palms of the hand.

Massaging these extremities sends an energy signal that stimulates reflexes, automatic nerve impulses connected to specific areas of the body. Other parts of the body are the ears, head, torso and back also contain reflexes corresponding to the whole of the body."

Here are some neat reflexology applications you can use Anytime Anywhere to reduce unwanted weight.

a) Thyroid Reflex Point: The thyroid gland is a 01-ounce gland located at the Adam's Apple. It secretes a hormone called thyroxine. Thyroxine is the body's main metabolic hormone that aids **the body to burn calories**. The thyroid reflex points are located at the pads on each palm below the thumbs. Apply firm kneading massage to both reflex points for a few minutes. Repeat a 2nd time.

b) Liver Reflex Point: The liver is a 03-pound, triangular-shaped organ that executes approximately 500+ functions for the body on a daily basis - 24-hours a day (filtering toxins, produces bile to <u>digest fats</u>, flush fat-attracting toxins, lubricate intestines, store sugar, producing hormones, forming blood cells, storing and using vitamins & minerals,...).

The liver is located at the upper right quadrant of the abdominal area. The reflex point is located at the palm of the right hand directly below the ring & small finger. Apply a kneading massage to these area for a few minutes and repeat a 2nd time.

REWARD YOURSELF: Once you and your doctor decide on a healthy diet for YOU, in the very near future, you're going to crave all those tasty foods and snacks that you once ate on a daily basis. So instead of giving in to those cravings and / or depriving yourself completely - REWARD YOURSELF with a small treat and not a smorgasbord of the unhealthy stuff. This way you won't "fall off the wagon" and fully regress back to your unhealthy ways. Eventually, once you see your great weight-loss progress - you may not touch any of those unhealthy foods and snacks.

RICE: Rice is not only delicious but filling and it's good for you. Rice contains only a trace of fat, a source of complex carbohydrates, is cholesterol free and has approximately 164 calories per cup. Brown rice still has the outer kernel or outer covering which makes brown rice higher in fiber and high in nutrients than white rice.

In the one study, Dr. Walter Kempner at Duke University, Durham, North Carolina, developed the *Rice Diet*. Rice was the staple food; fruits and then vegetables were later added to the diet. The Rice Diet **produced weight-loss, reversed and cured kidney ailments**, as well as helped **remedy high blood pressure!** If you desire to try the Rice Diet, read as much as you can concerning this diet and seek your physician's advice. Currently (Summer 2012) conducting research on the cancer-fighting Brown Rice Diet.

RUCKSACKING: One of the many discriminators or eliminating tools of the U.S. Army Special Forces Qualification Course (SFQC - Green Berets) was/is the rucksack. It's the SF candidate against himself (*"Fatigue Makes Cowards Of Us All."*) carrying his rucksack anywhere from 03 to 12-miles (timed) throughout the course and more during the patrolling phase. Speed walking, running and sprinting with a 45 - 55-pound rucksack (doesn't include the weight of weapon, water, and other gear) on hard dirt, pavement, sand and deep sand, **BURNS-UP A TREMENDOUS AMOUNT OF CALORIES**. Soldiers already in great shape still lost weight while trying out for US Army Special Forces – during Phase 01 with all the rucksacking and running.

One problem though, military style rucksacking **is for the young and already in good physical condition**. However, if you want to do some walking exercises and carry a small weighted backpack (10-pounds max), I'm sure you'll get a great workout and burn MORE calories than doing regular speed walking.

RUN-SWIM-RUCK-SHOOT: While in the U.S. Army and stationed at Fort Davis, Panama, every once in a while, the entire Battalion would do what we called a Run-Swim-Ruck-Shoot. From Ft. Davis, we'd run a couple miles to Dock #45, donn a life vest (safety) and swim 01-mile in open water to another location, donn our rucksacks an ruck a couple miles to the range and shoot our assigned weapons. A great workout, I estimate it burned a couple thousand calories. Consider something like this when you go on your next workout. Bottom line - mix-up your workout so you don't get bored. Heck, go to your local mall and start walking - checking-out everything as you fast-walk.

RUSSIAN ARCTIC WEED (RAW): What the heck is Russian Arctic Weed (RAW)? RAW is now surfacing as a potent herb to aid in longevity and you can look towards many "vibrant & sharp as a whip" Russian farmers as proof. RAW has a history of being fed to Russians that really needed to be at their very best for the Mother Land - astronauts and Russian World Class Athletes.

a) Brain Power: A test group ate an extract of RAW and in 24-hours their test scores shot up an amazing **88%!** The control group that took a placebo scored 84% lower.

b) Anti-Depression: RAW is also noted to boost the "feel good" hormone - serotonin - by 30%, thus fighting depression, thus avoiding binge eating.

c) Energy After-Burner: RAW is also noted to somehow boosts the energy levels. How it does this is unclear at the time of this writing.

d) Weight-Loss: As you just read if RAW could help boost energy levels it has to help you lose unwanted, unhealthy extra pounds. A test group that took RAW supplements lost 20-pounds in a few months while the control group gained weight. OK, I know what you're asking, where can you get more information on RAW? See *The Country Doctor's Big Bag Of Common Sense Cures* in the POC Section.

SCHEDULE AND PREPARE MEALS IN ADVANCE: To INSURE you stay on your diet, schedule and prepare your low-fat meals in advance (for freshness, 24-hours). This INSURES you keep your promise to yourself to stick to your healthy diet that will not only help you lose weight, save you money (eating out - high fat processed foods), but those premade meals will add plenty of healthy years to your life. Pre-made healthy meals will keep you from eating unhealthy fast-food meals, pastries, candy, sodas, snacks,...

SELF-HEALING: Sometimes you just gotta depend on yourself because nobody cares more about you than YOU! And I gave you plenty of examples of alternative self-healing throughout this Survival Book. You gotta BELIEVE that your body has the miraculous ability to heal itself via special diet, Mind-Over-Mater Applications, alternative therapies, exercises,... thus self-healing. Please re-read this Survival Book at your leisure.

SERE WEIGHT-LOSS PLAN: Here's the most radical and challenging weight-loss plan on Earth. SERE is a military acronym and it stands for Survival Escape Resistance and Evasion. I attended the 01-month U.S. Army SERE Instructor Course in the late 1980s in the jungles of Panama. The last week of the course was the evasion portion prior to individual hide site survival. Anyway, during the evasion, 02 platoons of infantry (80 soldiers) were searching for our team and several other teams throughout Panamanian jungle so that in itself kept us evading while eating hardly anything except for a few selected edible plants and water from streams.

The tail-end of the course was the isolation phase, located at our individual & isolated hide sites, we were tasked with several field-craft survival tasks we had to complete to pass the course. At this time of a few days I ate next to nothing and drank very little water. My mind was rapidly deteriorating (memory, calculating, decision-making,...). What I didn't know was deteriorating even faster was my weight.

After all that, the "survivors" (less than half the class) were rounded-up and we were evaluated by medical staff to include our weight. The last week of the course **I lost 25-pounds. That comes to 03 1/2-pounds a day!**

So if you go out in the woods on your next outdoor multi-day adventure and eat hardly anything - except drinking plenty of water (Fasting), I bet you'll lose some weight. See *Fasting*.

SHELLFISH: Shellfish are <u>**low in fat**</u> and furnish <u>**fewer calories than beef**</u>, furnish a source of calcium and are extremely tasty. Here are the calorie counts for four ounces of six types of shellfish. Shelled clams furnish only 86 calories. Cooked crab furnishes only 105 calories. A cooked lobster furnishes only 108 calories. Canned mussels furnish only 107 calories. Shelled oysters furnish only 103 calories. Cooked scallops furnish only 127 calories.

It was once thought that shellfish were hazardous to your cardiovascular system because they elevated blood cholesterol. Well it is just the opposite. Shellfish help protect arteries and blood vessels by significantly lowering bad-type blood cholesterol (LDL). Shellfish carry high concentrations of Omega-3 fatty acids that help prevent blood clots (thrombi) in blood vessels and are noted to be potentially beneficial to many diseases to include allergies, asthma, cancer, headaches, psoriasis and rheumatoid arthritis!

Are shellfish a brain food? Shellfish, as well as other seafood, do stimulate mental energy! According to Dr. Judith Wurtman, a leading researcher at MIT, shellfish and fish boost your mood and mental performance. Why? Shellfish are low in fat and carbohydrates and almost pure protein which delivers large amounts of an amino acid called tyrosine to the brain.

Tyrosine is then made into two mentally energizing brain chemicals called dopamine and norepinephrine. Research has proven in both animals and humans that when the brain produces those neurotransmitters, dopamine and norepinephrine, mood and energy are boosted! You have a tendency to think and react more quickly. You are more attentive, motivated and mentally energetic! To boost your brain power, a normal dosage would be approximately 04 ounces.

SIX STEPS FORWARD AND ONE STEP BACK: To stop cold turkey from eating all those delicious and unhealthy foods (candy, fast foods, Five Deadly Whites,...) and switching to a super healthy diet is very difficult. So do this, reward yourself on the 7th day. Stick to your super healthy diet for 06-days and on the 7th day go ahead and go to your favorite fast-food restaurant and reward yourself.

Get those urges, temptations,... out of your system and splurge on the 7th day. This should help keep you on track to meeting your weight-loss goals. YES, you can splurge on your Birthday too - I do. So take Six Steps Forward And One Step Back to meet your weight-loss goals.

SKIM MILK: One cup of skim milk has **only a trace of fat**. One cup of 02-percent-fat milk has 05 grams of fat, while 01 cup of whole milk has 08 grams of fat. Use Skim Milk to make tasty Smoothies - see *Smoothies* below.

SMOOTHIES: This may be the most tasty weight-loss meal (breakfast, lunch, dinner and snacks) you ever slurped. They're called smoothies. And when you make em' right (keep reading), compared to even weight-loss meals, smoothies are still lower in fat, lower in calories and they REALLY FILL YOU UP.

Smoothies are comprised of one or all of the following foods: fruits, vegetables, pure ice cubes, pure water, skim milk, spices, healthy oil [flax seed] and protein powder. Below are a few of my own Smoothie Recipes to help you get to your weight-loss goals. OK, let's get started with Pineapple Smoothie.

Pineapple Smoothie
Serving(s): 01

Ingredients: 1/4 cup of chopped frozen pineapple, 01 frozen banana, 06 frozen strawberries, 1/2 cup of skim milk, 02 cups of pure ice cubes, 01 teaspoon of flax seed oil, 01 scoop of peanut butter and 01 blender.

Directions: Place all ingredients in the blender and mix to a thick milk shake consistency.

Note: None

Peanut Butter Smoothie
Serving(s): 01

Ingredients: 1/2 cup of peanut butter, 3/4 cup of skim milk, 01 frozen banana, 02 cups of pure ice cubes, 01 teaspoon of flax seed oil, and 01 blender.

Directions: Place all ingredients in the blender and mix to a thick milk shake consistency.

Note: None

Goin' Nuts Smoothie

Serving(s): 01

Ingredients: 01 heaping tablespoon of pine nuts, 01 heaping tablespoon of chopped almonds, 01 heaping tablespoon of chopped walnuts, 01 scoop of peanut butter, 01 frozen banana, 1/2 cup of skim milk, 02 cups of pure ice cubes, 01 teaspoon of flax seed oil, and 01 blender.

Directions: Place all ingredients in the blender and mix to a thick milk shake consistency.
Note: None

OK, yes I got more smoothies for you, but you got the idea. Invent your own smoothies to your tasty liking; just make sure each ingredient is low in fat, low in calories, low in,... to get to your weight-loss goals. See *Right Size Smoothies* in the POC Section.

Hold the phone. You can purchase a variety of tasty "Smoothie" packets at your local grocery store. Concord Foods offers Chocolate Banana, Strawberry, Tropical Pineapple and Orange flavors. Just add the fruit, ice and or skim milk. Throw it all in a blender and you got a Smoothie! And yes, I checked the ingredients, they are all FAT FREE and they only cost about .88 cents per packet.

SNACKS: According to Jane Schultz of the Snack Foods Association, Alexandria, Virginia; the average American ate a whopping 22-pounds of salty snacks in 1994 compared to 17.5-pounds in 1988. No wonder the majority of Americans are overweight. I wonder what the stats are for this year - 2014!!!!

SOUP: Researchers have found that soup could actually **help you lose weight!** Why? First of all soup contains mostly water and second it fills you up. See *Jello* and *Water*.

SOYBEANS: Soybeans are inexpensive and nutritious. One-half cup of raw soybeans provides only 385 calories, while one-half cup of cooked soybeans provides only 150 calories. Soybeans are high in calcium, iron, potassium and protein.

The fat in soybeans is unsaturated and has a low content of sodium. Research indicates that soybeans may **lower serum cholesterol**, reduce triglycerides, help regulate blood sugar, relieve and prevent constipation and **lower the risk of cancer**. Research also indicates soybeans may prevent or dissolve gallstones.

Degenerative diseases from arthritis to cancer, are noted to be **substantially lower in Japanese men and women** than their American counterparts! Why? One reason is Japanese have **much less fat in their diet** **and Japanese eat a great deal more soy products** like miso, soy drinks, soy sauce and tofu. Soy beans contain phytochemicals called polysterols and saponins which are noted to **lower cholesterol**.

Other phytochemicals found in soybeans are called isoflavones, genistein and daidzein, also called phytoestrogens. Phytoestrogens are noted to **ease menopausal symptoms**, protect women against the effects of too much estrogen (breast and endometrial cancer), and may help protect men against **prostate cancer!**

Soybeans also contain anticarcinogens. Studies have noted that soy components have **inhibitory effects on leukemia** and cancers of the breast, colon, lung, prostate and stomach!

According to Japanese surveys searching for foods that protect against cancer, one of which was miso, a soybean-paste soup. Japanese men and women who consumed one bowl of miso a day had a one-third lower risk of stomach cancer than those who never ate miso! See *Haelan Products Incorporated* in the POC Section.

SPECIAL BREATHING EXERCISE: Special Breathing Exercise to instantly ENERGIZE yourself and help you **burn-up excess fat!**

Have you ever yawned? Sure you have. That's your body trying to tell you that you may need more oxygenated blood to your tired body, your tired hungry cells!

This subject should probably be titled *"Healing At The Cellular Level."* First let me tell you a bona fide fact. Most of us humans (99.9999999 percent) are shallow breathers. Unless you're a Yogi, Tibetan Monk, into meditation, or use Mind-Over-Matter applications like Visualization, you have no idea how to breathe better so it's more healthy & relaxing.

Every Mind-Over-Matter application that I've investigated since the mid 1990s has had some form of *"special breathing"* involved in the practice. So there's got to be something special about breathing - special breathing. First let me tell you why even a simple deep breath now and then is beneficial and healthy for you and I dare your doctor to say "that's BS, I don't want you to breathe differently, it's bad for you and everybody."

Every cell of your body needs nutrients and oxygen. and there are a lot of cells in your body aching for precious fuel it never really gets because you're a shallow breather! Are you ready for this - there are 100,000,000,000,000 (1-hundred trillion) cells in your body. Oxygen is one of those vital nutrients. **Your body has the innate ability to heal itself starting at the cellular level.** One cell in your body is a lot smarter for your health than any doctor. Let me give some eye-opening healing information about healing at the cellular level.

So here's one simple form of breathing and it's easy and FREE. In the POC Section are other POCs to get different and advanced healthy breathing techniques.

Step 01: Find a quiet time (30 minutes) & place in your home.

Step 02: Laying down or sitting-up, let out all the air in your lungs and inhale through your nose (filters air) real deep till you can't take-in any more air.

STEP 03: Hold the breath for 15 - 20 seconds and quickly force out all the air out through your lungs.

Step 04: Once all the air is expelled, again take a deep breath through your nose and hold it for 15-20 seconds and release.

Step 05: Repeat Steps 02 - 04 for a duration of 30 minutes.

Step 06: You can use visualization with your deep breathing to help heal your body. Close your eyes, when you exhale - imagine all the toxins from head to foot being forced out of your body through your mouth. Add color to the toxins like brownish red. When you deeply inhale imagine inhaling a bright white light that enters your nostrils, goes to your lungs and spreads throughout your body.

And as you hold your breath for 15-20 seconds that bright white light turns into shiny chrome fighting knights with chrome swords on white dressed-up stallions. The knights are fighting, slashing, stomping and killing disease, fat... and even fixing and repairing damaged parts of your body. You can even visualize the bright white light going to a specific part of your body when you deeply inhale for extra healing! Repeat for 30-minutes! Visualization must be used in a quiet and isolated place in your home.

Is this all there is? Is it that easy? NO! You can't expect results unless you practice this special breathing at least 30-minutes every day. So dedicate 30 minutes of your day to deep breathing exercises. Heck, you can do it while you're driving your car (do not use visualization). In a future AASN, you'll get several Visualization Scenarios you can use to heal yourself! Now let's cover an ancient practice that has healing benefits like deep breathing. You must read *Cellular Healing* in this book and see *"A Beginners Guide To Healthy Breathing"* in the POC Section. *Follow the recommended instructions only as per your doctor's approval.*

SPINACH: A cup of raw spinach furnishes only 12 calories, where as a cup of cooked spinach furnishes only 42 calories. Spinach is very low in fat, furnishes Vitamin A as carotene, Vitamin C, Vitamin E, calcium, iron and many other nutrients. Spinach provides that much needed fiber to **help prevent cancer and helps to lower cholesterol**, **lose weight** and control diabetes!

According to Dr. Richard Shekelle, an epidemiologist at the University of Texas, **spinach has it all**, including the ability to **rev up the metabolism**. According to the Journal of American Medicine, spinach is called *'King of Vegetables.'*

One of many dark green vegetables, spinach tops the list (along with carrots) of foods eaten most often by people worldwide with lower rates of all types of cancer, especially cervical, colon, endometrial, esophageal, laryngeal, lung, pharyngeal, prostate, rectal and stomach cancers.

Spinach provides high amounts of chlorophyll which is a noted cancer blocker. Italian studies, found that spinach, in test tube tests was dramatic at blocking the formation of one of the most powerful carcinogens known - nitrosamines. Of the foods tested (carrots, cauliflower, lettuce, strawberries...), spinach juice was by far the most potent! Spinach contains folic acid which is noted as a mood booster. Are you suffering from depression? Eat spinach!

SPIRULINA: The word Spirulina is derived from the Latin word for "helix" or "spiral" for the physical configuration of the organism when it forms swirling, microscopic strands. Spirulina is a simple, single-celled algae that can be found in warm, alkaline bodies of fresh water. The nutrient content of algae meets the food needs of every cell of the higher organisms and makes it one of the **most concentrated sources of pure food and nutrition in the universe**. It's one of the great unharvested pastures of the world. Spirulina is categorized according to predominating colorations: blue-green, green, red and brown. Spirulina is one of the **<u>BLUE-GREEN ALGAE</u>s because of the presence of chlorophyll (green) and phycocyanin (blue) pigments** in its cellular structure. Spirulina is not a sea plant even though it is distantly related to kelp.

Spirulina nutritional values are exceptional. Spirulina is approximately 65 to 71 percent protein which are biologically complete and **provide all eight essential amino acids in the proper ratios and supplies 10 of the 12 non-essential amino acids**. It also provides B-12, folic acid and chlorophyll.

The following are a fraction of noted diseases and ailments that have been studied in relation to the effects of Spirulina:

- **Anemia** -- The chlorophyll, B-12, folic acid and protein content of Spirulina was instrumental in increasing red blood cell volume and oxygen-carrying capacity **within 04 weeks**. Spirulina supplementation was most beneficial to those with long-term insufficient intake of trace nutritional elements. It also helped speed recovery from blood-loss anemias.

- **Diabetes** -- The sugars of Spirulina are easily assimilated and helped maintain blood glucose levels steady with reduced fluctuation in clinical test subjects. Spirulina's nutrient density helped to reduce food cravings which permitted **weight loss and reduced insulin need**. Diabetic condition improvement and overall vigor and sense of well-being increased.

- **Heavy Metal Poisoning** -- Supplementation of Spirulina has been noted to **stimulate the excretion of some contaminants**, notably cadmium. Lead as well as mercury are also excreted.

- **Liver Disease** -- When the liver is being assaulted by toxins or infections, it is dependent upon high-quality and easy-to-digest protein and concentrated Vitamins. According to Japanese studies, acute and chronic hepatitis and early liver damage via alcohol abuse, indicate that the nutritional content of Spirulina **boosts the liver's recuperative powers after 02 to 06 weeks of Spirulina supplementation** in both medicated and unmedicated patients.

- **Leukocyte Loss Prevention** -- Radiation and chemotherapy treatments may cause a reduction of those disease fighting white cells and Spirulina supplementation may help reduce that loss. Patients also reported **less nausea and lassitude from cancer treatment** when taking supplements of Spirulina.

- **Senility** -- According to Dr. Abram Hooffer, **most cases of true senility are caused by subtle nutritional deficiencies**. The concentrated minerals, proteins and Vitamins may potentiate restoration of normal function. Amino acids that stimulate brain catecholamine synthesis (mood regulators) and inositol (nerve nutrient) found in Spirulina **may help sharpen function in many people**.

- **Ulcers** -- According to 1965 test reported in the *"Japan Medical News,"* two grams of supplemental Spirulina **cured all symptoms of gastric ulcers!** Also, seven out of nine cases of duodenal ulceration were **completely cured**, while the other two cases noted marked improvement.

The chlorophyll coats the irritated stomach lining, inhibits maladaptive pepsin secretions and reduces tissue inflammation. Spirulina contains mesafirine which is a potent ulceration inhibitor. *Follow the recommended dosage and instructions from the label and as per your doctor's instructions.*

SPROUTS: Hey, I've grown plenty of sprouts and I'm going to tell you about it so you can do the same. First, what are sprouts? Sprouts are the young shoots from seed that were planted just a few days prior. Sprouts are loaded with nutrients and are exceptionally delicious.

If you have a St. Louis Bread Factory in your city, you may know they make all sorts of delicious sandwiches and they're complimented with delicious crunchy sprouts. Now you can make your own sprouts and it's super easy.

Ingredients: Pure water (not tap water), package of sprouts and Sprout Starter Kit. You can purchase a Sprout Starter Kit and sprout seeds at your local healthfood store, at www.amazon.com or take a look on the internet. Me, I got my kits and seeds from Gardens Alive   www.gardensalive.com   I actually purchased multiple kits cause I can stack 06 trays on top of each other and grow 06 trays of sprouts at the same time!

Step 01: Assemble all your trays. The trays are assembled so the top tray receives the water and drips the water to the multiple trays underneath. The tray underneath hold the small sprout seeds, receive the water and drip the unused water to the tray below. And the sprout trays underneath do the same. The bottom tray is the reservoir holds all the dripping water. Simply empty this tray once all the water has dripped down through all the trays.

Step 02: Sprinkle the small sprout seeds to each sprout tray so each tray is barely covered with seeds but NOT piled on.

Step 03: Place your assemble trays with seeds in a safe place and where the sun can shine on it.

Step 04: Carefully pour water on all sections of the top tray so the water drips on all parts of all the trays below.

Step 05: Continue pouring water on the top tray but be careful that too much water will not overflow from the bottom reservoir/

Step 06: Once the excess water has stopped dripping into the bottom reservoir, carefully disconnect the bottom reservoir tray and discard the water and reassemble it.

Step 07: Water the sprout trays 03 or 04 hours later and repeat Steps 02 thru Step 06.

Step 08: Water the sprout trays 03 or 04 hours later and repeat Steps 02 thru Step 06.

Your sprouts should be watered 03-times a days. In just 02-days, you'll already see your sprouts growing. In just a few days later, once you see the shoots growing and touching the tray above, your sprouts are ready to be harvested! Secure all your sprouts in a container with a lid and place in the fridge. Rinse all your trays and start the process all over. You can grow sprouts 365 days a year! You can eat them just like they are, add them to your sandwiches, add them to salads,…

STARCHES: Eat more starches (complex carbohydrates). Starches aren't fattening and can **lower your cholesterol** by diluting the fat you eat. Eat more starches like beans, grains and root vegetables. See Beans, Bean Diet and Baked Beans Weight-Loss.

STRESS BUSTERS: The everyday stresses of life could have you do some non-hungry eating to help comfort you, calm you down,... However, instead of turning to your comfort food even if it's healthy, try some of the following Stress Busters so to help you stay on your healthy diet. OK, let's get started with you Flaming Stress Buster.

a) Flaming Stress Buster: I've known it most of my life but had no scientific proof that flickering flames calm you down and here's proof. Have you ever stared into the flickering flames of your campfire or even into the flickering flames of your fireplace? How about just a regular candle flame? Sure you have. Bet you kinda got hypnotized didn't you? I've stared into the hypnotic relaxing flames kazillions of times since I was a kid. Anyway, recent studies have proven that flames may de-stress you. Experts state that focusing on the flickering colored flames induce a meditative state that aids to release your worries thus busting your stress. I bet even a single candle flame will do the job too.

b) Wabisabi Stress Buster: Here's a trick that could counter your stressed-out day. Japanese practice the stress-busting effects of a philosophy called wabisabi. It's a practice of appreciating nature. Research has proven that just looking at nature scenes INSTANTLY lowers heartbeat & respiration and calms the nervous system.

c) Color Therapy: Here's some recent scientific data on the colors blue and green that may help you out in stressful times. According to Carol Ritberger, Ph.D., author of "What Color Is Your Personality" states that the colors blue and green instantly slow down the pulse rate and slightly lowers the body temperature.

She states that the mind-brain associates the colors blue and green with cool things like cold streams and shady trees. So consider blue and green as a remedy to fight stress. Hey, on a clear day, take cover and stare at the beautiful blue sky.

d) Pet Therapy: Many studies have noted that pet owners have **less illness, recover from illness faster and are likely to live longer!** Pets actually take care of their owners in more ways than you know.

Can your cat, dog, bird, fish, King Snake... improve your health? It sure looks that way. Just the purring of a cat or the comfort of your dog laying in your lap or beside you can calm you, comfort you and a good chance your blood pressure - hypertension may drop a few points too!

Pets can also help support a strong immune system to fight-off disease! How? Because pets are great stress fighters! After a long day at work (if you don't work at home like I do), stress goes with the job and that stress drains your body of energy and that affects your immune system. But when you get home, you see that furry critter look up at you and you *"baby talk"* to him/her thus releasing your stress! Not as good as a warm bath and a massage but your pet calms you and comforts you continuously even when it's asking to be fed or let out for a while!

Yes, fish in their aquarium are known to lower blood pressure - hypertension. If you don't want a cat, dog... try some tropical fish! The whole set-up isn't that expensive and its presence (aquarium, floating bubbles and fish) will calm you continuously!

Did you know Pet Therapy is so convincing that it is now used in hospitals, convalescent homes, and nursing homes! Yep, Pet Therapy kills those lonely blues and great to fend-off depression too! If you have a pet, that's good, if you don't consider getting one or two...

SUGAR RESTRICTIVE DIET: Not all carbohydrates are the same. Some carbohydrates have your pancreas releasing more insulin which has your body storing more fat. These high-releasing insulin carbohydrates are high-glycemic carbohydrates. These high-glycemic carbohydrates should be AVOIDED to lose weight. Then of course there are better low-glycemic carbohydrates that will aid in weight-loss. And stay away from all candy, all sugar. If you want to eat something sweet, eat nature's candy - raisins. See High & Low Glycemic Carbohydrate Table below.

High & Low Glycemic Carbohydrate Table

High Glycemic Carbohydrates (should be avoided)	Low Glycemic Carbohydrates (preferred)
Bagel (white bread)	Apricots
Baked Potato	Black Beans
Beets	Butter Beans

High Glycemic Carbohydrates	Low Glycemic Carbohydrates
Black-Eyed Peas	Cherries
Carrots	Chick Peas
Cheerios Cereal	Grapefruit
Corn	Green Beans
Corn Chips	Kidneys
Corn Flakes Cereal	Lentils
Corn Meal	Lima Beans
Cream Of Wheat	Nuts
Flour (white)	Peanuts
French Bread	Pinto Beans
French Fries	Rye Grain
Grahan Crackers	Skimmed Milk
Grape Nuts Cereal	Soy Beans
Green Peas	Tomatoes
Instant Rice	Yogurt
Pasta	
Pita Bread	
Puffed Wheat Cereal	
Rice Cakes	
(should be avoided)	(preferred)
Shredded Wheat Cereal	
Spaghetti, White	
Sweet Potatoes	
TOTAL Cereal	
White Bread	
White Rice	
Whole Wheat Crackers	
Wild Rice	
Yams	

See *Glycemic Food Index (GFI)*.

SUPER BLUE GREEN ALGAE: Aphanizomenon flos-aquae, better known as Super Blue Green Algae, is a completely **wild algae** living in Upper Klamath Lake located in Southern Oregon **far from the pollution of the cities, their sewage and far from industrial and agricultural activities (pesticides and herbicides).**

Upper Klamath Lake is fed by 17 volcanic mountain streams and rivers shaping this high desert lake into an actual *nutrient trap*! Klamath Lake is protected by the high Cascade Mountains and fed by geothermal hot springs and 4000 square miles of melting snow.

All the minerals your body needs are contained here in the basin - in chelated form - to become food for the micro algae. Super Blue Green Algae has a **complete balance of Vitamins**, except for Vitamin D (sunlight) and Vitamin E (the algae's high chlorophyll contents help produce Vitamin E naturally in the body). It is **rich in the B Vitamins, including B-12 and it has the highest known source of chlorophyll, which is 300% higher than alfalfa!**

Blue Green Algae at Klamath Lake grows during the summer months. The Blue Green Algae is harvested fresh from the lake on a daily basis and flash frozen to preserve its vital nutrients. The nutrient rich soils of the Cascade Range support the enormous photosynthetic environment that **IS NOT DUPLICATED ANYWHERE ELSE IN THE WORLD. Algae may be the last complete basic food source remaining on the planet!**

- **Amino Acids** -- Essential (body is not capable of producing them) and nonessential amino acids, the building blocks of protein that comprise most of your body: brain, hair, muscles, skin... Amino acids are required for the orderly functioning of all body processes.

- **Carbohydrates** -- Carbohydrates are the main source of energy that help regulate protein and fat metabolism. Carbohydrates also assist in digestion and assimilation of foods as well as help lipids breakdown in the liver. Super Blue Green Algae has small amounts of carbohydrates. Eat complex carbohydrates like brown rice, oatmeal, whole grain... with Super Blue Green Algae.

- **Chlorophyll** -- Chlorophyll activates enzymes in the body to produce Vitamins A, E and K. Chlorophyll helps the quick assimilation of nutrients into the bloodstream and aids the digestive system.

- **Lipid\Fatty Acids** -- Required for the transportation and breakdown of cholesterol. Carriers of Vitamin A, E and K.

- **Minerals** -- Minerals to help build your body and regulate its systems.

- **Vitamins** -- Vitamins help transform food into energy for body maintenance. See McBarroon Diet and Going Green.

SUPER SWEET STEVIA: The Japanese developed a method of refining the sweet glycosides out of the stevia leaf creating a new product called Stevioside which is **300 times sweeter than sugar!**

At the time of this writing the FDA allows stevia to be used as nutritional\dietary supplement and not as a food additive (food manufacturing companies cannot use it). Stevia is noted to be superior to aspartame (brand names NutraSweet & Equal) which has been linked to health problems. Stevia may be a great alternative than using aspartame products. Stevia may be purchased at health food stores or from Body Ecology (1-800-4STEVIA) and Consumer Direct (1-800-947-6417). See *The Five Deadly Whites*.

SWIMMING: Swimming is a great exercise to burn that fat, whether you're just playing in the water, dog paddling, doing laps, or doing organized group exercises with or without pool equipment. And water exercises are easy on your joints. So consider adding water exercises to lose that unwanted weight, get in great shape and look good. Here are a few fun water exercises to rev-up your metabolism and help you lose weight: Frisbee, Volley Ball, Wading, Walking In Water, and Water Aerobics. See *Swimming Fat Burners* below.

SWIMMING FAT BURNERS: Here's a challenging workout I did many times while in the military and it burns piles of calories and fat to keep you slim. These exercises include swimming laps, stomach crunches and plain ol' pushups. Are you ready? OK here we go:

1st Set = Swim 50-meters as fast as possible.
  Get out and do 25 stomach crunches
  followed by 25 pushups
  followed by 25 04-count flutter kicks

with no rest

2nd Set = Swim 50-meters as fast as possible.
    Get out and do 25 stomach crunches
    followed by 25 pushups
    followed by 25 04-count flutter kicks

3rd Set = Swim 50-meters as fast as possible.
    Get out and do 25 stomach crunches
    followed by 25 pushups
    followed by 25 04-count flutter kicks
with no rest

4th Set = Swim 50-meters as fast as possible.
    Get out and do 25 stomach crunches
    followed by 25 pushups
    followed by 25 04-count flutter kicks

rest a few minutes

5th Set = Swim 50-meters as fast as possible.
    Get out and do 25 stomach crunches
    followed by 25 pushups
    followed by 25 04-count flutter kicks

with no rest

6th Set = Swim 50-meters as fast as possible.
    Get out and do 25 stomach crunches
    followed by 25 pushups
    followed by 25 04-count flutter kicks

7th Set = Swim 50-meters as fast as possible.
    Get out and do 25 stomach crunches
    followed by 25 pushups
    followed by 25 04-count flutter kicks

with no rest

8th Set = Swim 50-meters as fast as possible.
Get out and do 25 stomach crunches
followed by 25 pushups
followed by 25 04-count flutter kicks
BIG CONGRATS - you're done!!!!!

TANTRIC TONING: You've heard of healing yoga, Tai Chi, QiGong and aerobics haven't you? How would you like to do yoga, Tai Chi QiGong and aerobics at the same time and get all the healing and weight-loss benefits? It's called Tantric Toning and it combines all the above. You can learn Tantric Toning from a very affordable and easy to learn video.

THINK YOURSELF THIN: Mind Over Matter! That's right! You can *THINK YOURSELF THIN!* A book by Debbie Johnson, Think Yourself Thin, uses visualization techniques! Lose weight without diet or exercise! She is so sure that her book will work to take off that unwanted weight, she's offering a money-back guarantee! Does visualization really work? It sure does! Don't believe me, see *Vision Therapy*. See *Exercise Mind-Over-Matter Trick*.

THREE SQUARE MEALS IN A BOTTLE: Previously, I told you about nutritious peanut butter and here's another food - concoction you ought to know about. This food recipe substitute comes from my very dear friend Kimberly. It originally comes from a DETOX Diet that really works and the main food substitute while you're detoxing is "energy" in a bottle - pure organic maple syrup. Here's what you do:

Step 01: See your doctor before drinking the following concoction.

Step 02: Place 10-ounces of pure water in a clean plastic container.

Step 03: Add 02-tablespoons of pure organic maple syrup to the 10-ounces of pure water. Approximately a 10 to 02 ratio.

Step 04: Secure the plastic container with its top. Refrigerate till consumed (within a few days).

Step 05: You can pre-make larger portions or simply make your smaller Three Squares In A Bottle as you go.

Maple Syrup Nutritional Stats!
- Amino Acid
- Biotin
- Calcium
- Folic Acid
- Fructose
- Glucose
- Iron
- Magnesium
- Manganese
- Phenolic Compounds
- Phosphorous
- Potassium
- Riboflavin
- Sodium
- Sucrose
- Thiamin
- Vitamin B1
- Vitamin B2
- Vitamin B5
- Vitamin B6
- Vitamin B9

Now you know why nutrient-rich pure organic maple syrup may help you lose that unwanted weight and at the same time DETOX your body. See *Peanut Butter*, *Detoxification Therapy*, *Fasting* and *Cottage Cheese*.

THREE SQUARE MEALS IN A BOTTLE DETOX: Previously, I told you about *Three Square Meals In A Bottle*, now here's a *'twist to it'* (keep reading) - *Three Square Meals In A Bottle Detox*. This food recipe substitute comes from my very dear friend Kimberly. This is the original DETOX Diet that really works and the main food substitute while you're detoxing is *"energy"* in a bottle - pure organic maple syrup. You'll find this DETOX a great help to meeting your weight-loss goals.

When using this DETOX Concoction, you are to **abstain from ALL FOOD - EAT NO FOOD for 07 days**. All the while, drink the following concoction at least three (03) times a day. Here's what you do:

Step 01: See your doctor before doing any DETOX and any drinking of the following concoction.

Step 02: Place 10-ounces of pure water in a clean plastic container.

Step 03: Add 02-tablespoons of pure organic maple syrup to the 10-ounces of pure water. Approximately a 10 to 02 ratio.

Step 04: Take a fresh lemon and cut it up in quarters. Squeeze all the lemon juice from each quarter in your container. If you want place all the squeezed lemon quarters in your container.

Step 05: Add a pinch of cayenne pepper (100,000 SHU) or a teaspoon of cayenne liquid (100,000 SHU) in the container. Stir thoroughly.

Step 06: Secure the plastic container with its top. Refrigerate till consumed (within a few days).

Step 07: You can pre-make larger portions (gallon or more) or simply make your smaller Three Squares In A Bottle as you go.

Maple Syrup Nutritional Stats!
- Amino Acid
- Biotin
- Calcium
- Folic Acid
- Fructose
- Glucose
- Iron
- Magnesium
- Manganese
- Phenolic Compounds
- Phosphorous

- Potassium
- Riboflavin
- Sodium
- Sucrose
- Thiamin
- Vitamin B1
- Vitamin B2
- Vitamin B5
- Vitamin B6
- Vitamin B9

Now you know why nutrient-rich pure organic maple syrup may help you lose that unwanted weight and at the same time DETOX your body. See *Peanut Butter, Detoxification Therapy, Fasting* and *Cottage Cheese.*

TONIC OF LIFE: According to Dr. Jack Soltanoff, the tonic of life (garlic, honey and vinegar), taken three times a day quickly helps joint-stiffened arthritis patients loosen-up and move easily and painlessly. *"Garlic, vinegar and honey are incredible fighters of disease and the aging process,"* says health expert and cookbook author M.J. Smith.

The terrific trio of garlic, vinegar (Apple Cider Vinegar) and honey can cure everything from acne, arthritis, cellulite, cholesterol, hemorrhoids, high blood pressure, insomnia, to **dumping unwanted pounds!** The tonic of life taken three times a day can be made by combining three cloves of garlic, two tablespoons of apple cider vinegar and a tablespoon of honey in a blender. Add a generous amount of orange juice or unsweetened grapefruit juice, mix and you have the *"Tonic of Life."*

TROBRIAND SKINNY DIET: Since most Americans are overweight, I thought I'd add this diet. In the South Pacific lay the Trobriand Islands and **obesity is about non-existent**. Why? They eat no fried foods. As a matter of fact, their diet is mainly composed of fish, coconuts and steamed vegetables. It's that simple. (National Geographic - July 1992)

TURKEY: A protein-rich food that **elevates the brain's levels of dopamine and norepinephrine**, two neurotransmitters that help us to react quickly, feel motivated and mentally energetic.

Just 04 ounces of raw turkey provides **only 145 calories and only 05 grams of fat**. Compare this to an equal portion of ground beef that will provide a whopping 313 calories and 23 grams of fat. Replace that ground beef with turkey; like hamburger, meat loaf, spaghetti sauce... Eating turkey will help **lower your serum cholesterol**. See *Shellfish*.

TURNIPS: A cooked cup of turnips furnishes only 28 calories, 78 milligrams of sodium which is higher than most vegetables and **low in fat**. Turnips are **related to the cabbage family** (distant cousin) which comes with the **seal of approval from countless experts on cancer prevention**. Turnips provide a good source of Vitamins A and C, is rich in calcium and provides a modest source of iron and protein. Being a relative to the cabbage family, turnips are rich in nutrients known to **inhibit tumor formation!**

TV COMMERCIALS: You're watching another marathon of your favorite TV shows and you say you don't have time to exercise uh! Every time a set of commercials come on, you have a good 03 to 05-minutes to do some simple exercises like jumping jacks, stomach crunches, flutter kicks, push-ups, U.S. Army Rifle Drill Exercises, get on your treadmill, stationary bicycle, cross-country machine,... do something. I'll tell you, those few minutes add up. By the time the marathon of shows are over, you got a good workout. Yes, you can do some brief exercises while you're watching your favorite shows because it takes your mind off your *"boring"* workout.

U.S. ARMY RIFLE DRILL EXERCISES (07): If you want to tone-up and get in-shape, here are 07 Rifle Drill Exercises that will surprise you at their effectiveness. The 1st time you try them, I guarantee you'll be sore the next morning. These Rifle Drills were used during Phase 01 of the U.S. Army Special Forces Qualification Course (Green Berets) - early 1980s, for they gave the Special Forces candidate a great muscle strengthening workout.

Anyway, while teaching SROTC at Mercer University in Macon, Georgia - early 1990s, every once in a while, I had to discipline a cadet here and there. And the way I did it was with some extra PT (physical training). One day I had these 04 MS IIIs (College Juniors) who needed such discipline so I had them assemble in the large dayroom where the cadets formed-up for formations. I taught the 04 cadets 06 Rifle Drills and assigned each cadet a specific rifle drill to learn and copycat so they could each take their turns in repeating the Rifle Drills.

I taught all 06 Rifle Drills with 15 repetitions of each Rifle Drill - a good warm-up. Then each cadet took their own turn on their respective Rifle Drill and exercised the other 03 cadets. Instead of 15 repetitions, they each did 25 repetitions of each Rifle Drill. So now that's a total of 40 repetitions they exercised on each Rifle Drill. The next morning the cadets woke-up in their own rooms and were extremely sore. So sore they hurt all over their bodies. I just chuckled when I heard of their conditions.

Now each Rifle Drill has either a 04-count (movement) or 08 count (movement) to it. And each Rifle Drill is also done at a slow pace, moderate pace or fast pace. The following are instructions for each Rifle Drill and their sketches straight out of the Army's training manual FM 21-20 Physical Fitness Training. OK, let's warm-up with the 1st Rifle Drill - The Fore-Up, Behind Back.

Note: No, you don't have to have a weapon to negotiate the Rifle Drills. You can use other items that are thin, approximately 36-inches long and weighs approximately 07-pounds.

Rifle Drill Counting Of Each Movement And Repetition!

Now to properly count each repetition, count each 04-count movement for example like 1, 2, 3, **1**; 1, 2, 3, **2**; 1, 2, 3, **3**; 1, 2, 3, **4**; 1, 2, 3, **5**;...

And count each 08-count exercise like 1, 2, 3, 4, 5, 6, 7, **1**; 1, 2, 3, 4, 5, 6, 7, **2**; 1, 2, 3, 4, 5, 6, 7, **3**; 1, 2, 3, 4, 5, 6, 7, **4**;... And remember to adhere to the cadence for each exercise whether it's slow, moderate or fast pace.

Do at least 15 repetitions of each exercise and you'll get a great workout. NO weapon? No big deal. Improvise, just make sure the exercise tool you use is at least 07-pounds for a worthy workout.

Here's a photo of my 'home-made rifle.' I just got an old broom stick, added 02 sets of 03 ½-pounds of small rocks, put em' in 02 bags, secured them on each end of the broom stick and taped everything so it will last for years.

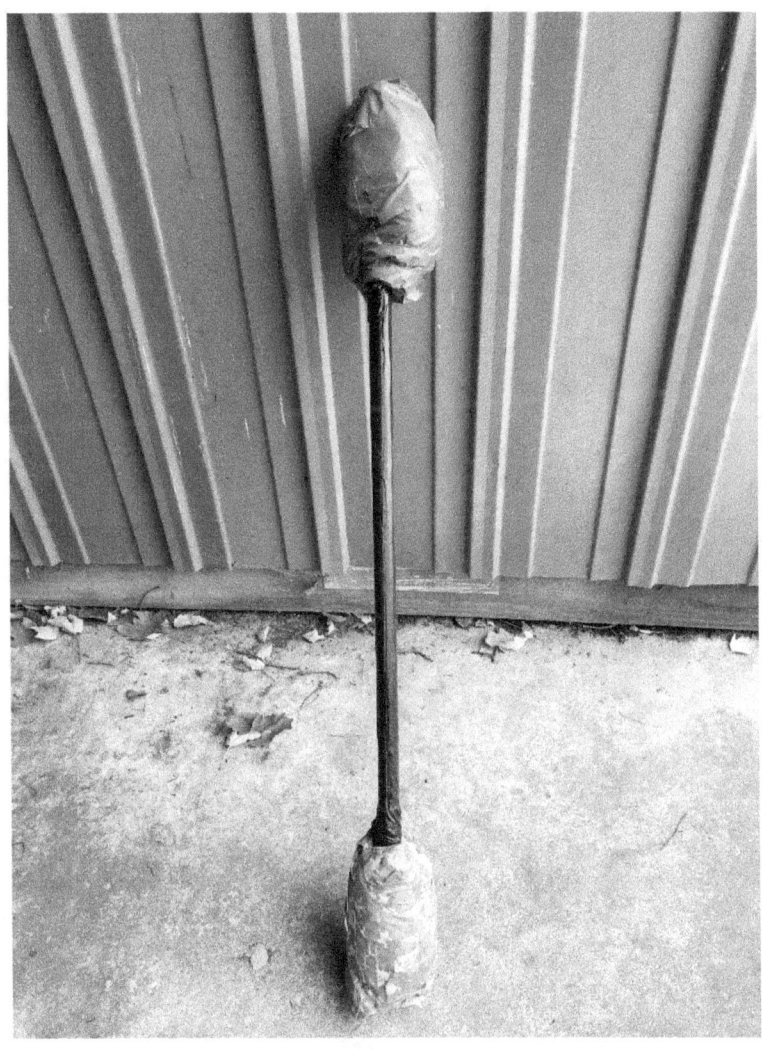

Rifle Drill #01
Fore-Up, Behind Back!

This is a four count exercise done at a moderate cadence.

The starting position, hold the rifle downward and feet together.

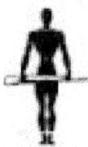

Swing arms forward and upward to overhead position.

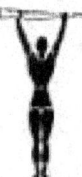

Lower rifle to back of shoulders.

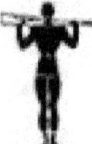

Move to first position.

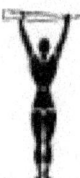

Recover to starting position.

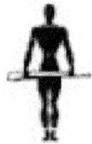

Rifle Drill #02
Fore-Up, Back Bend!

This is a four-count exercise done at a moderate cadence.

The starting position, hold rifle downward and feet together.

Swing arms forward and up to overhead position.

Bend backward, emphasizing bend in upper back. Keep face up and knees straight.

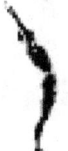

Move to first position.

Recover to start position.

Rifle Drill #03
Up And Forward!

This is a four-count exercise done at a fast cadence.

To starting position, hold rifle downward and feet together.

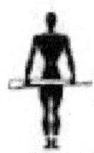

Swing arms forward and upward to overhead position.

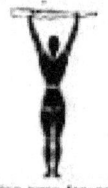

Swing arms forward to shoulder level.

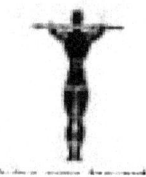

Move to first position.

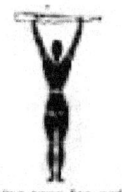

Recover to start position.

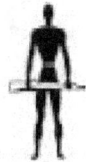

Rifle Drill #04
Fore-Up, Squat!

This is a four-count exercise done at a moderate cadence.
The starting position, hold rifle downward and feet approximately shoulder width apart.

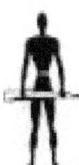

Swing arms forward and upward to overhead position.

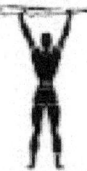

Swing arms down to shoulder level and assume a half-knee-bend position.

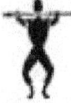

Move to first position.

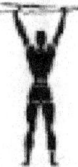

Recover to start position.

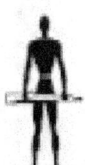

Rifle Drill #05
Fore-Up, Side Bend!

This is a four-count exercise done at a slow cadence.

The starting position, hold the rifle in front of you at eye-level with both arms locked in the horizontal position.

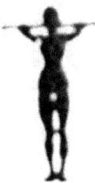

Bend the upper body to the left while keeping the arms horizontally locked and holding the weapon.

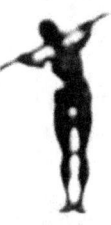

Return to the 1st position.

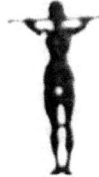

Bend the upper body to the right while keeping the arms horizontally locked and holding the weapon.

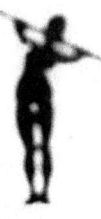

Return to the 1st position.

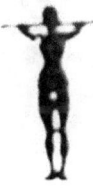

Rifle Drill #06
Fore-Up, Lunger!

This is a 08-count exercise done a moderate cadence.

The starting position, hold rifle downward and feet together.

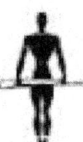

Step to the half-left with the left foot. At the same time, raise the weapon straight above the head with the arms locked vertically.

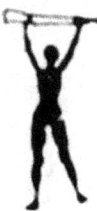

Bend downward keeping the arms locked and swinging the weapon downward so it's finally positioned outside the left ankle.

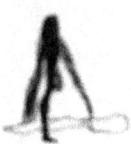

Straighten-up bringing the weapon straight above the head with the arms locked vertically.

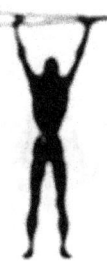

Return to the starting position.

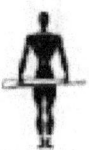

Step to the half-right with the right foot. At the same time, raise the weapon straight above the head with the arms locked vertically.

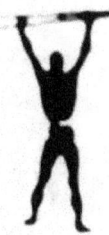

Bend downward keeping the arms locked and swinging the weapon downward so it's finally positioned outside the right ankle.

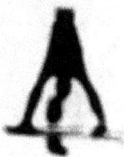

Straighten-up bringing the weapon straight above the head with the arms locked vertically.

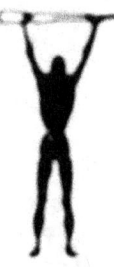

Return to the starting position.

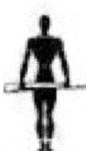

Rifle Drill #07
Horizontal Hold!

This static exercise should be done after completing all 06 Rifle Drills. It will hurt but it builds stamina and strength. Place feet shoulder width apart and your body erect. Raise your weapon up in front of you at eye level with your arms and the weapon in a "stiff" horizontal position.

Insure elbows are locked. Now hold the weapon in this position for a full 03-minutes. Each day you workout, add a little more time each time you do this last exercise. Yes, you'll feel the BURN but you're burning calories!!!! You must see *Military Weight-Loss Exercises*.

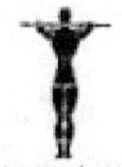

IMPORTANT NOTE: Check with your doctor before negotiating the *07 U.S Army Rifle Drills*.

VEAL: Veal is the **leanest form of beef**. It is a bit more expensive, but it provides the taste without the fat and is **loaded with protein, niacin and iron**. Four ounces of cooked veal has only 244 calories.

VISION BOARDS: You read Mind-Over-Matter Applications like Aroma Therapy, Exercise Mind-Over-Matter Trick, Hypnotherapy, Music & Sound Therapy, Mutt & Jeff Mind-Over-Matter, Past Life Therapy, Positive Affirmations, Prayer, Reflexology Blues Killer, Reflexology Weight-Loss Points, Self-Healing, Special Breathing Exercise, Stress Busters, Tantric Toning, Think Yourself Thin, Vision Therapy, Write Yourself A Contract, Writing Magic, Yoga, Your Picture, and now I want to tell you about an absolutely fascinating Mind-Over-Matter Application called Vision Boards.

What the heck are Vision Boards?
Vision Boards are a tool to consciously and subconsciously reach your goal(s). A Vision Board is a collection of pictures, phrases, words,... that are the epitome of what you want, what you desire, what your goal(s) is in the near and far future. Like all other Mind-Over-Matter Applications, a Vision Board is worthless if you don't believe. You must BELIEVE! A book that was recently published (December 2009) and is now available at book stores - it's called The Complete Idiot's Guide - Vision Boards, by Marcia Layton Turner.

This Survival Book is a great start to not only helping you meet your weight-loss goals but other goals you want in your life, no matter what it is like:
- Academics
- Athletics
- Bills (get out of debt)
- Education
- Freedom
- Friends
- Health
- Home Business or Business Success
- Home Improvements
- Marriage
- New Appliances
- New Baby
- New Boat
- New Car

- New Clothes
- New Home
- New Job
- Peace
- Pets
- Physical Appearance
- Physical Fitness
- Promotion
- Relationship Success
- Skin
- Skinny You
- Vacation
- Wealth ($$$$$$)
- Younger You

I think you got the idea. When you get a chance go to your local library or book store and get *The Complete Idiot's Guide - Vision Boards* so you can change your life for the better cause <u>you deserve only the best</u>. ***"I Deserve Only The Best."*** - cut this out for your personal *Vision Board*. OK, now let's get to the "$10,000.00 Weight-Loss Bet!"

VISION THERAPY: Vision Therapy and Guided Imagery are **HEALING POWERS OF THE MIND** and they work with the creative ability of your imagination. By utilizing Vision Therapy or Guided Imagery, you may be able to **heal yourself by building strong pictures in your mind of what you desire** to happen to you and BELIEVE that your creative mind pictures are REAL. The SECRET to building positive images in your mind is to visualize precise details. Imagine how your creative details FEEL, LOOK, SOUND, SMELL and TASTE! Trick your body into believing it is REAL!

In the past decade, Vision Therapy and Guided Imagery have been instrumental in **treating numerous illnesses including cancer, heart disorders and diseases of the immune system!** The following are some proven examples:

- A young boy with hemophilia confined to his wheelchair used his imagination to lower pain and ***"stop my bleeds."*** He imagined flying a diving fighter plane through the blood vessels in his body and dropping Factor 8 which is a much needed clotting substance.

- A 09 year-old boy diagnosed with inoperable and incurable brain tumor used a *Star Wars* scenario to defeat his deadly brain tumor. The young boy imagined himself as Luke Skywalker and his deadly brain tumor as the evil invader. The young boy's creative space battle was *so effective that 05 months later the deadly brain tumor was gone!*

- A woman diagnosed with breast cancer used her imagination to defeat this potentially life-threatening disease. She imagined small delicate birds searching her breast for crumbs, gold crumbs which represented her cancer. Each day the birds would eat the golden crumbs until they had their fill. She would then imagine a pure being of intense spiritual white light entering her body. Sometime later, the woman went in for a checkup. The **mammogram revealed that the BREAST CANCER DISAPPEARED!**

- A man diagnosed with throat cancer imagined his disease-fighting white blood cells as miners with pix axes, chopping away at the tumor and hauling it away to the dump. His **tumor shrunk to half its size** and the doctors were able to operate. The man left the hospital 02 days later as he imagined he would!

- A man **defeated his cancer** by imagining the cancer in his body as tiny creatures and his white blood cells as heroic white knights on horseback. Riding to his rescue, his white knights lanced and trampled the tiny cancer creatures until they were defeated!

Vision Therapy and Guided Imagery may be just as effective in healing other disorders and disabling injuries.

You just read some fascinating healings using Vision Therapy. Now think of what you can do with it for your weight-loss goals. See Think Yourself Thin, Write Yourself A Contract and Exercise Mind-Over-Matter Trick.

VITAMIN B1 (THIAMINE): Vitamin B1 enhances circulation and assists in the production of hydrochloric acid, blood formation and carbohydrate formation. Vitamin B1 **affects energy, growth disorders and learning capacity**. Vitamin B1 is needed for muscle tone of the intestines, stomach and heart. Thiamin is noted as a brain booster because it helps produce the messages your brain sends out to nerve cells. Thiamin is vital to memory and learning.

Sources of Vitamin B1 are asparagus, broccoli, Brussels sprouts, dried beans, brown rice, egg yolks, fish, organ meats (kidney, liver, heart), many nuts, oatmeal, peanuts, peas, plums, pork, poultry, dried prunes, raisins, rice bran, sardines, soybeans, turkey, wheat germ and whole grain.

Vitamin B1 is noted to repel bugs! Many testimonials of outdoors people have noted that mosquitoes simply want nothing to do with you. According to one study, Vitamin B1 did not prevent mosquito bites (controlled study), but may help in the prevention of the pain and itching brought on by the bites. Consuming sulfur like garlic, is also noted to have repelling effect on many insects including mosquitoes.

Follow the recommended dosage and instructions from the label and as per your doctor's instructions.

VITAMIN B2 (RIBOFLAVIN): Vitamin B2 is essential for red blood cell formation, antibody production, and cell respiration and growth. Vitamin B2 alleviates eye fatigue and important in preventing and treating cataracts. This Vitamin aids in the **metabolism of carbohydrates, fats and proteins**. Use Vitamin B2 with Vitamin A to maintain and improve the mucous membranes in the digestive tract.

Vitamin B2 facilitates oxygen use by body tissues like the skin, nails and hair as well as helping to eliminate dandruff. This Vitamin helps the uptake of iron and Vitamin B6.

Vitamin B2 is **important during pregnancy** because the **lack of this Vitamin may damage the fetus** even though the mother may be unaware of a deficiency. Vitamin B2 is needed for metabolism of tryptophan which is converted to niacin in the body.

Carpal Tunnel Syndrome may benefit from a treatment program that includes Vitamin B2 and Vitamin B6 (Pyridoxine). Cracks and sores at the corner of the mouth may indicate a deficiency of Vitamin B2 (Riboflavin). Sources of Vitamin B2 are asparagus, avocados, beans, broccoli, Brussels sprouts, cheese, currants, eggs, fish, meat, milk, nuts, poultry, spinach and yogurt.

WARNING: Increase intake of Vitamin B2 may be necessary when taking oral contraceptives and strenuous exercise. Vitamin B2 (Riboflavin) is easily destroyed by alcohol, antibiotics, cooking and light.

Follow the recommended dosage and instructions from the label and as per your doctor's instructions.

VITAMIN B3 (NIACIN, NIACINAMIDE, NICOTINIC ACID): Vitamin B3 is needed for circulation and healthy skin. This Vitamin aids in the functioning of the nervous system, **metabolism of carbohydrates, fats and proteins** as well as the production of hydrochloric acid for the digestive system. **Niacin lowers cholesterol and improves circulation**. It is also an effective treatment of schizophrenia and other mental illnesses. It is also noted as a brain booster and is vital to memory and learning. Sources of Vitamin B3 are beef, broccoli, carrots, cheese, corn flour, eggs, fish, milk, pork, potatoes, turkey, tomatoes tuna and whole wheat.

WARNING: A flush (usually harmless) may occur after ingestion of niacin. A red rash and tingling sensation may be experienced. Caution should be taken when consuming high amounts of niacin for pregnant women and people suffering from diabetes, glaucoma, gout, liver disease and peptic ulcers.
Follow the recommended dosage and instructions from the label and as per your doctor's instructions.

VITAMIN B5 (PANTOTHENIC ACID): Vitamin B5 is known as the anti-stress Vitamin. This Vitamin is instrumental in the production of the adrenal hormones, formation of antibodies, aids in Vitamin utilization and helps convert carbohydrates, fats and protein into energy.

This Vitamin is needed to produce vital steroids as well as cortisone in the adrenal gland. It's concentrated in the organs, essential to all cells of the body and an essential element of coenzyme A.

Vitamin B5 is also needed for functioning of the gastrointestinal tract. This Vitamin is also helpful in treating depression and anxiety. Sources of Vitamin B5 are beans, beef, eggs, salt-water fish, mother's milk, pork, fresh vegetables and whole wheat.

WARNING: To date, no side-affects have been noted.
Follow the recommended dosage and instructions from the label and as per your doctor's instructions.

WALKING EXERCISE: Walking is one of the best and FREE exercises. Walking doesn't pound your joints like running. Whether you slow walk or do speed walking - walking burns calories. Walking is very popular.

You'll see folks walking the mall corridors in the early morning hours. Many local parks have walking paths with folks using those paths at all daylight hours. You'll even see lots of folks walking during their lunch breaks. Activities That Burn Calories, you'll see that *Walking* for an hour clocks-in at 360-calories. See *Rucksacking*.

WATER: Drink clean water between meals. Water fills the stomach and helps decrease the appetite. It's a **natural appetite suppressant!** Pure clean water has **ZERO** **saturated fat,** **ZERO** **cholesterol, and ZERO** **calories.** See *Forced Hydration*.

WATER POLO: I consider myself a good swimmer (long distance). But the few times I participated in water polo (deep end of the pool), it kicked my butt and I knew I **burned a pile of calories in a short period of time**. Heck, I'd rather run 06-miles than play water polo. If you're a good swimmer, get a bunch of other folks together and consider water polo for a great workout.

WEIGHT-LOSS SUPPORT GROUP: You and your friends might want to consider starting-up your own Weight-Loss Support Group. Have a meeting and elect a committee (President, Treasurer,...). Give your group a name. Write a Mission Statement that details the goals of the group. Schedule regular get togethers so you can exercise together, eat together, exchange recipes,... Establish an alert roster so a member that needs support can telephone another member. A friend to talk to and weight-loss club is a great aid in weight-loss. It works great for alcoholics anonymous and it will work great for your weight-loss club so form a club today.

WEIGHT TRAINING: Weight training **BURNS FAT!** Have you ever seen a fat body builder? OK then, let's get started with this segment. Weight training really does burn fat. Why? Think of it this way. All those muscles that you're building through weight training are like little engines and those engines need fuel to run - fuel like fat! The more developed your muscles are - those kazillions of motors, the more fuel they need - fat.

You saw *Activities That Burn Fat*. Which of those activities burned the most fat? Go ahead look it up. Yes, Weight Training clocked-in at 850 calories during a 01-hour workout. For a weight-bearing workout, see *U.S. Army Rifle Drill Exercises*.

WHAT IS YOUR HEALTHY WEIGHT: Getting back to the basics, most experts, dieticians and doctors will tell you to lose weight, you'll have to **consume less calories, cut down on saturated fat and make exercise a part of your daily routine**. Even the simplest exercise like walking 30 minutes a day is an aid to lose unwanted pounds. Loosing 02 to 03 pounds a week is safe according to most experts. You have to exercise regularly and EAT THE RIGHT STUFF!

Before you see the Healthy Weight scale below, let me tell you about a landmark study. According to the New England Journal of Medicine, a 16-year study of 115,000 women revealed that women weighing 15% BELOW normal **lived longer** provided they didn't smoke! Meaning a 5' 5" women would have to weigh about 120 pounds. So may be the target weight isn't enough uh! Take a look at the height and weight chart below. SEE your designated physician for a healthy weight for YOU!

WHAT IS YOUR HEALTHY WEIGHT?

Height	Weight Upper Limits	Target Weight
4' 10"	119 pounds	109 pounds
4' 11"	124 pounds	114 pounds
5 feet	128 pounds	118 pounds
5' 01"	132 pounds	121 pounds
5' 02"	136 pounds	125 pounds
5' 03"	141 pounds	130 pounds
5' 04"	145 pounds	133 pounds
5' 05"	150 pounds	138 pounds
5' 06"	155 pounds	143 pounds
5' 07"	159 pounds	146 pounds
5' 08"	164 pounds	151 pounds
5' 09"	169 pounds	154 pounds
5' 10"	174 pounds	160 pounds
5' 11"	179 pounds	165 pounds
6 feet	184 pounds	169 pounds
6' 01"	189 pounds	174 pounds
6' 02"	194 pounds	178 pounds
6' 03"	200 pounds	184 pounds
6' 04"	205 pounds	189 pounds

Source: American Health Foundation.

If you're overweight or have any type of eating disorder, **YOU MUST SEE** the POC Section for many organizations and private companies that may help you concerning your weight problem or disorder. Below are some real quick references you can call according to your particular concern:

American Dietetic Association's Consumer Nutrition Hotline-----------1-800-366-1655
  (locate a Registered Dietician near you)

American Heart Association---1-800-AHA-USA1
  (ask for information on sensible eating)

Jenny Craig--1-800-775-JENNY
  (locate a center near you)

Take Off Pounds Sensibly (TOPS)--------------------------------------1-800-932-8677
  (locate a meeting near you)

Weight Watchers--1-800-651-6000
  (locate a meeting near you)

Can't lose that weight? SEE my **$10,000 WEIGHT-LOSS BET!**

Monitor obesity by using the Body Mass Index (BMI) Formula.

WARNING: Insure you see your doctor prior to any change of diet or implementing any exercise program.

WHEAT GERM WEIGHT-LOSS: Wheat germ is part of the wheat plant that's responsible for sprouting and making new wheat plants. The wheat germ is alive with life and is made-up of proteins, vitamins and minerals. Anyway, quite some time back, I interviewed a friend who told me their mother lost weight using wheat germ.

All she did was add wheat germ to EVERYTHING she ate. From breakfast to dinner meals and even snacks, wheat germ was always part of the meal. It was as simple as that. I use Kretschmer Wheat Germ. It's an excellent healthy food additive.

Note: Try a hefty combination of Wheat Germ (03 tablespoons), Sprouts (02 handfuls) and your favorite salad dressing for a super healthy meal. See Wheat Germ Oil For After-Burner Performance right below and see *Sprouts*.

WHEAT GERM OIL FOR AFTER-BURNER PERFORMANCE: Here's a health supplement worthy of your attention and it may give you that after-burner performance. This healthy supplement is called wheat germ oil. Again, wheat germ is part of the wheat plant that's responsible for sprouting and making new wheat plants.

The wheat germ is <u>alive with life</u> and is made-up of proteins, vitamins and minerals. Just a half-cup of wheat germ contains 24 grams of protein. It includes minerals like calcium, copper, manganese, magnesium and potassium. It also includes B Vitamins and Vitamin E.

Now wheat germ oil is pressed out of the wheat germ. The wheat germ oil is rich in fat soluble Vitamins. According to Dr. T. K. Cureton, head of the University of Illinois Physical Fitness Laboratory, wheat germ oil may help maintain endurance in athletic performance.

A single daily teaspoon of wheat germ oil along with exercise has shown **to increase men's physical endurance by as much as a whopping 51%!** This amazing find was based on Dr. Cureton's 04-year research that includes tests on 200 men including college men, middle-aged men, swimmers, wrestlers,...

According to Dr. Cureton, *"Wheat germ oil is a valuable dietary supplement to men doing hard exercise and it has possible application to competitive sports. We have tried it sufficiently to believe that this is true. It provides something that enables men to bear hard stress and continue to do hard labor without deteriorating. It particularly affects physical endurance and heart response."*

Note: All the B Vitamins aid to maintain healthy eyes, hair, liver, mouth, muscle tone in the gastrointestinal tract, nerves and skin. B-Complex Vitamins are coenzymes involved in energy production. B-Complex Vitamins may be useful to **combat depression or anxiety**. The B Vitamins should be taken together.

WILD BLUEBERRIES: Blueberries are not only super tasty they may be one of the top fruits that protect you when it comes to antioxidants. *"When research at Cornell University (Ithaca, NY) tested 25 commonly consumed fruits, they discovered that wild berries packed the most absorbable antioxidants. These antioxidants are vital for mopping up cell-damaging and disease inducing free radicals. Plus, some scientific data indicates that antioxidants help reduce muscle damage..."* - Muscle Mag (December 2009). See *Cellular Healing*.

WRITE YOURSELF A CONTRACT: Write yourself a contract - **a <u>promise</u> to lose weight**. Or you can write the contract to your spouse, child, friend, pet critter,... That contract obligates you to lose weight and will give you that "kick in the butt" to "lose it or else" and this is the Survival Book that will help you keep your contract to your loved one(s). You can write the contract so it's broken-up in phases like:

Phase 01: Starting tomorrow, I'll completely stop eating candy, salty snacks,... I'll completely stop eating high-fat foods, high cholesterol foods,...

Phase 02: Starting tomorrow, I'll start eating fruits, vegetables and start juicing.

Phase 03: In a few days, I'll start walking a little bit.

Phase 04: In 02-weeks I'll work up to walking 02-miles a day and at a faster pace.

Phase 05: In 02-weeks I'll lose a total of 04-pounds.

Phase 06: In 03-weeks I'll lose a total of 06-pounds.
You got the idea ---

And **most important** about the contract, write the unhealthy consequences of not completing your part of the contract like, high cholesterol (LDL), heart disease, diabetes, high blood pressure, stroke,... - early DEATH!!!

OK, tonight before you go to bed, draft-up a contract for starters. And after that *"Visualize yourself thin"* and vibrantly healthy. And while you're at it *"Visualize"* a battle going on in your body of good guys travelling throughout your heart and circulatory system destroying killer artery-blocking plaque.

And another group of good guys travelling throughout your ENTIRE body and especially organs (lungs, liver, pancreas,...) killing cancer cells, bad bacteria, bad fungi, hook worms,... See Vision Therapy and Writing Magic.

WRITING MAGIC: This is one Mind-Over-Matter application that is rarely used cause it's unknown and not proven to work for the same reason. Handwriting (not typing) your specific goals on paper gives the writer the unique magical power to achieve their goals. Handwriting your specific goals on paper accesses the subconscious of the writer which has the writer implement minute and major actions (direct and indirect) to achieve progressive goals. So go to a quiet place, get some paper and a pencil and start writing your weight-loss goals or plan of action to achieve your weight-loss goals. C'mon get going. Do it "write" now. See Write Yourself A Contract.

YOGA: Yoga to improve your health, **lose weight**...! Before I go over this subject let me tell you a story. I really believe yoga can help you lose weight. Why? Several years ago, I purchased a yoga VHS tape for beginners. The yoga tape was about 50-minutes.

Anyway, I put the tape in and I followed it step-by-step. **I'm not a stretchy person**, but I tried every movement the best I could do along with the instructors on the tape. I gotta tell you, that 50-minute yoga tape **kicked my butt so bad**, I never did it again. Yes, there are yoga tapes specifically for weight-loss - good luck!

Yoga may be your key to a healthier and tranquil life. Also called Hatha Yoga, yoga is an ancient Hindu system of health and longevity which employs various physical postures, breathing exercises, meditation and lifestyle considerations to achieve a state of balanced health and wellbeing.

Numerous studies have shown that Yoga and meditation have **positive health effects on a wide variety of conditions including asthma, headaches, high blood pressure, pain and stress**. I just read an article about a yoga practitioner who attributes yoga to her **weight-loss** & sustained great shape and not to high-impact aerobic exercises or a starvation diet.

What is Yoga?

Before I answer this question, let me tell you this - YOU DON'T have to turn into a monk, yogi, or live in a cave to benefit from practicing yoga OK! Yoga is a set of non-impact exercises that make you fitter, improve your mind therefore the mind - body -spirit connection. Yoga with its postures, stretches, movements and breathing (non-shallow) improves your circulation (remember I told you - *"the blood rules"*), tones your body, **improves metabolism**, reduces stress and it gives your body a chance to heal itself!

Why does Yoga work?

I strongly believe in the placebo affect which is one word "faith"! Besides Yoga, there are 60 Alternative Health Practices in lieu of conventional medicine of drugs and surgery. Yes, it has its place but folks all over the world are being healed by Alternative Health Practices from Prayer, Reike, Target Nutrition, Visualization, QiGong, Yoga... Why? The Alternative Practice like Yoga does have merit like 60 other Alternative Practices but the person practicing it *"believes, knows, wants"* it to work and it does! Even if Yoga were to be scientifically proven worthless 100 years from now - guess what? It still worked because of the placebo effect - *"faith"*!

Yoga has been practiced for more than 6,000 years, so doesn't that tell you there is something to it! Yoga has one common ingredient found in other ancient *"exercises"* and Mind-Over-Matter applications and that is breathing (called Pranayama)! No, not shallow breathing but deep breathing. Did you read *"Special Breathing Exercise To Instantly ENERGIZE Yourself And Help You Burn-Up Excess Fat!"*

Breathing is so important, not only for yoga - for EVERYTHING. Even if you're laying there on your recliner like a slacker slug watching TV - you need fuel, so deep breathe even a few times, you have the time so do it! Remember when involuntarily yawning, that's your body telling you that you need more oxygen to re-energize yourself, to fight that *"time to take a nap"* feeling!

I've been deep breathing while writing this segment! Now it's YOUR TURN! Take a DEEEEP BREATH through your nose, HOLD IT for 15 - 20 seconds and force it out and do it 05 more times! Don't you feel better!!! Sure you do - it's fuel for your body. Again, most of us are shallow breathers. Our bodies - our 100,000,000,000,000 cells are not getting that vital fuel it needs to function properly. **Yes, to even help your body heal itself too!** Seriously, DEEP BREATHE 05 or 06 times right now! Do it for you. If you're smoking a cigarette, put it out and give me 50 (push-ups)! See *Smoker's Body Starts Healing Itself.*

,

Yoga starts off with breathing exercises in the difficult lotus position or a position comfortable for the practitioner. It has to be a comfortable position - posture. Most beginners are stiff and couldn't bend-over if there was a $100 in front of them! NO PROBLEM - in the POC Section, you'll have access to folks that offer beginner, intermediate and advanced yoga videos! **There are different breathing practices besides deep breathing.** Once the practitioner has warmed-up with proper breathing, he/she then goes into a relaxation period - again proper breathing is practiced.

Next the practitioner negotiates Asanas. Asanas are stretches, movements and positions to redevelop and improve the functioning of the body, mind and spirit. Asanas reawaken **muscle strength** and flexibility, dramatically improves blood flow, wakes-up the body at the cellular level which helps to clear the mind and improve its power to think and solve problems due to increased blood flow and healthier oxygenated cells and finally boosts the spirit to positive tranquil thinking.

There are basic and advanced Asanas. Depending on which book you read or video you view, Asanas may be different but all are designed to improve Mind, Body and Spirit! Meditation is another advanced part of a serious Yoga practitioner.

Yoga, Tai Chi, Qi Gong, Tantric Toning, Chi Exercises... are all designed to improve Mind, Body and Spirit and in many cases have **actually done the impossible** with respect to health, martial arts and Mind-Over-Matter applications. Insure you go over the POCs I give you and request their FREE information today! See *Special Breathing Exercise*.
Follow the recommended instructions only as per your doctor's approval.

YOGURT: One-half cup of plain yogurt provides between 45 to 80 calories depending on the brand you purchase. Yogurt could be a great way to **lose weight**; just be careful which brand you purchase. READ the Nutrition Facts!

Yogurt with its active cultures, make it digestible for people with lactose intolerance. Yogurt with its active cultures are also noted for their **anti-bacterial properties**. Eating yogurt helps increase your body's levels of interferon, which is a **powerful immune-enhancing hormone**. Yogurt contains L-acidophilus. L-acidophilus has been noted to significantly decrease the incidence of vaginal infections in women who are prone to them. **INSURE** the yogurt you purchase states the following on the label: *"made with live and active cultures."* To guarantee healthy intestinal flora, see *Prevail Corporation*. See *Zulu Super Food*.

YOUR PICTURE: Here's another Mind-Over-Matter application to help you lose weight. Find a picture of yourself when you were thin - the weight you want to be in the near future. Place this picture and a few like it or several like it when you have no choice but to see it all the time throughout the day. Put one on the fridge, all mirrors, in your wallet, in your car, your debit card (keep you from buying fast-food). Looking at that "thin" picture over and over again will go to your subconscious. You may not notice, but you'll start doing little things here and there that will help you lose weight. Your everyday pattern of things that made you overweight will be altered. If you don't have a picture of yourself, attach a picture of your face to a thin body out of a magazine.

And do this, take a picture of yourself at your heaviest - a picture you don't like - you hate and paste it to your fridge - that will keep you from snacking!!!! See *Mutt And Jeff Mind-Over Matter*.

ZULU SUPER FOOD: Odds are, you're throwing away whey all the time. Each time you reopen the same carton of yogurt, you'll notice there's always a milky watery substance that gathers at the top of the yogurt. Most folks discard the milky watery substance - whey. As you already read, whey is not only edible, it's surprisingly super nutritious. Curds are soured congealed milk used to make cheese and other products.

Whey - The Super Food: No whey. Yes whey! Zulus warriors (1800s) were in absolutely phenomenal shape, able to cover 50-miles in a single day and do fierce battle afterwards! Was it because of their diet of whey? Recent research shows that whey is a super food. It's touted as **turning off the aging process**.

Whey is loaded with protein, it's **low in fat & calories**, and its loaded with several amino acids (leucine, isoleucine, valine,...). It builds muscle by 50% **to burn fat and helps <u>turn off your appetite</u>**. It helps **<u>raise the metabolism</u>** by as much as 68%! It helps drop stress hormones while increasing the amino acid - tryptophan that helps produce serotonin - the feel good hormone. It also helps boost mental alertness by 15%.

It's also an immune booster and anti-oxidant that fights free radicals that cause the human body to age, become sickly,... It helps increase the body's glutathione - the master antioxidant. German research shows that whey prevents cancers and most important, slows the aging process by 32%!

Tests demonstrated that animals on a whey diet lived 50% longer than their counterparts not on a whey diet! The best part is you don't have to go to Zululand to get whey, you can get a quality whey product at your local health food store.

Look for whey products in powdered form. I conducted my own research on quality whey products and started drinking delicious whey every day (01 August 2003)! No whey? Yes whey, this is what I found: French vanilla). It contains 24 grams of protein per serving (16 serving total), high in essential (body doesn't provide) and branch chain amino acids (18), ion exchange whey and stevia (sweetener).

Ultra Whey Protein Powder *24* cost about $16 for a 02-week supply. However, I turned it into a 30-day supply by taking 1/2 scoop (scoop provided) and pouring it into an empty small *Arrowhead* half-pint water bottle. I pour in cold pure water about 3/4 full and shake vigorously for my daily Zulu drink. NO, I ain't running 50-miles and pickn' fights with Brits (may be the French). I'm still in the R&D phase. Just thought you should know about *Whey - The Super Food!*

YES, I found several other powdered whey products. If you're interested, look into whey as a supplement to your diet AFTER your doctor's OK.
Follow the recommended dosage and instructions from the label and as per your doctor's instructions.

$10,000.00 Weight-Loss Bet!

I've had a standing *$10,000.00 Weight-Loss Bet* **since the 1990s** and have yet to have any takers, not one single challenge. I am so confident in my ability to lose weight so fast and so safe (for me), here's my *$10,000.00 Weight-Loss Bet* to YOU and ANYBODY out there to include the media (Radio, TV, YouTube,...). OK, here it is:

"I challenge and bet YOU, anyone that I (Joseph A. Laydon Jr.) can lose 45 pounds in 45 days or less; using only the writings from "169+ Lose It Or Else Accelerated Weight-Loss Facts, Tricks & More!' If I fail, I will pay my challenger $10,000.00 CASH! When I lose 45 pounds in 45 days or less, the challenger owes me $10,000.00 cash."

1st Note: I have the opportunity to gain weight to a weight of - 210 - 225+- pounds prior to starting the *$10,000.00 Weight-Loss Bet*.

2nd Note: At the time of this writing (26 June 2012) the *$10,000.00 Weight-Loss Bet* is no longer up for any challenge.

PS See *$10,000.00 Weight-Loss Bet Diet*.

$10,000.00 Weight-Loss Bet Diet!

You've just read the majority of *"169+ Lose It Or Else Accelerated Weight-Loss Facts, Tricks & More!"* And here's my simple personal plan to lose weight - in fact - lose '45 pounds in 45 days or less.'

Consume at least 03 12-ounce glasses of carrot juice by Juicing or V8 Juice each day. Drinks are supplemented with any 'green powder' of my choice. Cayenne pepper (100,000 SHU rating or higher) may be used with each drink. Unlimited fresh water may be consumed at any time.

Consume 03 to 06 large portions of <u>raw</u> chopped-up cabbage and/or any other large portions of <u>raw</u> fruits and/or <u>raw</u> vegetables each day.

Exercise 60-minutes to 120-minutes each day via walking, running, push-ups, stomach crunches, swimming and/or use of any exercise machine.

PS See *$10,000.00 Weight-Loss Bet*.

Why The $10,000.00 Weight-Loss Bet Diet Works!

Here's why my Special Diet works. Each food and supplement that you **read on the previous** page works to lose weight all by itself. But TOGETHER - they work synergistically, meaning they are more powerful together - getting the most results together than individually. OK, let's take one of them at a time. Let's start with *Cabbage*.

Cabbage: I like Green Cabbage (sliced) and it's the main entre of my Special Diet. You read <u>all the healthy benefits of raw cabbage</u>. It has to be raw cause you need the nutrients and especially the enzymes to help you lose weight. It supplies nutrients and at the same time helps to DETOX your body.

Other Vegetables: I like adding other raw vegetables to the raw cabbage. Like carrots, radishes, olives, celery, cucumbers, minced garlic,... It's delicious and especially weight-loss nutritious.

Garlic: You read a MOUNTAIN of healthy benefits of *Healing Garlic* and it's part of my Special Diet. I've read testimonials where folks used only garlic as their weight-loss supplement. Garlic, also known as *Russian Penicillin* is just plain SUPER healthy. Me, I don't have the time nor the patience to chop-up fresh garlic so I purchase a 32-ounce jar of the *Spice World Minced Garlic*. I use about tablespoon per meal.

Cayenne Pepper: Cayenne Pepper undoubtedly has a bounty of healthy benefits but the main reason I use it for this Special Diet is because it revs-up my metabolism for weight-loss. And when the metabolism is revved-up, I burn fat. I add just a tiny bit (a small pinch - rating of 100,000 SHU) of cayenne pepper to a big bowl of sliced raw cabbage, other raw vegetables,... Insure you close it all up with Bragg ACV & Bragg Liquid Aminos (keep reading) and shake it all up to spread the hot cayenne pepper throughout the meal of cabbage, vegetables,... If it's too hot, make a 2nd meal without the cayenne pepper and add it to the 1st batch. Divide it all in-half and eat one meal and fridge the other half for the next meal. See *Cayenne Company Inc.* and *Frontier Cooperative Herbs* in the POC Section.

Note: <u>DO NOT</u> purchase any cayenne pepper at your local grocery store. It's absolutely worthless. Get a *"HOT"* cayenne pepper at your local health food store with a Scoville Heat Unit (SHU) rating of 100,000 SHUs or more.

Bragg Apple Cider Vinegar (ACV): DO NOT use the apple cider vinegar (ACV) at your local grocery store. That ACV is worthless when it comes to this Special Diet. Get your Bragg ACV at your local health food store. And don't forget to hold the bottle above your head and look at the bottom of it. You should see a goldish colored sediment. This will tell you that you got the good stuff. Just shake it real good before each use. You read a bounty of healthy benefits of ACV to include weight-loss. Plus, I especially like the taste when it's combined with *Bragg Liquid Aminos* (keep reading). I add a good squirt to the meal, close it up and shake it so it's all thoroughly mixed-up together (especially the cayenne pepper).

Bragg Liquid Aminos: I know there are other amino acids out there but I prefer the salty taste of *Bragg Liquid Aminos* (provides 16 amino acids) especially when it's mixed with Bragg Apple Cider Vinegar. As you read previously, amino acids provide a bounty of health benefits and I add a good squirt to the meal, close it up and shake it so it's all thoroughly mixed-up together (especially the cayenne pepper). In my humble opinion, *Bragg Liquid Aminos* directly and indirectly aids in weight-loss.

Juicing: Juicing alone is a SUPER SUPER HEALTHY meal. It's loaded with nutrients and gets into your system quicker cause it's in a liquid form. And without all the other bulk foods made-up of fats, sugars, salts,... your body detoxifies itself and you lose unhealthy weight by detoxification and lose weight by eliminating *The Five Deadly Whites* from your diet. I mostly use carrots when juicing. If not juicing, I use a 46-fluid ounce bottle of *Spicy Hot V8 Tomato Juice* or *High Fiber V8 Tomato Juice* (saves time & cleaning up). Juicing alone will help you lose weight but why only juice (keep reading).

Green Powder: I use a 'Green Powder' supplement (most or all types are loaded with nutrients) to my juicing. The 'Green Powder' I'm using are *Essential Greens* (local health food store) and *All Day Energy Greens* (see *Institute For Vibrant Living* in the POC Section). Both, especially *All Day Energy Greens* are **LOADED** with vital nutrients your body needs for vibrant health. And I've found that when taking 'Green Powder' the cravings for the sweets, the salts, and the other unhealthy foods and snacks goes away - thus weight-loss! Plus, the 'Green Powder' will provide that fuel you need when you exercise (weight-loss). I HIGHLY recommend 'Green Powder' to any weight-loss plan.

When I don't juice, I just add 03 heaping tablespoons of 'green Powder' to a 46-fluid ounce bottle of *Spicy Hot V8 Tomato Juice* or *High Fiber V8 Tomato Juice*. Insure you shake it up real good initially and between uses cause the 'Green Powder' has a tendency to clump-up. YES, I may add some cayenne pepper too so my metabolism is revved-up. Plus, it keeps my back in good shape (no muscle spasms).

Water: The body requires water all the time. And an extra amount of water each day may be an additional key to lose weight cause it fills you up and water has no fat, no calories, no sugar, no salt, no nuthin' except the pure water your body requires to be vibrantly healthy. Many many different types of diets have water as part of their successful weight-loss plan and rightly so for again, water fills you up and your body requires it all the time. Me, I use a Brita Pitcher & Water Filter for purified water. See *Four Star Books in the POC Section* for a book called *Your Body's Many Cries For Water*.

Exercise: Using my Special Diet above, you'll no doubt lose weight. But if you want to kick your weight-loss into ultra-high gear, exercise will do it. Yes, even yoga (see *Yoga* in the Itemized List) and other non-cardio exercises I listed in this Survival Book. I'm telling you, exercise every day while doing this diet and weigh yourself daily. You'll drop the unhealthy pounds so fast, you'll say what I said *"This weight scale must be broken. I'm losing weight real fast."*

Five Deadly Whites: Using my Special Diet, do you know what you're doing? You're AVOIDING *The Five Deadly Whites*. You already read about *The Five Deadly Whites* and I hope it helps you rethink about what you eat from this day forward even after you meet your weight-loss goals.

Yes, I've said go ahead and eat & splurge now and then but not all the time. See *Six Steps Forward And One Step Back* in the Itemized A-Z Index.

OK, here's an extra thing I do to feed my body the good stuff. I grow sprouts and I grow sprouts all the time. I make a salad using sprouts instead of cabbage. I add other raw vegetables (radishes, carrots, celery, green peppers,...) and then I may splurge and use *Wish Bone Chunky Blue Cheese Dressing* instead of Bragg ACV, Bragg Liquid Aminos,... Pound for pound I'm still eating healthy and mostly AVOIDING *The Five Deadly Whites*.

You can grow a BOUNTY of sprouts every single day (multiple sprouters). I use multiple 'Sprouters' and have fresh sprouts ready-to-go just about every day. What I don't use I place in a sealed container and refrigerate for the next day or so. See *Gardens Alive* for a Sprouter and a variety of sprout seeds in the POC Section. Just a single pack of sprouts (from *Gardens Alive*) contains approximately 45,000 seeds and that's a lot of super healthy food!

Most Important Note: What you just read is my core Special Weight-Loss Diet. However, in this Survival Book - you have so many many other different options that YOU can use for YOUR OWN Special Diet. You eat what you like, you eat what's tasty & healthy for YOU so you stick with it!

Points Of Contact

A Beginners Guide To Healthy Breathing----------------------------------**by Ken Cohen**
In this audio book, qigong expert - Ken Cohen teaches you how to *"instantly breathe energy and healing qi (life force) into your body every minute of the day,..."* This 73-minute audio book is very worthy of your super vibrant health.

American Board of Medical Specialist (ABMS)------------------------------**1-800-776-2378**
As competition in health care increases, some doctors are advertising themselves as specialist in areas in which they haven't received training. The ABMS Hotline will inform you *whether the physician is certified by a recognized* board and in what specialty. Board-certified doctors have completed training and passed written and oral exams in their areas of expertise. Call Monday through Friday from 9 a.m. to 6 p.m., Eastern Standard Time. See Joint Commission on Accreditation of Healthcare Organizations in this section.

American Diabetes Association National Center----------------------------**1-800-232-3472**
American Diabetes Assoc., 1660 Duke St., Alexandria, VA 22314. The American Diabetes Association National Center is staffed during regular business hours. Call Monday through Friday from 8:30 a.m. to 5 p.m., Eastern Standard Time. If you would like *information concerning diabetes* call their Patient Information Line at 1-800-DIABETES. If you want information about General Membership and newsletters call 1-800-806-7801.

American Dietetic Association's Nutrition Hot Line----------------------**1-800-366-1655**
Registered dietitians will answer your questions. Call Monday through Friday from 9 a.m. to 4 p.m. Call 8 p.m. to 8 a.m. for recorded seasonal messages in English and Spanish. TDD service for the hearing impaired is available from 9 a.m. to 4 p.m. weekdays.

American Heart Association--**1-800-242-8721**
If in the Chicago area 1-312-342-4675
To talk to a staff member in Illinois, call Monday through Friday from 8:30 a.m. to 5 p.m., Central Standard Time. Request information according to your concern.

American Society of Clinical Hypnosis, The-------------------------------**1-708-297-3317**
The American Society of Clinical Hypnosis, 2200 East Devon Ave., Suite 291, Des Plaines, IL 60018-4534. Call or write for a *qualified hypnotherapist* in your area. If you locate a hypnotherapist on your own, insure that he\she received their graduate degree from an accredited university and is licensed by the state. Some hypnotherapist listed in your yellow pages have a worthless degree and may use the term "certified registered." Cost of hypnosis may run approximately $100. Insurance may cover hypnosis described as "psychotherapy" and not cover it under preventive therapy -- smoking cessation. See *Hypnotherapy*.

Arbico Organics--**1-800-827-2847**
www.arbico-organics.com
Arbico Organics, P.O. Box 8910, Tucson, AZ 85738-0910. Arbico Organics offers natural products for your home, garden, farm, pets,... Instead of using cancer-causing chemicals, use far safer applications so now and in the future you and your family, pets, property are healthier, cleaner and non-toxic. Call or write their FREE, all-color 52-page catalog. See *Gardens Alive* in this Section.

Aromatherapy--**1-800-877-6889**
                                                                              1-303-443-1433
P.O. Box 17155, Boulder, Colorado 80308. Precious Collection Aromatherapy was founded in 1990 with the intention to present the public with unique, informative and affordable introductory essential oil packets. Aromatherapy has many avenues of exploration, whether it be the Medical, Aesthetic, Psychological or Holistic approach. Call or write and ask for free information.

Ask Cooking Light Hot Line - Nutrition Information Service---------**1-800-231-3438**
The University of Alabama at Birminghams's Department of Nutrition Sciences answers questions for Cooking Light readers. The University's information service also gives brief answers to nutrition questions posed by anyone. Call Monday through Friday from 8:30 a.m. to 4:30 p.m.

Aspartame Consumer Safety Network (ACSN)----------------------------**1-214-352-4268**
Aspartame Consumer Safety Network (ACSN), P.O. Box 780634, Dallas, TX 75378. First of all, stop right now and go to Section 26 and read about a *sweet poison* called aspartame which is a *serious health threat to everyone!* Now that you know about the dangers of aspartame, it's time to do something about it. Call the Aspartame Consumer Safety Network and get involved by eliminating aspartame all together!

I talked to Mrs. Mary Stoddard who's been involved with revealing the health threat of this *sweet poison* for more than 10 years! An expert in her field, she appeared on the National TV Series *HARDCOPY* (October 1996)! She speaks throughout the U.S. and is an international speaker as well! A very busy and dedicated spokeswoman against aspartame, she'll send you valuable information (200+ page book) concerning aspartame for only $25!

   Please send your remittance to the address above. Read much more about this *sweet poison* - aspartame in Section 11. See Aspartame Victims & Their Friends, Food & Drug Administration (FDA) Product Complaint & Emergency Operations Line and NUTRIVOICE in this section. See ACSN in World Wide Web addresses in this section.

Aspartame Victims & Their Friends---------------------------------------# unavailable
Aspartame Victims & Their Friends, Attention: Joyce Wilson, P.O. Box 1424, Forest Park, GA 30031. First of all, stop right now and go to Section 26 and read about a *sweet poison* called aspartame which is a serious health threat to everyone! Now that you know about the dangers of aspartame, it's time to do something about it. Write to the address above and get involved by eliminating aspartame all together! See Aspartame Consumer Network, Food & Drug Administration (FDA) Product Complaint & Emergency Operations Line and NUTRIVOICE in this section.

Association for Research Enlightenment, Inc. (ARE)-------------------1-800-333-4499
                                             1-804-428-3588
                                             1-804-422-4631(fax)
Association for Research Enlightenment, Inc., (ARE) continues the work of a man named Edgar Cayce who founded the ARE in 1931. ARE is an international network of people and volunteers who are interested ancient civilizations, dream interpretation, ESP & psychic development, holistic healing, meditation, reincarnation, spiritual growth, the purpose of life, and much more. There are many benefits to ARE members such as: ARE Camp, ARE Conferences and Seminars, ARE books by mail, The *New Millennium Journal*, *Venture Inward* Magazine, and much more. Call Monday through Friday from 8:00 a.m. to 5:00 p.m., Eastern Standard Time, for your free information packet!

Barlean Organic Oil---1-800-445-3529
Barlean Organic Oil, 4936 Lake Terrell, Ferndale, WA 98248. Barlean Organic Oil offers a cookbook of recipes for flax seed and flax oil called *Flax for Life* ($5.95 plus $1.70 shipping). This company also offers the very health enhancing flax oil products. INSURE you read about flax seed in Section 14. Please write "Order Department" when ordering your book. Included with your book, you'll receive a price list on their other healthy products. See Heintzman Farms in this section. See *Flax Seed*.

Blessed Herbs--**1-800-489-HERB**

1-508-882-3755(fax)

Blessed Herbs, 109 Barre Plains Road, Oakham, Massachusetts 01068. Blessed herbs is a nine-year old, family owned business that provides 200 premium quality bulk herbs and herbal products to herbalist, health professionals, herbal manufacturers, health food stores and individuals in the U.S. and abroad. Their herbs mainly come from organic growers and wildcrafters. *Certified organic growers cultivate without the use of synthetic fertilizers, herbicides or pesticides and take care to enrich the soil naturally!* Call or write for their free 24-page catalog. Their catalog covers multitudes of herbs, Aromatherapy products, spices, and wide variety of healthy reading booklets & books and a price list.

Bragg--**www.bragg.com**
See *Health Science* in this Section.

Butterball Turkey Talk-Line, The--**1-800-323-4848**

1-800-833-3848(TDD)

The Butterball Turkey Hotline, Swift and Company, Inc., 115 W. Jackson Boulevard, Chicago, IL 60604-3505. The Butterball Turkey hotline is staffed by experts in buying, basting, stuffing, carving and storing your Holiday bird. These experts will also answer your questions about chicken, geese and Cornish hens! Hours of operation:
* November 18 and 19, from 8 a.m. to 6 p.m.
* Weekdays through November 22nd, from 8 a.m. to 8 p.m.
* Thanksgiving Day, from 6 a.m. to 6 p.m.
* November 24th to December 22nd, from 8 a.m. to 6 p.m.

Cayenne Company Inc.--**1-800-CAYENNE**
Cayenne Company Inc., 2235 East 38th Street, Minneapolis, MN 55407. Cayenne Company Inc. offers cayenne pepper - a 'powerful circulation stimulant.' I've used cayenne pepper for years and it really works. See *Three Square Meals In A Bottle Detox*, *Capsicum (cayenne)*, and *$10,000 Weight-Loss Bet Diet*.

Complete Guide to Exercise Videos, The---------------------------------**1-800-433-6769**
Collage Video, Collage Video Specialties, Inc., 5390 Main Street N.E., Minneapolis, MN 55421. If you can't motivate yourself to exercise, then try *exercise videos! Choose from 286 workouts!* Exercise videos are fun, they're private and they're convenient! Call or write for your free 71-page, all color and very informative catalog. See Dynamix Music Service in this section.

Complete Idiot's Guide - Vision Boards, The----------------------------by Marcia Layton Turner

Country Doctor's Big Bag Of Common Sense Cures, The------------by Dr. LaMar's Products Inc.-----------------1-800-941-2889
www.drlamarsproducts.com
Dr. La Mar's Products Inc., P.O. Box 1461, Emporia, KS 66801. If you didn't read about Dr. LaMar's super healthy products, shame on you. Re-read about several super healthy products now. Then come back and call or write for a packet of super healthy information. I believe the lady at Dr. LaMar's company told me the packet cost $2.50.

Department of Agriculture Meat & Poultry Hotline-----------------1-800-535-4555
(Washington DC) 1-202-720-3333
Do you have questions about preparing that turkey or other poultry? Call during regular business hours to talk to a registered dietician. Call Monday through Thursday 9 a.m. to 4 p.m. from November 1st through the holidays. To listen to recorded messages on most frequently asked questions, simply follow the recorded instruction. Listen to the recorded messages 24-hours a day.

Diabetes Information Center--1-303-468-2162
National Diabetes Information Clearinghouse (NDIC), Box NDIC, Bethesda, MD 20892. Ask for many publications too numerous to list.

Diabetes Self-Management--1-800-234-0923
Diabetes Self-Management, P.O. Box 51125, Boulder CO., 80321-1125. The Magazine for your whole life. Call and ask for a free issue. If you like what you see and read, discount subscription rate of $9.97 for a full year (6 issues in all) a savings of over 50% OFF the cover price.

Diatomaceous Earth (food grade)---------------------------------------www.arbico-organics.com

Diatomaceous Earth (food grade)---------------------------------------www.dirtworks.net

Diatomaceous Earth (food grade)---------------------------------------www.earthworks health.com

Diatomaceous Earth (food grade)--------------------------------------Perma-Guard

Diatomaceous Earth (food grade)--**www.wolfcreekranch.com**

Most Important Note: When you get to these websites, search for *Diatomaceous Earth (food grade)*. See *Diatomaceous Earth (food grade)*.

Doctor Julian Whitaker, Health & Healing-----------------------------**1-800-777-5005**

(Subscription)---1-800-539-8219

Dr. Julian Whitaker Health & Healing, 7811 Montrose Road, P.O. Box 59745, Potomac, Maryland 20897-5904. Undoubtedly, *one of the most valuable, extremely informative, health related newsletters you can possibly obtain anywhere!* Each month, you'll receive information that may enhance your health as well save your life. Dr. Julian Whitaker, editor of *Health & Healing*, is a well qualified and knowledgeable physician who will share the healthiest information available each and every month. I've (author) been a subscriber for over three years and the subscription is worth every penny and then some. Call or write today, and ask for the latest subscription prices. If you want some *very powerful and healthy reading*, call 1-714-851-1550 to order these health enhancing books authored by Dr. Julian Whitaker: *A Guide to Natural Healing, Is Heart Surgery Necessary?, Reversing Diabetes, Reversing Health Risk and Reversing Heart Disease*. See Doctor Atkins' Health Revelations in this section.

Dynamix Music Service--**1-800-843-6499**

1-410-243-9755

1-410-243-9759

Dynamix Music Service, 733 West 40th Street, Suite 10, Baltimore, Maryland 21211. "Music for Fitness." Why buy Dynamix? Selection, Customer Service, Energy, Knowledge, Original Artist, Flawless Mixing, Quality Reproduction, 100% Satisfaction, & The Best! Ask for their free, all color, 24-page catalog. Dynamix Music Service also offers exercise videos. See *The Complete Guide to Exercise Videos* in this section.

East Park Research, Inc.---**1-888-374-2363**

East Park Research, Inc., 2709 Horseshoe Drive, Las Vegas, NV 89120-3337. Call or write East Park research, Inc., and ask to be put on their mailing list. In particular, ask for their 96-page booklet *Indium - The Missing Trace Mineral*, written by Dr. Robert Lyons. Once you receive their material, decide if Indium is for you then see your doctor for a final go-ahead.

Eating Disorders---**1-301-443-3170**

Office of Public Affairs, Food and Drug Administration, 5600 Fishers Lane, HFE88, Rockville, MD 20857. Ask for free pamphlet: *Eating Disorders: When Thinness Becomes an Obsession* (#86-2211).

Eating for the Elderly---**1-703-821-8955**

National Clearinghouse for Primary Care Information, 8201 Greensboro Dr., Suite 600, McLean, VA 22102. Ask for free collection of recipes: *Easy Eating for Well-Seasoned Adults*.

Eating for Two---**1-301-443-3170**

Office of Consumer Affairs, Food and Drug Administration, Public Inquires, 5600 Fishers Lane, HFE88, Rockville, MD 20857. Ask for free booklet: *All About Eating for Two* (#84-2183).

Elderly and Exercise--**1-301-495-3455**

National Institute on Aging Information Center, 2209 Distribution Circle, Silver Spring, MD 20910. Ask for the booklet *Don't Take It Easy - Exercise!*

Elderly and Menu Ideas---**1-301-495-3455**

National Institute on Aging Information Center, 2209 Distribution Circle, Silver Spring, MD 20910. Ask for *Food: Staying Healthy After 65, Be Sensible About Salt, Hints for Shopping, Cooking and Enjoying Meals and Dietary Supplements: More Is Not Always Better*.

Enzymatic Therapy---**1-800-783-2286**
1-414-469-1313
1-414-469-4400(fax)

Enzymatic Therapy, P.O. Box 22310, Green Bay, WI 54305. In 1981, Enzymatic Therapy started with 10 products designed to support the specific body functions. In the last 13 years, Enzymatic Therapy has become one of the fastest growing companies in the natural health industry. Enzymatic Therapy offers more than *130 nutritional and herbal formulas*. "You need to experience for yourself the difference between an excellent product and one made from inferior ingredients." Call or write and ask for their free information. I received *Essential Formulas for Health* magazine, *Discover the World of Natural Medicine*, their price list and a free sample. They may also refer you to a local stores in your area.

Family News, The---**1-800-284-6263**
1-305-759-8710

The Family News, 9845 N.E. 2nd Avenue, Miami Shores, Florida 33138. This news catalog offers information you probably won't find anywhere else. The publication is dedicated to presenting thought provoking articles on health, nutrition and the environment. The Family News, Volume VI No.II had a great deal of information concerning *Ozone Therapy*. Call or write for your free sample subscription.

It's packed with information, products and sources of other information in support of your health and well-being. Call today!

Featherspring International Corporation------------------------------------**1-800-628-4693**
Featherspring International Corporation, 712 North 34th St., Seattle, Washington 98103. I (author) can vouch for this company. Suffering from great pain from both feet (flat feet), I purchased these arch supports in 1980. The pain went away almost immediately and I've been wearing them ever since. Call or write for free information.

Federal Health Information Catalog-------------------------------------**1-800-336-4797**
ODPHP National Health Information Center, P.O. Box 1133, Washington, DC 20013. For a $2 fee, ask for *Health Information Resources in the Federal Government.*

FitnessWarehouse--**1-800-FW-STORE**
FitnessWarehouse, 8205 Clayton Road, Clayton, MO 63105. FitnessWarehouse offers great fitness equipment. They offer:
* Low Impact Treadmill.
* Total Body Treadmill.
* Climber Machines.
* Exercise Bikes.
* Weight Training Equipment and more.
Write or call for their free 20-page, all color catalog today! Call Monday through Friday during regular business hours! You'll receive store locations nearest you so you can see and feel their exercise products!

Fitmix---**1-888-4-FITMIX**
                                                            1-410-243-9755
                                                            1-410-243-9759(fax)

Fitmix, 733 West 40th Street, Suite 10, Baltimore, Maryland 21211. Fitmix offers "Motivating music just for fitness!" Fitmix offers a wide variety of audio as well as video products previously available only to professional fitness instructors. Their products include Walking Tapes, Running and their Fitmix Series. Great motivating music for cross-country, cross-training, cycling, general fitness, in-line skating, jump roping, running, stair stepping, walking, weight training and X-country skiing. For a music preview, call their Music Preview Line at 1-410-243-2671 and simply pick your choice of music! Call (Monday through Friday from 9 a.m. to 8 p.m., Eastern Standard Time) or write and ask for your free 16-page, all color product catalog.

Fleischmann's Yeast Baker's Helpline--**1-800-777-4959**

The Fleischmann's Yeast Baker's Helpline provides advice to bread bakers. Call Monday through Friday from 9 a.m. to 7 p.m.

Flora Inc.--**1-800-446-2110**

Flora, Inc., P.O. Box 950, 805 East Badger Road, Lynden, WA 98264. Flora, Inc., provides a good source for *unrefined oils made from certified organic seeds* the old fashioned way. Pressed in small batches and protected from damaging light and heat, and processed without chemicals or preservatives. The taste of their fresh, pure oils is incomparable. Great for healthy cooking needs. Flora Inc., also offers herbal teas, food products, body care products, and appliances (fermentation crocks and juice extractors). Write or call for free product information. You'll receive a letter and a full-size 8-page catalog.

Foundation for Education About Eating Disorders (FEED)-------------**1-410-467-0603**

Foundation for Education about Eating Disorders (FEED), P.O. Box 16375, Baltimore, MD 21210. Call or write for information pertaining to your concern.

Four Star Books--**1-800-350-2350**
                                                                    1-541-955-2742
                                                                    1-541-955-2745(fax)

Four Star Books, 128 SW "I" Street, Grants Pass, OR 97526. Four Star Books offers the book, *Your Body's Many Cries for Water*, which reveals the simple benefitting effects of drinking plain ol' water (uncontaminated). You'll read why hydration works versus drugs for many common diseases and ailments. Four Star Books also offers a wide variety of other reading materials that may change your life for the better and satisfy your reading pleasure. Call or write the friendly people at Four Star Books today. They'll send you free information on their assortment of books and videos!

Frontier Cooperative Herbs--**1-800-786-1388**
                                                                    1-800-717-4372(fax)

Frontier Cooperative Herbs, 3021 78th Street, P.O. Box 299, Norway, IA 52318. At Frontier Cooperative Herbs, quality is taken seriously. The Quality Control Department is staffed with botanists, herbalists and specialists with Ph.D.s who carefully monitor every step in product handling to maintain Frontier's high quality standards. Frontier is one of the largest buyers of organic herbs in the United States. ALL of their organic herbs have been certified by an independent third party organization. Certification papers are available on request. Frontier has a 170-page, full size catalog listing thousands of products. They may ask you for your business name and license to receive this free catalog. Call Monday through Friday from 7 a.m. to 6 p.m., Central Standard Time.

Fusion Video--**1-800-959-0061**

1-708-799--8375(fax)

Fusion Video, Fulfillment Services, Inc., 17311 Fusion Way, Country Club Hills, IL 60478-3113. If you like Science Fiction, Battle Films, Cinema's Best, Comedy Classics, Music and so much more, look into Fusion Video. I received 3 great catalogs that offer great videos at affordable prices. Discount coupons and free video offers are also included. See many other "movie - video" offers in this section!

Future Medicine Publishing, Inc.---**1-800-990-9499**

Pacific Highway East, Suite 6, Tacoma, Washington 98424. The *Alternative Medicine* book and *Alternative Medicine Yellow Pages* is *a must for every family*. Ask for Mr. Bob McLaughlin.

Tell Bob, you want to know about their Promotion Package: *Alternative Medicine: The Definite Guide* (1,068 pages) with three free issues of Alternative Medicine Digest, a FREE Alternative Medicine Yellow Pages (a $12.95 value) packed with Alternative Medicine sources throughout the U.S. and a free audio cassette tape. This huge reference book is worth every penny - from Acupressure to Yoga. Future Medicine Publishing, Inc. offers a 30-Day Money Back Guarantee.

Gardens Alive--**1-513-354-1482**

www.gardensalive.com   1-513-354-1484 (fax)

Gardens Alive, 5100 Schenley Place, Lawrenceburg, IN 47025. I was impressed when I browsed then read in detail each page of Gardens Alive all-color, 50-page catalog. Why? They offer environment-SAFE products that work. Safe products for your lawn, pets, gardens (fruit, vegetable, plants,...), wildlife,... Call or write them today for your FREE catalog. Yes, you'll read testimonials and see color photos from very happy customers who are long-lasting Gardens Alive customers like me (author). See *Arbico Organics* in this Section.

Garlic Information HOTLINE--**1-800-330-5922**

The Garlic Information Center, The New York Hospital-Cornell University Medical Center, P.O. Box 2506, Stuart, FL 34995. The New York Hospital-Cornell Medical Center now operates a *Garlic Information Hotline*. Call Monday through Friday, from 9 a.m. to 5 p.m., Eastern Standard Time and speak directly to a nutritionist. Ask for your free *Is Garlic Beneficial For Health* booklet. They'll send you this very informative booklet.

General Mills Holiday Helpline--**1-800-793-0464**
The staff will troubleshoot baking and cooking problems; provide lost recipes for General Mills products, including Gold Medal Flour and Bisquick baking mix; answer questions about General Mills products. Call Monday through Friday from 7:30 a.m. to 5:30 p.m., and on Saturday from 9 a.m. to 4 p.m. Line is staffed November 18th to January 13th.

GERD Public Information and Education Program - American College of Gastroenterology--**1-800-HRT-BURN**
GERD Public Information and Education Program - American College of Gastroenterology, P.O. Box 3099, Alexandria, VA 22302. Do you have heartburn or GERD (see GERD in Section 26)? For much more information concerning GERD and a list of specialist in your area, call or write today for a free information packet!

Gilroy Garlic Festival--**# unavailable**
Gilroy Garlic Festival, P.O. Box 2311, Gilroy, CA 95020. People all over the world have celebrated garlic with feasting, festivals and celebration for thousands of years. Since 1978, Gilroy, California the granddaddy of U.S. garlic festivals, is held the last weekend of July each year. The Gilroy Garlic Festival is complete with food booths, a golf tournament and many kinds of contests and exhibitions. The Gilroy Garlic Festival may be the healthiest fun you may have all year. Write for free information.

Grain and Salt Society, The--**1-800-867-7258**
                                                                                         1-916-873-0294
                                                                                         1-916-873-4186(fax)
The Grain and Salt Society, P.O. Box DD Magalia, CA 95594. The Grain and Salt Society published a 4-page article on *The Value of Real Sea Salt*. Coarse grained and finer ground Celtic Seal Salt can be purchased through this company. While investigating whole salt, I purchased a 4-page report for $6 through another source, but you can call get this same report and a *whole lot more* directly from The Grain and Salt Society at *no-charge!* They even sent free samples (3) of their healthy products! Ask for your free information packet and samples. Call Monday through Friday from 8 a.m. to 5 p.m. Pacific Standard Time for free information and ordering Celtic Sea Salt. SEE *Whole Salt*.

NOTE: As of December 1996, The Grain and Salt Society is offering a new product! If you like drinking clean, good for healthy water, could you be spending up to 1,000 times the cost of regular tap water for bottled water? Outrageous isn't it? I'm here to save you money so here it is: The Grain and Salt Society is offering a "portable Water Filtration Unit in a Sports Bottle!"

It provides more than 1,500 refills (200 gallons) of *99% superior water* for about a lousy .05 cents a gallon instead of the *mega bucks you pay at your local grocery store!* This filtration unit in the Sports Bottle removes: bad taste, odor, sediment, suspended items, pathogens like giardia and cryptospordium and bacteria, chlorine, volatile organic compounds, lead, heavy metals, pesticides, detergents.... It fits almost anywhere! Folks I'm not getting a single dime to relay this information to you. You need to know about this product as well as all the other healthy information throughout this book! CALL NOW and request free information about ALL their healthy products!!!

GREENS+ Pro-N-30---**1-800-643-1210**
1-407-562-2766
1-407-562-9848(fax)

GREENS+ Pro-N-30, 2183 Ponce de Leon Circle, Vero Beach, FL 32960. GREENS+ is an affordable *whole living food* containing concentrated sources of Vitamins, organic covalent minerals, essential amino acids, phytochemicals, enzymes, co-enzymes, cell salts, chlorophyll, standardized herbal extracts, unique botanical extracts and soluble and insoluble plant fibers from high quality, organic, nutrient-rich foods.

* Improves Mental Acuity   * Strengthens Immune System
* Increases Energy Naturally   * Emulsifies & Metabolizes Fat
* Cleans and Rejuvenates Cells & Colon

   You would not believe all the Superfoods that are in one bottle of GREENS+! It's all annotated in their free brochure and other free brochures about Pro-N-50+(the strongest antioxidant from grape seed extract), you'll receive by calling or writing today. Look into this company! You'll even receive a $5 discount coupon for your first order and a free sample!

Haelan Products Incorporated---**1-800-5HAELAN**
1-504-885-2776
1-504-885-3272(fax)

Haelan Products Incorporated, 3200 Severn Avenue, Suite 120B, Metairie, LA 70002. If your afflicted with a degenerative disease like cancer or any wasting-away disease, a soy drink used in China for 15 years, has *demonstrated great success!* Haelan Products Inc., offers a product called Haelan 851 which is a concentrated soy drink. Haelan may be available at your local health food store. Call or write for free information. You may also order Haelan 185 from this company by calling their toll free number.

Health Science & Live Longer Products------------------------------------**1-800-446-1990**

fax 1-805-968-1001

1-805-968-1028

Health Science & Live Longer Products, P.O. Box 7, Santa Barbara, CA 93102. This company offers a 75-page book *Apple Cider Vinegar Health System* (very informative). The book also offers many other informational books as well as Bragg All Natural Liquid Aminos and Bragg Organic Raw Apple Cider Vinegar. Call or write for product price list. Call the top 2 phone numbers for credit card orders. Call Monday through Friday 8:30 a.m. to 4 p.m., Pacific Standard Time.

Heintzman Farms---**1-888-333-5813**

Heintzman Farms, Rural Route 2 Box 265, Onaka, SD 57466. If you haven't read the health-enhancing benefits of flax seed oil, *STOP* right now and go to Flax Seed in Section 14. Mr. Rick Heintzman owner of Heintzman Farms offers a kit that includes three 1-pound bags of Dakota Gold flax seed, an electric grinder and two home cholesterol test kits for only $70. If you want a free sample of flax seeds send a SASE! Heintzman Farms also offers 1-pound bags of flax seed or in bulk. See *Barlean Organic Oil* in this section.

Hitchcock Shoes--**1-781-749-3571**

1-781-749-3576(fax)

Hitchcock Shoes, Inc., 225 Beal Street, Hingham, Massachusetts 02043. If you're a man and need those hard to find *W I D E   S H O E S*, this is the company to order from. From *EEE to E E E E E!!!* All kinds of footwear!!! After looking and looking for wide shoes for my feet (author), this is the *ONLY* company that had my size.

I've ordered shoes from Hitchcock for several years now. Call or write for their free, all color, 48-page catalog. *STOP the pain* and get the correct pair of footwear. Call their Customer Service at the number above.

Home Health Products for Life--**1-800-278-7092**

Home Health *Products for Life*, P.O. Box 2219, Virginia Beach, VA 23450-2219. Call or write and ask for their free, 48 page, all color and very informative catalog on many health enhancing products. They offer natural remedies, natural skin care, pain relief, Vitamins & herbs and weight loss products. Call 24 hours a day for their free catalog!

Institute For Vibrant Living---**1-800-218-1379**
Institute For Vibrant Living, P.O. Box 3840, Camp Verde, AZ 86322-3840. Institute For Vibrant Living offers some the best healthy products I have ever come across. Besides *All Day Energy Greens*, they offer another powerhouse *Go Ruby Go* and they also offer Apple Cider Vinegar Extra, CoQ10 Supreme, LifeForce Rejuvinator, Osteo K2, Pain & Brain Rescue Formula, Vision Clear,... to name a few. Call and get on their mailing list today. STOP reading this segment and call them NOW!

Intensive Research Information Service And Products (IRISAP)----**1-618-790-3235**
Intensive Research Information Services And Products (IRISAP), P.O. Box 48, Cutler, IL 62238-0048. IRISAP was founded by Joseph A. Laydon Jr. in August 1991. In 1991, IRISAP began his "intensive research" and R & D (Research & Development) for Anytime Anywhere Survival - (international wilderness survival - Wilderness Survival) in order to help all his subscribers far more self-reliant in all aspects of their life besides being in an outdoor's environment. IRISAP also conducts "intensive research" and R & D (Research & Development) in the other 'survivals' - Health Survival (one example is this Survival Book), Crime Survival and Money Survival.

IRISAP's Mission: *"Greatly reduce or eliminate the multitudes of minor to unforgiving everyday threats & risks to you and those under your care. Reduce life's threats & risks through International Wilderness Survival and complimented by Health, Crime & Money Survivals so you're ready Anytime Anywhere."* See **https://www.survivalexpertblog.com**

International Hotline Juvenile Diabetes Foundation---------------------**1-800-223-1138**
International Hotline Juvenile Diabetes Foundation, 60 Madison Avenue, New York, NY 10010-1150. The staff at the Juvenile Diabetes Foundation will answer questions on juvenile diabetes and offer referrals to physicians and clinics. Office hours are Monday through Friday from 8 a.m. to 6 p.m., Eastern Standard Time.

International Nutrition, Inc.---**1-800-899-3413**
International Nutrition, Inc., P.O. Box 43422, Baltimore, MD 21236. International Nutrition offers "Targeted Nutrition Intervention for Down's Syndrome" called Nutrivene-D. Call or write for your packet of very informative information (product brochure, Health & Healing reprint and detailed information). See Cognitive Enhancement Research Institute's (CERI) and especially Trisomy 21 Research, Inc. in this section.

Jenny Craig--**1-888-Jenny-Go**

www.jennygo.com

Jenny Craig, a weight-loss company, is dedicated to help its customers lose weight. Consider Jenny Craig.

Kelley Bean Company--**# unavailable**

Kelley Bean Company, P.O. Box 457, Morill, NE 69358, Attn: Marty Ritz, Consumer Services. Do you like beans? Sure they're healthy for you but do you like beans? Discover great tips on how to prepare dry beans for cooking. Write and ask for their free *Cookbook for Beans & Peas* recipe booklet! See AkPharma Inc., Frankly Beans and Beano Bulletin in this Section. Insure you read about the amazing health-enhancing benefits of beans in Section 01!

Land O'Lakes Holiday Bakeline--**1-800-782-9606**

Land O'Lakes Holiday Bakeline offers advice to homebakers from home economists. Callers will get a free recipe and tips leaflet. Call daily through the Holidays up to December 24th, from 8 a.m. to 6 p.m.

L & H Vitamins Inc.--**1-800-221-1152**

1-718-361-1437(fax)

L&H Vitamins Inc., 32-33 47th Avenue, Long Island City, New York 11101. Ask for free complete catalog featuring name brand Vitamins and Health Products at discount prices. I received their 80-page catalog and their 56 page "Health Newsline." It's very informative. You'll learn the benefits of supplements just browsing through their Newsline. Call today! Call Monday through Friday from 8:30 a.m. to 8:00 p.m., Eastern Standard Time and 9:00 a.m. to 5:00 p.m. on Saturday.

Life Fitness--**1-800-877-3867**

Life Fitness, 10601 West Belmont Avenue, Franklin Park, IL 60131. Life Fitness offers you to "Take the First Step to a Better Body." I was very impressed with their literature and brochures which reflects their products and customer service! Life Fitness offers a very well-built and unique stairclimber that will help you get in shape and stay in shape. I even received a free video! Their 5500 Stairclimber is impressive! Don't believe me, call them during regular business hours and request your free literature and video on their 5500 Stairclimber. You'll get a great workout!

Linus Pauling Institute--**1-415-327-4064**

Linus Pauling Institute, 440 Page Mill Road, Palo Alto, CA 94306. During World War II, Dr. Pauling worked with the Office of Scientific Research and Development and developed artificial plasma called Oxypolygelatin. At the end of World War II, he was awarded Presidential Medal for Merit for his wartime contributions. Dr. Pauling won his first Nobel prize in 1954. He was awarded his second Nobel prize for peace (he campaigned against atmospheric testing of nuclear weapons in the late 1950s and early 1960s - on August 5, 1963 the ban on atmospheric testing of nuclear weapons was signed). Why is this important?

It's important to know something about Dr. Pauling, author of *Live Longer and Feel Better* and *Cancer and Vitamin C*. Both books are available at the time of this writing. Call or write for recent price and shipping cost.

Luke Chan---**1-513-777-0588**
                                                                          1-513-755-5722(fax)

Luke Chan, 9676 Cinti-Columbus Road, Cincinnati, OH 45241. If your interested in QiGong - Chi-Lel, the author of *101 Miracles of Natural Healing* will send you a free copy of the Chi-Lel newsletter, workshop & retreat schedule, information on Chi-Lel instructor certification program, and dates for trips to the Chi-Lel Center in China! It's all free, so call, write or fax Monday through Friday during regular business hours.
SEE QiGong in Section 22 and read Luke Chan's amazing book as annotated above. It includes 101 real testimonials (Chinese) and I hear he's working on an American version at the time of this writing! His book is being sold in most health food stores right now! Keep a lookout for the American version!

National Centre for Padre Pio, Inc., The,----------------------------------**1-610-845-3000**
                                                                          1-610-845-2666(fax)

The National Center for Padre Pio, Inc., 2213 Old Route 100, Barto, PA 19504. The National Center for Padre Pio, Inc., is an Affiliated Centre, authorized by the Capuchin Friary, San Giovanni Rotondo, Italy. First of all let me give you a brief history of Padre Pio. Padre Pio was born on 25 May 1887 in Pietrelcina, Italy. He entered the priesthood at the age of 15 and was ordained a priest in 1910. On 20 September 1918, the five wounds of Our Lord's Passion appeared on his body, making Padre Pio the first stigmatized priest in the history of the Church.

Countless numbers then and to this day come from all over the world to seek Padre Pio's spiritual blessings. On 23 September 1968, Padre Pio was called to his heavenly reward which attracted almost 100,000 people. Padre Pio was entombed in the crypt of Our Lady of Grace Church.

If you would like much more free information concerning this *Chosen One* call Monday through Friday from 9 a.m. to 5 p.m. and Saturday from 10 a.m. to 2 p.m. Eastern Standard Time. If you would like to make known graces or favours received through Padre Pio's intercession see Our Lady of Grace Capuchin Friary in this section.

NATR Inc. of California---**1-800-422-4716**
1-707-443-3885

NATR Incorporated of California, 2806 Broadway, Suite #2, Eureka, CA 95501. Have you ever heard the saying *"Death Begins in the Colon?"* Look into this company if you suffer from body odor, bowel problems, Crohn's Disease, colitis, colon problems, constipation, diarrhea, diverticulitis, gastritis, headaches, hemorrhoids, obesity... and much much more! Some users of this formula have *reported changes in their eye color, hair becoming straighter & shinier!* REMEMBER - TOXINS in your body affect your entire body! If you want to *DETOXIFY* your body, look into this company today. I talked to the owner and he demonstrated a sincere desire tell me about his company and his products. Call during regular business hours to receive your free informative *Special Report Letter* with many testimonials. Yes, I even tried their product and their published testimonials are true, I lost weight (debris in colon, became slimmer in the stomach area and felt more energy!

Nature's Distributors, Inc.,--**1-800-624-7114**
1-602-837-8420(fax)

Natures Distributors Inc., 16508 E. Laser Drive, Suite 104, Fountain Hills, AZ 85268. You have to look into this company. Not only do they have great products, but their advertisement reads "place your first order with us, you will automatically receive the next 12 monthly issues of *The Healthy Cell News.*" I simply called them and asked for any literature about their products (to protect you from the bad companies). Nature's Distributors Inc., sent me *The Healthy Cell News*! One of the *most informative health orientated subscriptions* I have ever read! *The Healthy Cell News* is a full-size, 36-page, colorful, and *extremely informative newspaper*. Throughout the newspaper, you'll find and read about their healthy products. *CALL* them today! Call Monday through Friday from 8:00 a.m. to 4:00 p.m., Mountain Standard Time.

Nature's Gate--**1-800-327-2012**
1-818-882-2951

Levlad Inc., 9200 Mason Avenue, Chatsworth, CA 91311. Nature's Gate Herbal Fresh Natural Roll-On Deodorant. Did you read Section 11 with respect to the health hazards of aluminum? If you're troubled about aluminum that is found in most antiperspirants\deodorants which is linked to Alzheimer's Disease, then call the number above about their aluminum-free deodorant products.

NordicTrack--**1-612-205-5243**
1-952-361-5575

Important Note: I'm not sure if the original NordicTrack is still in business. However, here's the write-up I did more than 10-years ago. The numbers above go to a company that sells "woodfen ski machine" parts. You must see *Exercise*.

NordicTrack, 104 Peavey Road, Chaska, MN 55318-2355. Folks, I can vouch for this company! If your doctor says it's OK to exercise, and I mean EXERCISE, then you better look into this company! I've used their cross-country ski machine many times and I always got a sweat-pouring workout! These machines are well built and they last! If it's OK with your doctor and you want to get in shape and stay that way, call for free information now! Their lines are open 24-hours a day! You'll receive full-size color brochures on their cross-country ski machines, accessories, price list and testimonials! Their guarantee is 2nd to none! CALL MOW! They also offer a "30-DAY IN-HOME TRIAL." CALL NOW!!!! NordicTrack offers many other exercise machines. Ask them for their catalog on all their products. Hold-up! Nordic offers other quality built workout machines other than their cross-country machines. Below s a partial list: AbWorks, Arnold Palmer Life Walker Treadmill, Firm Thighs and Hips, NordicFlex, NordicRider, NordicTrack Walkfit 3500 Exerciser, Revolution Cycle, Step Up to Fitness, Total Body Exerciser, Vitamaster Elite Treadmill, Voit Ladder Climber, Voit Programmable Exercise Bike.... and more! Call and ask for their free 32-page, all-color catalog on all their exercise and health equipment today!

Obesity and Energy Metabolism---**1-301-496-2563**
Office of Clinical Center Communications, Warren G. Magnuson Clinical Center, NIH, Building 10, Room 5C-305, 9000 Rockville Pike, Bethesda, MD 20892. Ask for free publication: *Obesity and Energy Metabolism* (#86-1805). A video tape can be purchased or loaned.

Old Well Corporation---**1-800-296-0506**

Old Well Corporation, P.O. Box 19351, Raleigh, NC 27619. Old Well Corporation offers an *Australian bush medical discovery for those who suffer from arthritis*. This medical discover has been used by Aborigines for hundreds of years. This successful discovery is called Emu Oil and is sold as Emu Arthritic Formula 7. No folks this ain't no witchcraft brew, it's been *scientifically studied and proven to work!* Talking to one of the customer representatives, she stated one of the main ingredients in the formula is capsaicin.

Members from the following medical organizations endorse the ingredients in Emu Arthritic Formula 7(partial list):
- Arthritis Foundation of Australia
- Australian Rheumatism Association
- Orthopedic Research Society of the USA
- New York Academy of Science

Call or write today and ask for their free literature on this amazing product. Research data and testimonials are included!

Older Adults and Nutrition---**1-617-556-3330**

Human Nutrition Research Center on aging at Tufts University, 711 Washington St., Boston, MA 02111. Ask for information according to your concern.

Omega Nutrition U.S.A. Inc.,--**1-800-661-3529**

Omega Nutrition, 6505 Aldrich Road, Bellingham, Washington, 98226. Omega Nutrition, provides a good source for unrefined oils made from certified organic seeds the old fashioned way. Pressed in small batches and protected from damaging light & heat and processed without chemicals or preservatives. The taste of their fresh, pure oils is incomparable. Great for healthy cooking needs.

Omega Nutrition has other health related products like flours, body care products, apple cider vinegar (not the grocery store kind), water filters and books you'll want to read (cancer, fats, Omega-3, nutrition...). Write or call for free 16-page product catalog and a handful of other healthy and informative brochures.

Overeaters Anonymous---**1-310-618-8835**

Overeaters Anonymous, P.O. Box 92870, Los Angeles, CA 90009. Call or write for information pertaining to your concern. See *Binge Eating*.

Paramount---**1-800-721-2121**

1-888-PARAFIT

1-213-721-8841(fax)

Paramount, 6450 E. Bandini Blvd., Los Angeles, CA 90040-3185.
You'll not only be impressed with their multiple all-color brochures but very excited about their exercise equipment that will begin to get you in shape like never before! Their fitness line is must be seen! Call or write today for a very professional package of their fitness line and price list. You'll be impressed by their brochures, their fitness equipment and your new body!

Physical Fitness Awards for Adults--**1-202-272-3421**
President's Council on Physical Fitness and Sports, 450 5th ST., NW, Suite 7103, Washington, DC 20001. The Amateur Athletic Union administers this program. Upon meeting the qualifying standards, participants receive a personalized Presidential Certificate of Achievement and a sports award lapel pin. Categories (51) are too many to list. For additional information contact Tom Leix, Presidential Sports Award, P.O. Box 68207, Indianapolis, IN 46268, Ph: 317-872-2900.

Physical Fitness Awards for Youngsters-------------------------------**1-202-272-3421**
President's Council on Physical Fitness and Sports, 450 5th ST., NW, Suite 7103, Washington, DC 20001. Conducts two award programs for youngsters from ages 1-17. Call or write and ask for information.

Physical Fitness--**1-202-272-3421**
President's Council on Physical Fitness and Sports, 450 5th ST., NW, Suite 7103, Washington, DC 20001. Ask for quarterly newsletter and for a small price ask for several informative publications to promote, encourage and motivate the development of physical fitness.

Plants for Clean Air Council--**# unavailable**
The Plants for Clean Air Council, 10210 Bald Hill Rd., Mitchelville, MD 20721. The Plants for Clean Air Council is a non-profit organization dedicated to expanding the role of green plants in improving the quality of human life through knowledge, research, education and information. Clean-up indoor air pollution! Read the NASA study on the effectiveness of plant air purification. Send a large SASE and $1 for your report. You'll receive a two-sided fact-filled brochure on everything you need to know to *start breathing much cleaner 24-hours a day!*

Prevail Corporation--**1-800-248-0885**

1-503-667-5527

Prevail Corporation, 2204-8 N.W. Birdsdale, Gresham, OR 97030. "PLANT ENZYMES: The Missing Link to Optimum Health?" Even with a wholesome, balanced diet, deficiencies in the bodys' digestive enzymes can lead to illness and disability, as nutrients from foods remain undigested and unabsorbed. Malabsorption of nutrients causes malnutrition and robs the body of building blocks needed for maintenance of health and repair tissue. Enzymes aid the breakdown of foods into smaller building blocks which can be easily absorbed from the intestines and assimilated into the body. Enzymes help to release and deliver the nutrient content which would otherwise remain locked in foods. Prevail Corporation offers several plant enzyme products to enhance your health in specific areas and general health. Call or write today. You'll receive 17 all color, full size & very informative brochures and a price list on their health enhancing products.

Purity Farms--**1-800-568-4433**

Purity Farms, 14635 Westcreek Road, Sedalia, CO 80135. CERTIFIED Organic Clarified Butter! The Charak Samhita, the ancient Ayurvedic Text on health and medicine regarded Ghee as a very important food supplement for healthy skin, mental alertness, good digestion and improved memory. Ghee is a form of butter. Milk solids have been removed to form clarified butter. It's noted to have healing properties. So don't sludge-up your arteries, look into this product! Purity Farm's Ghee is salt-free, lactose free and has a shelf life of many years! Call or write and ask for free information. The people at Purity Farms are very helpful!

Quinton Fitness Equipment--**1-800-426-0337**

Quinton Fitness, 3303 Monte Villa Parkway, Bothwell, WA 98021-8906. Quinton Fitness Equipment "A Workout for Your Other Half." This company offers a stairclimber that works "your other half!" It's a *Cross Country Climber!* This company also offers their SkeeCros II. Get all the data and see these machines for yourself. Call or write to receive your free literature!

Real Goods--**1-800-762-7325**

1-707-468-9486(fax)

Foreign Orders---1-707-468-9214

Real Goods, 555 Leslie Street, Ukiah, California 95482-5507. Real Goods has an 80-page, all color catalog for those who *care about their environment, their health as well as their immediate surroundings and enhancing the pleasures of life!* Real Goods offers camping, kitchen, leisure, household, pet, solar and yard products.

One amazing product called *Clean Power Laundry Disks* actually *cleans your laundry without any detergent!* The laundry disks *last 500 to 700 washes without polluting the environment!* Real Goods was skeptical at first so they gave the laundry disks a test. "...we found that they really do work!"

Three (3) *Clean Power Laundry Disks* costs only $49. Buy $49 worth of laundry detergent. How many loads can you wash, 100 or 150 at best. Will these laundry disks *save you big-money* on laundry detergents help your environment or what (see phosphates in Section 26)? How do they work? It's high-tech science! Call or write and order your catalog today and read how these laundry disks work as well as browse and read about many other great products in the Real Goods catalog!

Reflexology---**1-816-444-2239**
Progressive Reflexology Institute, P.O. Box 22501, Kansas City, Missouri 64113-2501. Call or write and ask for information according to your concern. See Reflexology in Section 22.

Reconstructive Therapy (RT) Doctors---**1-805-544-3126(fax)**
Thomas A. Dorman, M.D., 171-A, North Santa Rosa St., San Luis Obispo, CA 93405-1322. Write or fax Dr. Dorman to obtain a nationwide list of RT doctors.

REGATTA SPORT---**1-800-567-CREW**
                                                                              1-905-937-5130
                                                                              1-905-937-4941(fax)
REGATTA SPORT, 38 Lakeport Road, St. Catharines, Ontario, Canada L2N 4P5. If you like the exercise or sport of *ROWING*, then this is the source for all your "rowing specialty" needs! REGATTA SPORT catalog offers a wide variety of apparel and many other products for yourself or your team! Call today for your free 25-page, all-color catalog.

Republic of Tea in San Francisco, The---**1-800-354-5530**
                                                                              1-415-382-3401
The Republic of Tea in San Francisco, 8 Digital Drive, Suite 100 Novato, CA 94949. The Republic of Tea in San Francisco offers Teas, Teaware and Gift Sets. The reason I added this company in this section like hundreds of other companies, organizations and agencies is because this company will *enhance your health, safety, welfare and save you money!*

This company offers the amazing Green Tea products which have been noted to help *fight against cancer, heart disease, aging and help lower your cholesterol!* Call Monday through Friday from 9:00 a.m. to 5:00 p.m., Pacific Standard Time. Ask for their free catalog 32-page all color catalog. After hours, dial 03 to get their free catalog.

Reynolds Turkey Tips Line--**1-800-745-4000**
Reynolds Turkey Tips Line, offers recorded tips on three ways to roast turkey. If you want additional free information just follow the recorded instructions. Call 24-hours a day from November 1st up to December 31st.

Right Size Smoothies---**1-800-500-0507**
Right Size Smoothies offers smoothies for weight-loss. You might have heard their advertising on your radio. They were offering FREE smoothies so you can see if they help you lose weight. Call today for more information.

R Pur-Aloe International--**1-800-888-2563**
                                                                                      1-303-451-1803
R Pur-Aloe International, Northglenn, Colorado. R Pur-Aloe Whole Leaf Aloe Vera Beverage Concentrate. A 16-ounce bottle cost $29.95. Ask for free information.
WARNING: Quality of their aloe vera products is unknown. Ask for a MPS\ml count!

Runners World Magazine--**# unavailable**
Runners World Magazine, P.O. Box 366, Subscription Department, Mountainview, CA 94042. Ask for subscription information. If you're a runner or wannabe, write today!

Safe Drinking Water Hotline--**1-800-426-4791**
                                                                                      1-202-544-2600
Call and ask about getting a copy of *Do You Have Lead in Your Drinking Water?* and *Preventing Drinking Water Contamination.* Call between 9 a.m. 5:30 p.m., Monday through Friday.

Safe Exercise, Nutrition, Medicines For Seniors----------------------------**1-800-336-4797**
                                                              In Maryland---1-301-565-4167
ODPHD National Health Information Center, P.O. Box 1133, Washington, DC 20013. Education program on health promotion and aging. Ask for information according to your concern.

Salt and Low-Sodium Diets--**1-301-443-3170**

Office of Public Affairs, Food and Drug Administration, 5600 Fishers Lane, HFE88, Rockville, MD 20857. Ask for free pamphlet: *A Word About Low-Sodium Diets* (#87-2179). See *Whole Salt* on page 258.

SelfCare Catalog--**1-800-345-1848**

                                                                          1-800-345-3371

                                                                          1-800-345-4021(fax)

SelfCare Catalog, 104 Challenger Drive, Portland, TN 37148-1716. I was impressed with their all-color catalog that is full of products that will enhance your health, beauty, and save you money! The Self Care Catalog offers products for: allergy relief, back care, dental, nutrition, pain relief, personal care, remedies and weight control. Call (first number) or write for your free 39-page all color catalog.

Shape-Up America--**1-800-U SHAPE IT**

Shape Up America, 6707 Democracy Boulevard, Suite 107, Bethesda, MD 20817. Shape-Up America was founded by C. Everett Koop who is a noted Public Health Authority and former U.S. Surgeon General. Write to Shape Up America to receive your free *On Your Way To Fitness* booklet, and *How to Lose a Few Pounds, Sensible Eating, & How to Increase Your Physical Activity* brochures! You'll read some very health-enhancing information when you receive your free packet!

Smokenders--**1-800-323-1126**

                                                                          1-616-241-3604

                                                                          1-616-248-4322(fax)

Smokenders, P.O. Box 3146, Glen Ellyn, IL 60138. Smokenders will send you free information on the oldest, largest and most successful smoking cessation program in the United States. *Smokenders brags they have an 80% success rate!* No cold turkey or much will power is required. Smokenders offers their world-famous seminar in their *"Learn How to Quit Kit"* for those who really want to quit smoking! Call this very second. Call Monday through Friday from 9 a.m. to 5 p.m., Central Standard Time. After hours leave your name and phone number and a staff member will return your call.

Smoking Cessation and Cancer Prevention-------------------------------**1-800-4-CANCER**

Office of Cancer Communications, National Cancer Institute (NCI), Bldg. 31, Room 10A-18, 9000 Rockville Pike, Bethesda, MD 20892. Ask for many publications to include: *Smoking Programs for Youth* (#81-2156).

Smoking Cessation Methods--**1-404-488-5705**

Office on Smoking and Health, Centers for Disease Control, 1600 Clifton Rd., NE, Mail Stop K-50, Atlanta, GA 30333. Ask for *Review and Evaluation of Smoking Cessation Methods*.

Smoking and High Blood Pressure--**1-301-951-3260**

High Blood Pressure Information Center, 120/80 National Institutes of Health, Bethesda, MD 20892. Ask for free 24-page, *The Physician's Guide: How To Help Your Hypertensive Patients Stop Smoking* (NIH #84-1271).

Sound Nutrition--**1-800-844-6645**

Sound Nutrition, P.O. Box 555, Dover, ID 83825. Sound Nutrition's Thin Oil, packs 14 grams of medium-chain triglycerides (MCTs) per tablespoon which is approximately 350% more MCTs than the emulsified products. Sound Nutrition also has a formulated Thin Oil-Butter Flavor for *popcorn lovers*, to put on bread, cooking... Sound Nutrition also offers olive flavored and garlic flavored thin oils. Write and enclose a large SASE for an order form & brochure. They'll send you a very informative Question\Answer brochure about MCTs and their products. Call between 8:30 a.m. to 5 p.m., Pacific Standard Time, Monday through Friday.

Sounds True---**1-800-333-9185**

1-303-665-3151

Sound True, P.O. Box 8910, Boulder, CO 80306-8010. Sounds True offers some great Mind-Over-Matter products and they're backed with a 01-Year Money Back Guarantee. Sounds True offers products like: *Unlocking Your Intuitive Power*, *Self-Healing With Energy Medicine*, *The Self-Hypnosis Diet*, *Self-Hypnosis Home Study Course*, Reiki Meditations For Self-Healing, The Essential QiGong Training Course,... Call or write today to get your own 40-page, all-color catalog. Yes, it *"sounds too good to be true."* Get their catalog, you won't be disappointed. Last catalog I received, Sounds True also offers Diatomaceous Earth (food grade).

Sports Music--**1-800-878-4764**

Sports Music Inc., Box 769689, Roswell, GA 30076. "Make your workout fun & easy with music." If you want to get in shape or stay in shape, look into this company. They offer music tapes for a variety of workouts like: aerobics, cycling, power walking, rider machines, rowing, running, skiing, step aerobics, treadmill, walking and even tapes for your relaxation!

Their free 90-page booklet will even give you data of specific walking tapes with respect to *"steps per minute along with the miles per hour,"* so you get the proper beat and music to the type of workout you desire! yes, they even have testimonials! Call Monday through Friday from 9 a.m. to 6 p.m., and on Saturday from 9 a.m. 2 p.m., Eastern Standard Time for your free booklet. Turn-off that TV and get going!

StairMaster--**1-800-782-4799**
StairMaster, Home Sales Division, 12421 Willows Road N.E., Suite 100, Kirkland, WA 98034. StairMaster is "Shaping the Future of Fitness." Folks, StairMaster offers some very impressive exercise equipment! Impressive machines like the StairMaster 4000 PT, FreeClimber 4400PT, Stepmill 7000PT, Crossrobics 1650 LE, and more! Testimonials are included in their packet of information which includes several brochures and a video! Serious about getting in-shape, then call StairMaster today! I've (the author) used the StairMaster 4000 PT many times and received graet workouts!

Starwest Botanicals, Inc.--**1-800-800-4372**
                                                                                1-916-638-8100
                                                                                1-916-638-8293(fax)
Starwest Botanicals, Inc., 11253 Trade Center Drive, Rancho Cordova, CA 95742. Starwest has been a leader and innovator in quality botanical products for 20 years. Starwest is a primary importer, processor and supplier of botanicals, culinary spices, teas, essential oils, aromatherapy and other all natural products. Starwest offers over 500 of the finest botanicals in various forms; from whole cut and sift, tea bag cut and powder.

Starwest works with *reputable growers, wildcrafters, organic farmers and suppliers* from around the world. To order their free 131-page, wholesale catalog, you must have a business license. The customer service representative will ask you the name of your company! The catalog has multitudes of healthy products far too numerous to mention. Everything to satisfy your needs, your pets needs and then some! *Everything from A to Z!*

Take Off Pounds Sensibly (TOPS)--**1-800-932-8677**
www.tops.org
TOPS may be an organization that may help you take-off that stubborn excess weight. Call them or see their web page for more information.

Tamarind Tree LTD., The--**1-201-818-7300**

1-201-818-4768

The Tamarind Tree LTD., 55 Grant Street, Ramsey, NJ 07446-9998. Tamarind Tree LTD., offers a variety of tasty and nutritious vegetarian cuisines (The Taste of India). Tamarind Tree LTD., products are available in many grocery stores, health stores and ethnic stores. If they are not available at a local outlet, call or write for a free information packet.

Total Gym--**1-800-308-5800**

Total Gym, 1230 American Blvd., West Chester, PA 19380. I was amazed by this exercise machine so I thought it was worthy of your attention. The Total Gym utilizes your own body weight (46% at the lower incline and 60% at the highest incline) for resistance to do myriad of exercises for your entire body!

Chuck Norris (black belt in Martial Arts and famous actor) has been using the Total Gym for over 16 years and its very portable! The Total Gym also helps with Rehabilitation Therapy and is used in 4,000 hospitals and Rehab Centers throughout the United States! The cost of the Total Gym is $649 and that includes shipping! The price is up there, but remember this: What you pay for is what you get! I got a Total Gym for less than $200 bucks so please do shop around instead of paying full price.

Trotter---**1-800-677-6544**

1-508-533-4300

1-508-533-5500(fax)

Trotter, 10 Trotter Drive, Medley, Massachusetts 02053. "Every piece of TROTTER equipment is engineered and built up to a standard, not down to price." The Trotter exercise equipment really impressed me! The offer: Trotter 3300 Climber, Trotter 510 Treadmill, Trotter 535 Treadmill, Trotter 2100 & 2300 Fitness equipment (weight training). Their color brochures of all their equipment is impressive! Call or write to receive a free packet of information today so you can start looking and being your best tomorrow!

Tunturi---**1-800-827-8717**

1-206-881-8156

1-206-881-7178(fax)

Tunturi, Inc., P.O. Box 97047, Redmond, WA 98073-9747. Tunturi is known all the world! Tunturi is a leading name in fitness equipment! Tunturi offers treadmills, exercise cycles, climbers, muscle trainers, rowing machines and many accessories! Look into this company today and start getting in shape tomorrow! Call today for your free literature!

University of Natural Healing Inc., The------------------------------------**1-804-973-0262**

1-804-973-8352

The University of Natural Healing Inc., P.O. Box 8113, 355 West Rio Road, Suite 201, Charlottesville, Virginia 22906. *"Information that can CURE the Incurable - after Medicine and Nutrition have failed."* Folks I highly recommend that you look into this company! The University of Natural Healing Inc., offers some "can't stop reading" books about the amazing benefits of *natural healing through herbalism!* Not the stuff you buy at the health franchises but at locations listed below.

The books *Cures from the Last Chance Clinic*, *Vision Problems* and the *Save Your Life Herbal Video Collection* (12 videos - approximately 1 hour each and a 600+ -page User Manual) are some of the *best alternative health information and products* I've come across in the 03 years it has taken me to put this book together. I purchased both books and a *two-year subscription* of *The Last Chance Health Report* for $60.00. If you're curious about their healthy informational products, give them a call.

They even have a free video offer after purchasing their books! They even have an incredible herbal formula that helps correct vision problems! Don't believe me read their many testimonials! I (author) tried this herbal formula and after the very *first application, my sight went from 20\200 to 20\70!*

NOTE: Listen folks, I've already reviewed their *Save Your Life Herbal Video Collection!!* It is nothing less than *GREAT* healing information! I'm not getting a dime for this recommendation OK! If you are not satisfied with your progress no matter your diagnosis - YOU must look into these *"natural methods that cured thousands of incurable patients who were sent home to die."* Twelve videos and a 600-page book of GREAT healing information! The Master herbalist will tell you like it is and relate many testimonials of patients and even doctors who have turned to him for a solution because conventional medicine simply failed! *Full-blown last-stage AIDS, cancers, heart disease, severe burns, terminal cases...* This Collection will stay with you for a lifetime! DON'T BELIEVE ME - do yourself a favor and look into this company and their products! They've worked for me! CALL today!

Vitamins and Recommended Dietary Allowances------------------------**1-301-443-3170**
Office of Public Affairs, Food and Drug Administration, 5600 Fishers Lane, HFE88, Rockville, MD 20857. Ask for free pamphlet: *Some Facts and Myths of Vitamins* (#82-2164).

Vitamin Shoppe---**1-800-223-1216**

                                                                      1-800-852-7153(fax)

Vitamin Shoppe, The, 4700 Westside Avenue, North Bergen, New Jersey 07047. The Vitamin Shoppe offers a large selection (over 14,000 items in stock) of Vitamins, herbs and homeopathic remedies. "Compare and Save! 20% to 40% Off Nationally Advertised Brands." Call or write to get their latest seasonal all color, 100-page catalog. Vitamin Shoppe's catalog is very informative. You'll learn by simply browsing through their pages eye-catching and healthy products.

Vita-Mix TNT---**1-800-848-2649**

Vita-Mix Total Nutrition Center (TNT), 8615 Usher Rd., Cleveland, OH 44138-2199. Before you but a regular juicer machine, you'll want to read the Vita-Mix Special Report. Vita-Mix TNT is a "whole food" juicer that delivers more than *9 times the very valuable nutrients* than regular juicer machines. The Vita-Mix TNT doesn't discard the very valuable and extremely nutritious peel, pulp and skin in those healthy fruits and vegetables. Don't *lose the vital nutrients and disease-preventing phytochemicals missing in the American Diet!* The Vita-Mix does much more! Call or write for their free impressive report. Ask for their *Vita-Mix Special Report*!

Walking and Fitness--**1-202-272-3421**

President's Council on Physical Fitness and Sports, 450 5th St., NW, Suite 7103, Washington, DC 20001. Ask for free 16-page manual titled *Everybody's Walking For Fitness and Walking for Exercise and Pleasure.*

Walking Tapes--**1-404-993-4233**

Walking Tapes, Box 767364, Roswell, GA 30076. Just plain ol' walking is a great exercise for your health and lose those unwanted pounds! Walking Tapes offers a free catalog covering music from the 40's, 50's. 60's, 80's, Marches, Latin, Country, swing, Classical, New Age... Call or write for your free *The Walking Music Catalog.*

WaterRower Inc.---**1-800-852-2210**

                                                                      1-401-728-1966

                                                                      1-401-728-1968(fax)

WaterRower Inc., 453 Cottage Street, Pawtucket, RI 02861.

WaterRower Inc. offers one of the best rowing machines in the world! Their rower machine is constructed of the finest materials to insure you get a great workout each and every time for years into your healthy future! Their unique rower machine uses water for resistance instead of air like all other rowing machines.

Call or write today for your free, all-color, fold-out brochure on one of the finest if not the best rowing machines you've ever seen! Call today and start getting in-shape tomorrow!

Waterwise Inc.,--**1-800-874-9028**
1-352-787-5008
1-352-787-8123(fax)

Waterwise Inc., 26200 U.S. Highway 27 South, Leesburg, FL 34748-9026. Waterwise Inc., is a member of the National Water Quality Association. "Be Waterwise Drink Pure Water!" Waterwise Inc., interest and concern with the quality of drinking water is both personal and professional. Waterwise Inc., has been in business for over 15 years.

They offer solutions to possible unhealthy water in your home, whether for drinking, cooking or bathing. Call for free information! You'll receive several full-size, all color, and very informative brochures about Waterwise Inc. and their healthy products. Call Monday through Friday from 8 a.m. to 5 p.m., Eastern Standard Time.

Weleda--**1-914-268-8572**
Weleda, 175 N. Rt. 9W, P.O. Box 249, Congers, NY 10920. Weleda Natural Citrus Deodorant Spray. Did you read Section 11, with respect to the hazards of aluminum? If you are troubled about aluminum that is found in most deodorants and is linked to Alzheimer's Disease, then call the number above about their aluminum-free "Sage Deodorant and Citrus Deodorant" products as well as many other consumer health and beauty products that are all natural.

Whirlpool Holiday Help-Line--**1-800-953-7434**
The Whirlpool Holiday Help-Line offers help on cleaning your refrigerator, eliminating odors and using leftovers. Whirlpool has declared November 15th as *"Clean Out Your Refrigerator Day."* Call during the Holidays, from 9 a.m. to 5 p.m., Monday through Friday up to December 15th.

Wilderness Society, The--**1-202-429-2637**
The Wilderness Society, 900 Seventeenth Street, N.W., Washington, D.C. 20006. "Protecting America's wilderness Since 1935." The Wilderness Society urgently needs your support to ensure that future generations will not be deprived of their heritage of wild lands and wildlife. Call for free information and become a Wilderness Society member today!

Wileswood---**1-419-433-3355**

1-419-433-7781(fax)

Wileswood, P.O. Box 328, Huron, OH 44839. You can make healthy popcorn at home by using *Country Store Popcorn's No. 500 Stove Popper Kit* (a stove popper, popcorn, popcorn salt and coconut oil). Cost is $38.95. Produces fluffy, tender popcorn in only five minutes. Call or write for free catalog.

World Famous Catalogs---**1-800-444-7366**

1-800-555-4053(fax)

World Famous Catalogs, Publishers Inquiry Services, 951 Broken Sound Parkway NW, Building 190, P.O. Box 5057, Boca Raton, FL 33431-0857. Too many catalogs to mention! This catalog offers very low prices of catalogs to enhance the quality of your life (art, collectibles, computers, crafts, fashion, fish supplies, fitness wear, gardening, herb teas, home decor, lingerie, men's wear, military, music, pets, tools, toys, videos (many specialized selections and much more)!

Call or write for your free 63-page all color catalog of catalogs. See The Complete Catalog Guide and The Great Directory of Undiscovered Catalogs in this section.

Yeast Connection, The---**by William G. Crook, M.D.**

Your Body's Many Cries For Water--**by**

439+ DOCTOR WORDS AND OTHER INFORMATION YOU SHOULD KNOW!

Thank you for reading this far. Once you read this entire Survival Book, I guarantee you'll know more about your health than 99.999% of folks walking this Earth. I hope it enhances your decision-making to be more vibrantly healthy from this second forward. OK, let' start this segment with the beneficial ingredients to Aloe Vera - Acemannan.

Note: These are hand-picked 'doctor words' from the Glossary of the 667-page Gettysburg Program.

Acemannan -- Beneficial ingredients in Aloe Vera. One percent of the Aloe leaf consist of more than 200 nutritional substances called mucopolysaccharides. The remaining 99 percent of the aloe leaf is water. The trade name for mucopolysaccharides is acemannan.

Acetic Acid -- Acetic acid is an inorganic acid in which a 5 percent solution and water makes vinegar.

Acetylcarnitine -- Acetylcarnitine is a natural substance produced by your body. According to a clinical test at the Mario Negri Institute for Pharmacological Research in Milan, Italy, acetylcarnitine taken orally significantly improved attention span, memory, verbal capacity and other mental functioning in 130 Alzheimer's patients. Throughout the United States, 27 centers are in their final stages, (if they haven't already been completed), of human trials using acetylcarnitine. Food & Drug Administration approval is near at hand if it hasn't already been approved at the time of this writing. See Alzheimer's Disease.

Acidosis -- Acidosis is a pathological condition resulting from accumulation of acid or depletion of the alkaline reserve (bicarbonate content) in the blood and body tissues and characterized by an increase in hydrogen ion concentration.

Acids -- Acids are compounds often found in plant tissues (especially fruits) that prevent secretion of fluids and shrink tissue. Nine important acids are: acetic acid, ascorbic acid, hyaluronic acid, hydrochloric acid, lactic acid, retinoid acid, sorbic acid and sulfuric acid. See this section for definitions.

Acute -- Acute meaning having rapid onset, severe symptoms and short duration. Acute is opposite of chronic.

Adipose Cells -- Adipose cells are also called fat cells.

Adjuvant Therapy -- Adjuvant Therapy is treatment given to supplement the primary treatment.

Aerobic -- Aerobic means occurring in the presence of oxygen.

Aerobic Conditioning -- Aerobic exercise is a fat burner. Exercise aerobically like a brisk walk, jogging, swimming... Exercise at least 30 minutes four times a week.
WARNING: Consult your doctor prior to any exercise.

Aging -- Aging is a degenerative process of the breakdown of cellular matter.

AIDS -- AIDS stands for Acquired Immuno Deficiency Syndrome, a condition in which the immune system cells have been infected with the human immunodeficiency virus. The body can no longer fight off illnesses caused by bacteria, fungus, virus or other pathogens because the compromised immune system is unable to defend it. AIDS compromises the competency of the immune system, characterized by persistent lymphadenopathy and various opportunistic infections, such as Pneumocystis carnipneumonia, cytomegalovirus, disseminated histoplasmosis, candidiasis and isosporiasis, and malignancies such as Kaposi's sarcoma; the etiologic agent is HTLV-III, transmissible by blood fluids such as blood and semen. Early symptoms include diarrhea, fatigue, fever, headache, heavily coated white tongue, lung infection, night sweat, swollen lymph glands and weight loss.

Alkaloid(s) -- One of a group of organic alkaline substances obtained from plants. Alkaloids react with acids to form salts that are used for medical purposes.

All Bran -- See Bran in this section.

Allergin -- Allergin is a substance that is capable of producing an allergic response in the body.

Allergy -- An allergy is an immunologic response (inappropriate or harmful) to substances like drugs, foods, infectious agents, inhalants, pollen or other contaminations. These substances are harmless to most people. Conventional treatment like antihistamines, cortisone, decongestants and desensitizing injections are established therapies.

Allicin -- Allicin is the active ingredients in garlic. Allicin is a bacteriostasis; meaning it inhibits further growth of bacteria. Read the very health enhancing beneficial effects of garlic.

Aloe Vera -- SEE Acemannan.

Alternative Medicine -- Alternative Medicine is different from established conventional medicine.

Alzheimer's Disease -- Alzheimer's is a degenerative disease of the brain, often occurring in middle age, causing progressive loss of mental faculties. It is also called "presenile dementia," previously classified as senile dementia. Alzheimer's disease is characterized by tangled nerve fibers surrounding the hippocampus. When the nerves surrounding the hippocampus become tangled , nerve impulses no longer carry information to or from the brain. The brain's circuits are now disconnected, information cannot be retrieved. This entanglement does not destroy the memory stored information, it prevents the information from being transferred. See acetylcarnitine in this section.

Deprenil is not a cure for Parkinson's Disease, but is a promising treatment. A natural enzyme called monoamine oxidase (MOA) is a natural scavenger of excess dopamine. However, in Parkinsonism, MOA depletes the already deficient dopamine and leaves the afflicted Parkinson's individual seriously inhibited in all types of muscular movement. Deprenil has the ability to block MOA's action without raising blood pressure and preserves the remaining dopamine. It has dramatic effects in early Parkinsonism. Deprenil halts progression of the disease in later stages and even reverses some effects in advanced cases.
Deprenil is also noted as a life extension, increases sexual activity, and an anti-depressant.
Deprenil is available by prescription from your doctor.

American Diet -- The American diet is no doubt an unhealthy mixture of refined starches & sugar, saturated fats (30%), salt and too low in fresh fruits, vegetables, whole grains and ample amount of good clean water.

American Medical Association (AMA) -- The AMA is a partnership of physicians and their professional associations that promotes the art and science of medicine.

American Red Cross -- The American Red Cross is a name for people in your community who can help you prevent, prepare for and cope with emergencies, whether those emergencies involve blood, disaster, health and safety, social services or tissue transplants. There are a few million well-trained and dedicated volunteer and paid staff members who serve in every American community through thousands of chapters.

Amino Acids -- Amino acids are a name given to the ultimate products of digestion of protein foods and from which protein materials of the body are again built up. See Amino Acids.

Anecdotal -- Characterized by, containing, or given to telling a short account of some interesting incident.

Anemia -- Anemia is any condition in which the number of red blood cells per mm3, the amount of hemoglobin in 100ml of blood, and the volume of packed red blood cells per 100ml of blood are less than normal. Clinically, anemis generally pertains to the concentration of oxygen-transporting material in a designated volume of blood, in contrast to total quantities.

Anemic -- Anemic is relating to or suffering from anemia.

Anesthetic -- An anesthetic is a substance that causes loss of sensation or feeling in a part or all of the body.

Angina Pectoris -- Angina Pectoris is a chest pain which occurs when a coronary artery becomes partially blocked which causes an oxygen debt in the heart muscle. More often than not, angina pectoris is brought on by a sudden exertion or vigorous exercise. Blood flow to the heart is insufficient to meet the oxygen demand. A Framingham Heart Study has estimated that 2.5 million people suffer from angina pectoris with 350,000 new cases each year.

Angioplasty -- Angioplasty is a medical procedure in which a balloon is inflated at the location of a blockage in the artery. This procedure is supposed to open the vessel allowing normal blood flow. This procedure has been used since 1983. Approximately 400,000 angioplasty procedures are conducted each year.

According to my research, angioplasty eventually fails 30% to 50% of the cases which may lead to another angioplasty, atherectomy or coronary-bypass surgery. Patients arteries often reclog with scar tissue, this is called restenosis.

According to a study based on 400,000 patients in each group (angioplasty & atherectomy), to patients that had no heart procedure done, those patients had an annual death rate of 4,000 (1%) while an angioplasty group had a six month death rate of 18,400 (4.6%)!

Anorexia Nervosa -- Anorexia nervosa is an eating disorder usually associated with young females who have a morbid fear of being overweight, even slightly overweight.

Antacid -- An antacid neutralizes acid in the stomach, esophagus, or first part of the duodenum.

Antibacterial -- Antibacterial refers to a substance which has the property of destroying or stopping the growth of bacteria. Next time you go to your local grocery store, look for many products (hand soap, dishwashing detergent, laundry detergent, cleaning detergents...) that KILL bacteria!

You'll have peace of knowing that your home environment is cleaner and healthier for you and your family! One good habit for a healthier environment is to simply wash your hands on a regular basis.

Antibiotic -- An antibiotic is any of various substances, such as penicillin and streptomycin, produced by certain fungi, bacteria, and similar organisms, that are effective in inhibiting the growth of or destroying microorganisms and are widely used in the prevention and treatment of diseases. See *Antibiotic-Resistant Infections* below.

Antibiotic-Resistant Infections -- Bacteria may remain in the body, growing stronger and more deadly. If illness recurs or a new one begins, the infection is more difficult to beat because the bacteria has now learned to fight off the antibiotics. According to Stuart Levy, M.D., author of Antibiotic Paradox: How Miracle Drugs are Destroying the Miracle, when people start to feel better, they stop taking their medicine only to begin it again when symptoms resurface.

By not finishing the prescription, the bacteria remain in the body, growing stronger and more deadly. Dr. Levy recommends the following:
* Even if symptoms subside or you feel better, finish all prescribed drugs.

* Don't ask for antibiotics if you have the cold or flu. Antibiotics are meant to fight bacteria and not viral infections.

* Do not take leftover pills. The present infection may be different from the one for which the pill were originally prescribed.

Antibody -- An antibody is a protein molecule from the immune system that counteracts the effects of invading organisms and other foreign substances.

Antidote -- An antidote is an agent that neutralizes a poison or counteracts its effects.

Antihistamine -- Antihistamines are drugs having an action antagonistic to that of histamine.

Antioxidant -- An antioxidant is a substance that slows oxidation which include Vitamins C and E as well as the minerals selenium, germanium, superoxide dismutase (SOD), Coenzyme Q10 (CoQ10), catalase and some amino acids. Antioxidants are chemical substances that stop the uncontrolled production of harmful free radicals in our bodies and help to protect our bodies' cells. See *Pycnogenol*.

Antiseptics -- Antiseptics are substances which have the property of preventing or arresting putrefaction in dead animal or vegetable matter.

Antiviral -- An antiviral is any substance which bears the properties of opposing the action of a virus.

Anxiety Disorder -- General Anxiety Disorder (GAD) is a chronic and exaggerated worry and tension, even though nothing seems to provoke it. Having this disorder means always anticipating disaster, often worrying excessively about health, money, family or work.

Aorta -- The aorta is a large artery that is the main trunk of the systemic arterial system, arising from the base of the left ventricle and ending at the left side of the body of the fourth lumbar vertebra by dividing to form the right and left common iliac arteries.

Apple Cider Vinegar -- See *Apple Cider Vinegre*.

Aroma Therapy -- See Aroma Therapy.

Arrhythmia -- Arrhythmia is an abnormal heartbeat rhythm.

Arteries -- Ateries are vessels which convey oxygenated blood away from the heart to the tissues of the body, limbs, and internal organs. In the case of most arteries, the blood has been purified by passing through the lungs, and is consequently bright red in color, but in the pulmonary arteries which carry it to the lungs it is unoxygenated, dark and like the blood in the veins.

Arteriosclerosis -- Arteriosclerosis is arterial or vascular sclerosis or hardening of the arteries. Types generally recognized are: atherosclerosis (also known as artery clogging process), Monckeberg's, hypertensive and arteriolosclerosis.

Arthritis -- Arthritis is articular rheumatism or inflammation of one or more joints.

Artificial Respiration -- This is the process of breathing air into the lungs of a person who has stopped breathing. Mouth-to-Nose and mouth-to-stoma breathing are types of rescue breathing.

Artificial Sweetener -- See The Five Deadly Whites.

Ascorbic Acid -- Ascorbic Acid is an inorganic acid. It is also called Vitamin C. It is used as a cosmetic and antioxidant.

Aspartame -- Aspartame, a synthetic sweetener (brand names NutraSweet & Equal) has been linked to many health problems.

Aspirin -- The American Indians have been treating aches and pains for hundreds of years using a herbal brew made from white willow bark. The synthesized and refined willow bark, acetylsalicylic acid, is known as Aspirin! Aspirin was first made commercially in Germany at the turn of the century. Acetylsalicylic acid is a widely used analgesic, antipyretic and anti-inflammatory agent. The Physicians Health Study revealed that a one-half group - aspirin group of over 22,000 doctors had 44% fewer nonfatal heart attacks than that of the placebo group. However, aspirin increased the risk of hemorrhagic strokes - bleeding into the brain, sudden cardiac death was almost twice as high in the aspirin group and the incidence of gastric and duodenal ulcers was also about twice as high.

WARNING: Seek consultation from your designated physician prior to using aspirin as a preventive medicine.

Asthma -- Originally, asthma was a term used to mean "difficult breathing." Now it is used to denote bronchial asthma. Asthma is a treatable disease. Approximately 21 to 25 million Americans have been diagnosed with asthma.

Atherectomy -- Atherectomy is a medical procedure in which a "Roto-Rooter" device is used to open up blocked arteries. Atherectomy uses a high-speed circulating knife that shears away the cholesterol from the artery wall.

According to a study based on 400,000 patients in each group (angioplasty & atherectomy), to patients that had no heart procedure done, those patients had an annual death rate of 4,000 (1%) while an atherectomy group had a six month death rate of 34,400 (8.6%)! Approximately 1 out of 12 atherectomy patients dies within six months. Read about the amazing benefits of Coenzyme Q10 (CoQ10).

Atherosclerosis -- The build-up of fatty deposits in the arteries. The build-up of plaque in artery walls that narrows the artery opening. Narrowing of the arteries.

Atrial Fibrillation -- Atrial fibrillation makes the heart beat rapidly and erratically which increases the a person's chances to dangerous and deadly blood clots that can lodge in the arteries leading to the brain.

Atrophy -- The emaciation or wasting of tissues, organs or the entire body. A wasting away due to nonuse.

Auricular Therapy -- It is also called Auriculotherapy. Auricular Therapy or ear acupuncture is a sophisticated treatment using an electronic instrument called Stim Flex. The Stim Flex stimulates specific points on the ear with undetectable microcurrents.

Auricular Therapy is pain-free and no puncture is involved. This therapy is noted to relieve pain, all kinds of pain in minutes! It is noted to have other amazing benefits like reversing stroke symptoms!

Autoimmunity -- Autoimmunity is a broad category of related diseases in which the person's immune system attacks its own tissue. Approximately 50 million Americans suffer from Autoimmunity. It includes Autoimmune Diseases like Behcet's, Crohn's, Graves', ITP, Juvenile Diabetes, Lupus, Multiple Sclerosis, Myasthenia Gravis, Myositis, Pemphigus, Rheumatoid Arthritis, Sjogren's, Thyroiditis (Hashimoto's) and over 70 more!

Bacteria -- It is plural of bacterium. They are microscopic germs. Some bacteria are harmful and can cause disease, while other friendly bacteria protect the body from harmful invading organisms. There is more bacteria in your body than all the people that were ever on the earth! White blood cells are in constant defense against diseases every minute of every day by engulfing germs and neutralizing their unhealthy effectiveness. See Antibacterial in this section.

Bariatric -- A Bariatric is a weight-loss physician.

Baroque Music -- Music by the sixteenth to eighteenth century composers, Bach, Vivaldi, Telemann, Corelli and Handel is often called Baroque music. Baroque music often has a very slow bass, beating like a slow human pulse. According to Superlearning Inc., their Superlearning Subliminal cassette tape which has slow Baroque Music has been *"experimentally proven to relax the body, lower heart beat and blood pressure and calm the mind."*

Benign -- It means relating to not malignant, not cancerous. See *Benign Tumor* below and see *Malignant*.

Benign Tumor -- Benign tumors are not cancer. They can usually be removed and, in most cases, they do not come back. Most important, cells from benign tumors do not spread to other parts of the body. Benign tumors are rarely a threat to life.

Beta Blockers -- Beta blockers are any of a group of drugs that slow down the action of the heart by blocking the action of nerve endings called betareceptors. They are used to treat abnormal heart conditions and high blood pressure.

Beta-Carotene -- It is a derivative of Vitamin A. Beta-Carotene is widely accepted today as a cancer preventative. Beta-Carotene is partially converted into Vitamin A in the body. It's an antioxidant that can be found in dark-green vegetables and some deep-yellow and orange vegetables and fruits.

Bile -- Bile is a substance released by the liver into the intestines for the digestion of fats.

Binge Eating Disorder -- It is an illness that resembles bulimia nervosa except the sufferers DO NOT purge their bodies of excess food. Individuals with binge eating disorder feel that they lose control of themselves when eating. They eat large quantities of food and do not stop until they are uncomfortably full. Binge eating disorder is found in 02 percent of the general population and more often with women than men.

Bio-Availability -- It refers to that proportion of a drug which reaches the systemic circulation unchanged after a particular route of administration.

Bioflavonoids -- Bioflavonoids are not true Vitamins in the strictest sense, but are referred to as Vitamin F. Bioflavonoids enhance Vitamin C and should be taken together. The human body cannot produce bioflavonoids, therefore they must be supplied by your diet. Bioflavonoids are used in athletic injuries because they relieve pain, bumps and bruises.

Bioflavonoids act synergistically with Vitamin C to protect and preserve the structure of capillary blood vessels. Bioflavonoids have an antibacterial effect and promote circulation, stimulate bile production, lower cholesterol levels and treat and prevent cataracts.

Bioflavonoids and Vitamin C taken together reduce the symptoms of oral herpes. A supplement called Quercetin may effectively treat and prevent asthma symptoms. Bromelain and Quercetin are synergists (work together better than separately). 1,000 to 2,000 milligrams of Quercetin daily in 03 to 06 divided doses for asthma or allergies.

Sources of Bioflavonoids are the white material just beneath the peel of citrus fruits, apricots, buckwheat, black currants, cherries, grapes, grapefruit, lemons, oranges, peppers, prunes and rose hips.
WARNING: Extremely high doses of Bioflavonoids may cause diarrhea.

Biological Therapy -- Biological Therapy is treatment with substances that can stimulate the immune system to fight disease effectively. It is also called immunotherapy.

Biopsy -- A biopsy is an excision of tissue from a living being for diagnosis. For example, a piece of tumor may be cut out and examined to determine whether it is cancerous.

Biotin -- Biotin aids in cell growth as well as fatty acid production, and in metabolism of carbohydrates, fats, proteins and in the utilization of B-Complex Vitamins. Significant quantities are needed for healthy hair and skin. Biotin may prevent hair loss in some men.

Biotin promotes healthy sweat glands, nerve tissue and bone marrow. A deficiency of this B Vitamin is rare because it can be produced in the intestines from food. Sources of Biotin are cooked egg yolks, salt-water fish, meat, milk, poultry, soybeans, whole grains and yeast.

WARNING: Raw egg whites contain a protein called ovidin, which combines with Biotin in the intestinal tract depletes the body of this nutrient. A dry, scaly scalp or face in infants, called seborrheic dermatitis, may indicate a deficiency of Biotin. Consumption of rancid fats or saccharin inhibits Biotin absorption. Use of sulfa drugs and antibiotics threatens the Biotin.

Black Vomit -- Due to the presence of blood in the stomach.

Bladder -- The urine passes from each kidney and is stored in the bladder until elimination. A sphincter muscle around the exit from the bladder prevents urine from escaping. Once the bladder is half full, the body feels an urge to empty the bladder. At this time the sphincter muscle is relaxed voluntarily to release the urine.

Blood -- Blood is the "circulating tissue" of the body. (The fluid and it's suspended formed elements that are circulating through the heart, arteries, capillaries and veins by the means of which oxygen and nutritive materials are transported to tissues, and carbon dioxide and various metabolic products are removed for excretion). Blood consists of plasma in which are suspended red and white corpuscles, platelet, fat globules and a great variety of chemical substances including carbohydrates, proteins, hormones and gases such as oxygen, carbon dioxide, and nitrogen. Blood consists of approximately 78% water and 22% solids.

Blood Cholesterol -- See Cholesterol.

Blood Clot -- It means to coagulate. It is a soft, non-rigid, insoluble mass formed when blood or lymph gels. Heart attacks usually occur when a small blood clot lodges in an artery that is already blocked with cholesterol and other materials. This blood clot may be the final strike to one that has blocked or partially blocked arteries.

Blood Count -- A blood count is the number of red and white blood cells and platelet in a sample of blood.

Blood Sugar -- It is sugar in the form of glucose present in the blood, normally 60 to 100 milligrams/100 milliliters of blood. The blood sugar may rise to as much as 150 milligrams/100 milliliters of blood, but this may vary.

Blood Vessels -- They are any elastic, tubular canal, such as an artery, vein or capillary, through which blood circulates. Blood vessels form a network of passages that transport blood throughout your body. See *Circulatory System* in this section.

Body Mass Index (BMI) -- A standard measure of body fat in order to monitor obesity. Are you obese? See the BMI Formula.

Bone -- A bone is a hard connective tissue consisting of cells in a matrix of ground substance and collagen fibers. The fibers are impregnated with mineral substance, chiefly calcium phosphate and carbonate, which comprises about 67% by weight of adult bone.

Bones form the framework upon which the rest of the body is built up. There are 206 bones in the human skeleton. Bones collect calcium for the entire body, storing 99% of the body's supply of calcium. Inside some of the bones is a substance called marrow. Marrow produces red and white blood cells and platelets.

Brain -- Your brain is a 03-lb. maze of nerves and tissue and a lab of chemicals that control everything! The brain is the portion of the central nervous system in the vertebrate cranium that is responsible for the interpretation of sensory impulses, the coordination and control of bodily activities, and the exercise of emotion, memory and thought.

Brain Infarct -- Medical term for stroke, also called a brain attack.

Brain Tumor, Primary -- Primary brain tumors are those that arise in the brain which will appear in approximately 17,000 Americans this year, of which 13,000 Americans will die, according to the American Cancer Society. The most common brain tumors are called gliomas, which develop from the glial cells that protect and nourish nerve cells in the brain. The most malignant glioma is also the most common primary brain tumor of middle-aged adults, which accounts for 30 percent of all primary brain tumors. Patients rarely live more than 02 years after a diagnosis of malignant glioma.

Bran -- Bran is a by-product of the milling of wheat, containing approximately 20% of indigestible cellulose. It is a bulk cathartic, usually taken in the form of cereal or special bran products.

Breast Self-Examination (BSE) -- See your doctor for the best technique and advise on a BSE. Between visits to your doctor, you should do a BSE once a month.

Bromelain -- Bromelain is a natural enzyme found in pineapples. This nutrient increases the body's ability to break down fats and protein promoting body metabolism. You'll find Bromelain advertised on some "Fat Burning" products sold at your local health and nutritional stores.

Bronchial Asthma -- It is a condition of the lungs in which there is widespread narrowing of the airways, varying over short periods of time either spontaneously or as a result of treatment, due in varying degrees to contraction (spasm) of smooth muscle, edema of the mucosa and mucus in the lumen of the bronchial and bronchioles. It is caused by the local release of spasmogens and vasoactive substances in the course of an allergic process.

Bronchitis -- Bronchitis is a respiratory illness characterized by inflammation and swelling of the main airways connecting the windpipe to the lungs.

Brown Spots -- Brown spots are noted to be caused by free radicals. Toxic oxygen molecules are a major cause of aging and most degenerative diseases. The best way to prevent brown spots is to supplement your diet with antioxidants like Vitamins A, C, and E and zinc and selenium.

Bruxism -- Bruxism is nocturnal tooth grinding.

Bulimia Nervosa -- Bulimia Nervosa is a eating disorder in which the bulimic person consumes large amounts - high calorie foods only to later purge their systems by vomiting, using laxatives, diuretics or a combination of these.

Caffeine -- Trimethylxanthine; an alkaloid obtained from the dried leaves of Thea sinensis, tea, or the dried seeds of Coffee arabica, coffee; used as a diuretic and circulatory and respiratory stimulant.

Caffeinism -- Caffeinism is chronic coffee poisoning, characterized by palpitation, dyspepsia, irritability and insomnia.

Calcium -- According to the Food and Nutrition Board of the National Research Council, it has determined the Recommended Dietary Allowance of calcium is 1200mg per day for male and female adolescents up to the age of 24 years old. For adults 25 years of age and older, the Board's recommendation is 800mg per day.

Calcium is the most abundant mineral in the body. Ninety-nine percent is lodged in the teeth and skeleton and the remaining portion makes up the soft tissue. To metabolize calcium, magnesium, phosphorus and Vitamins A, C and D must be present in their proper proportions. The major role of calcium in the body is to build blood and maintain bone structure. Calcium assists in the process of blood clotting, muscle contraction, muscle growth, prevents accumulation of excess alkali in the blood, regulates the heart rate and transference of nerve impulses.

Calcium is a useful therapeutic agent in acne, aging, allergies, anemia, celiac disease, colitis, common cold, constipation, diabetes, fractures, gum disorders, hemophilia, kidney disfunction, Meniere's syndrome, mental illness, nail trouble, obesity, Parkinson's disease, pernicious anemia, rickets, stomach ulcer, tuberculosis, worms....

Calorie -- Kcal is a measure of energy. Just one pound of body fat equals 3,500 calories of stored energy. Calories are units of measure used to calculate the amount of energy contained in foods. One calorie equals the amount of heat required to raise the temperature of 1 gram of water from 14.5 degrees to 15.5-degrees Centigrade.

Cancer -- Cancer is a group of more than 100 different diseases. Cancer occurs when cells become abnormal and keep dividing and forming more cells without control and order. All organs of the body are made up of cells. Normally, cells divide to produce more cells only when the body needs them. This order process helps keep us healthy. If cells keep dividing when new cells are not needed, a mass of tissue forms. This mass of tissue, called a growth or tumor, can be benign or malignant. Approximately 1/3 of all cancer deaths may be related to what we eat.

Cancerous Tumor -- Cancer Carcinoma and Sarcoma are general names for forms of tumor to which the term 'malignant' is applied.

Carbohydrates -- Carbohydrates are all, chemically considered, derivatives of simple forms of sugar and are classified as disaccharides (eg. cane sugar), monosaccharides (eg. glucose) and polysacchrides (eg. starch). Carbohydrates are classified as either complex carbohydrates (starches) or simple carbohydrates (sugars), providing energy.

Carcinogen -- A carcinogen is any agent that is known to cause cancer.

Carcinoma -- A carcinoma is a cancer that begins in the epithelial tissue that lines or covers an organ.

Cardiologist -- A cardiologist is a heart specialist.

Cardiology -- Cardiology is the medical specialty concerned with the heart and it's diseases.

Cardiomyoplasty -- Cardiomyoplasty is detaching a portion of the patient's back muscle, wrapping the back muscle around the unhealthy heart and implanting a pacemaker. The pacemaker delivers calibrated burst of electricity to the back muscle, which stimulates it to contract like a heart muscle. The back muscle eventually learns to pump like a heart muscle. As of February 1994, more than 150 patients have undergone a cardiomyoplasty

Cardiopulmonary Resuscitation (CPR) -- CPR is an emergency procedure used for a person who is not breathing and whose heart has stopped beating (cardiac arrest). It is used to keep the body's cells from dying until advanced medical help arrives. The procedure involves a combination of rescue breathing and chest compressions.

Cardiovascular System -- Relating to the heart and the blood vessels or the circulation. Your blood is pumped by your heart through 60,000 miles of blood vessels so to nourish nutrients and oxygen to every cell.

Carotid Pulse -- This is the beat which is felt at the side of the neck when the carotid artery is pressed. Located between the windpipe and the neck muscle, the carotid pulse is checked to determine the presence or absence of heartbeat.

Cartilage -- Cartilage cushions and protects bones with the help of various joint fluids and bursae (small sacs of lubricating fluid that encompass the joint).

Cell -- The cell is the basic unit of all living things. Many HEALING ASPECTS that you read throughout this book BEGAN AT THE CELLULAR LEVEL! Through proper nutrition, exercise, supplements, your thoughts and other treatments (alternative and conventional), YOUR BODY HAS THE ABILITY TO HEAL ITSELF! See Cellular Healing.

Cellulose -- Cellulose is a nondigestible carbohydrate found in the outer layers of fruits and vegetables.

Centers for Disease Control and Prevention (CDC) -- The CDC, a federal agency that protects the nation's health, was formed in 1946 and is located in Atlanta, Georgia. The CDC's work force consists of 7,000 employees, of which 1,000 highly trained specialists and researchers battle infectious diseases. Of their $2 billion budget, $130 million is for infectious diseases.

The CDC consist of seven centers, dealing with threats like AIDS, childhood vaccination, environmental health, injury prevention and control.

The CDC has contributed an overwhelming abundance of successes and ongoing battles in fighting and warding off catastrophes throughout the U.S. and the world during its existence. The CDC helped to wipe out smallpox on a global scale and polio in the U.S. and tracked down E. coli O157:H7 bacteria in undercooked fast-food hamburgers. The list of past and ongoing threats to the public health are too many to list.

Certified Organically Grown -- The grower went to extremes to produce a chemically free plant. In some areas of the United States, this also means no chemicals could have been used on the soil in the past 10 years.

Chelation Therapy -- Chelation Therapy uses EDTA (Ethylene Diamine Tetraacetic Acid) or other supplements that carry out heavy metals like lead, cadmium and arsenic, as well as other foreign substances, from the body. In the process of chelation, a larger protein molecule surrounds or encloses a mineral atom. The purpose of chelation is to increase the flow of blood to the vital organs and tissues of the body by reducing calcium deposits in the arteries and blood vessels. Chelation agents are used to bind with heavy toxic metals such as cadmium, lead and mercury and to excrete them from the body.

Chelating agents are available in over-the-counter formulas that can be taken orally at home or administered intravenously under the supervision of your doctor. Chelation Therapy has been used effectively to treat arteriosclerosis for over 40 years in the U.S.

Chemotherapy -- Chemotherapy is a treatment of disease by any chemicals. It refers to the chemical treatments used to combat cancer cells. Chemotherapy not only destroys cancer cells, but it also destroys other fast growing cells like bone marrow, hair and intestinal cells. Side effects of chemotherapy are digestive problems (constipation, diarrhea, nausea, vomiting), loss of appetite, peeling of skin and sores in the mouth.

Chinese Restaurant Syndrome -- Development of chest pain, feelings of facial pressure, and sensation of burning over variable portions of the body surface after ingestion of food containing Monosodium L-glutamate (MSG) by persons sensitive to this food additive. See MSG in this section.

Chiropractic -- Over 15 million Americans a year turn to chiropractic care for drug-free treatment of backaches, injuries, pain, trauma and certain internal disorders. The core or foundation of chiropractic's approach is the relationship between the spinal column\musculoskeletal structures of the body and the nervous system.

When misalignments (subluxations) in the spine occur, they may cause nerve interference. These interruptions cause pain and lower body defenses. Removing misalignments and restoring normal nerve function, OPTIMIZES THE BODY'S INHERENT ABILITY TO HEAL ITSELF!

Chiropractor -- A Chiropractor is practitioner of Chiropractic.

Chlorine -- Chlorine is a yellowish green, gaseous element, of suffocating odor. It is a disinfectant, decolorant and irritant poison. It is used for disinfecting, fumigating and bleaching, either in aqueous solution or in the form of chlorinated lime. It is found in almost all public water sanitation systems.

Cholesterol -- Cholesterol is a waxy, fat-like substance. It is implicated experimentally as a factor in atherosclerosis.

Chromium -- Chromium plays a role in glucose metabolism. It is considered essential in trace amounts in nutrition.

Chromium Picolinate -- See Chromium Picolinate.

Chronic -- Chronic is of long duration. It denotes a disease of slow progress and long continuance.

Chronic Fatigue Syndrome (CFS) -- CFS is a daily fatigue to the degree of incapacitation. The patient does not have the energy to exist in a normal everyday fashion.

Circulatory System -- The circulatory system is composed of 60,000 miles of arteries, veins, and capillaries. Five to six quarts of vital fluid (blood) continuously travel through your circulatory system.

Citric Acid -- Citric acid is an organic acid in citrus fruits. It is used in cosmetics to lower the pH of a product. See *pH* in this section.

Clinic -- A clinic is an establishment where patients are admitted for special study and treatment by a group of physicians practicing medicine together.

Clinical Ecology -- Clinical ecology is a relatively new and unknown study of environmental causes of disease. This branch of medicine is concerned with the process of adverse reactions from environmental insults to the human body and the consequent reactions and adaption to such insults by the susceptible individual.

Clinical Trial -- A clinical trial is research conducted with cancer patients, more often than not to evaluate a new treatment. Each trial is designed to answer scientific questions and to find better ways to treat patients.

Clove -- A clove is any of the small sections of a separate bulb, such as that of garlic.

Cobalt 60 -- Cobalt 60 is a radioactive isotope of the element cobalt which is widely used in radiation therapy.

Co-carcinogen -- A co-carcinogen is an environmental agent that acts with another to cause cancer.

Coenzyme -- A coenzyme is a *"helper"* enzyme. A substance that enhances or is necessary for the action of enzymes; coenzymes are of smaller molecule size than the enzymes themselves; are dialyzable and relatively heat-stable, and are usually easily dissociable from the protein portion of the enzyme; several Vitamins are coenzyme precursors. SEE Coenzyme Q10 below!

Coenzyme Q10 - Coenzyme Q10 (CoQ10) is a Vitamin-like substance that resembles Vitamin E which may be more powerful as an antioxidant. Of the 10 common coenzyme Qs, only CoQ10 is found in human tissue. CoQ10 declines with age and should be supplemented in the diet. CoQ10 plays a crucial role in the effectiveness of the immune system and the aging process. The New England Institute reports that CoQ10 alone is effective in reducing mortality in experimental animals afflicted with tumors and leukemia.

Colitis -- Colitis is inflammation of the colon.

Collagen -- Collagen is the protein substance of the white fibers of skin, tendon, bone, cartilage and all other connective tissue.

Collagen Disease -- Collagen disease is a term applied to diseases which involve the connective tissue system like lupus erythematosus, scleroderma and rheumatoid arthritis.

Colloidal Silver -- Colloidal Silver is electrically charged particles of silver that are 0.01 to about 0.001 microns in diameter and suspended in distilled water. According to medical literature, the best quality of Colloidal silver is actually gold in color and has the quality for injection use. According to medical journals from around the world, therapeutic value of Colloidal Silver is annotated as a powerful wide-spectrum antibiotic that disables the enzyme that all one-celled bacteria, fungi and viruses use for their oxygen metabolism causing them to suffocate in six minutes or less upon contact which was recently tested at UCLA Medical Labs.

Colon Cancer -- Colin cancer is cancer of the large intestine which extends from the cecum to the rectum. In 1994, the number one cancer for men and women was colon cancer.

Complex Carbohydrate -- It includes indigestible molecules of fiber (starch and glycogen). It slowly releases sugar into the bloodstream and also adds the fiber.

Complications -- A complication is a morbid process or event occurring during a disease which is not an essential part of the disease, although it may result from it or from independent causes.

Concussion -- A concussion is an injury to the brain caused by a violent jar or shock, like a strike to the head. The force of the strike causes the brain to strike against the inside of the skull which produces temporary brain swelling and malfunctioning and often loss of consciousness. The strike may cause cerebral contusion (bruising of the brain tissue), cerebral hemorrhage (bleeding between the covering of the brain and the skull or inside the brain covering) or formation of a hematoma (collection of clotted blood). Symptoms of a concussion may be feeling nauseated, irritable, dizzy, unconsciousness and even coma. Any violent strike to the head should be followed-up with immediate medical attention.

Congestive Heart Failure -- A congestive heart failure is a condition characterized by abdominal discomfort, breathlessness, weakness and edema in the lower portions of the body, resulting from venous stasis and reduced outflow of blood from the left side of the heart. It is the inability of the heart to pump all the blood returned to it.

Constipation -- Constipation is infrequent or difficult evacuation of the feces. The bowels should move at least once a day and three movements, one after each meal, would be better. Toxins that accumulate without being evacuated cause an imbalance in the bacterial flora of the colon and may stimulate disease.

Consumption -- Consumption is wasting away of the body, especially as caused by tuberculosis of the lungs. See tuberculosis in this section.

Contaminated -- It means the presence of or reasonably anticipated presence of potentially infectious materials on any item or surface.

Contusion -- A contusion is a bruise. It is an injury in which the skin is not broken.

Convulsion -- A convulsion is uncontrollable contraction of the voluntary muscles that results from abnormal cerebral stimulation.

Convulsive Disorder -- A convulsive disorder is a violent involuntary contraction or series of contractions of the voluntary muscles.

Coronary Artery Disease -- Coronary artery disease is a narrowing of the coronary arteries which prevents adequate blood supply to the myocardium. Narrowing is usually caused by atherosclerosis and may progress to the point where the heart muscle is damaged due to lack of blood supply.

Coronary Bypass Surgery -- Coronary Bypass Surgery is performed on one or more of the coronary arteries, which lie on the outer surface of the heart and supply the heart muscle with oxygen and needed nutrients. The purpose of the operation is to bypass the obstructed area to permit free blood flow. The operation may be required because of the coronary artery a section or sections of the arteries gradually become obstructed by a buildup of cholesterol, calcium and scar tissue. Without the operation, heart muscle beyond the obstruction is starved for blood and oxygen. If one or more of the coronary arteries become completely blocked, the result may be a heart attack, in which a portion of heart muscle becomes so starved for blood that it dies.

Coronary Heart Disease -- In coronary heart disease\coronary artery disease, a section or sections of the arteries gradually become obstructed by a buildup of cholesterol, calcium and scar tissue.

Coronary Occlusion -- It is a blockage (clot) in a coronary artery that prevents blood from reaching the heart for its own purpose.

Couch Potato -- See *Sedentary* in this section.

221

Cranial -- Cranial is relating to the bones that cover the brain.

Crohn's Disease -- Crohn's disease is a chronic granulomatous inflammatory disease of unknown etiology, involving any part of the gastrointestinal tract from the mouth to the anus, but commonly involving the terminal ileum (the distal portion of the small intestine extending from the jejunum to the cecum), with scarring and thickening of the bowel wall. It frequently leads to intestinal obstruction and fistula (an abnormal passage) and abscess formation (a localized collection of pus caused by suppuration buried in tissues, organs or confined spaces) and has a high rate of recurrence after treatment.

Cruciferous -- Cruciferous is a group of vegetables named for their cross-shaped blossoms (broccoli, Brussels sprouts, cabbage, cauliflower, turnips and rutabagas), which may prevent colon cancer.

Cryptosporidium Parvum -- This waterborne parasite caused 104 deaths and caused more than 400,000 people to become sick in Milwaukee in 1993. This organism is a microscopic protozan which exist in surface water sources of supply.

Cures -- A cure is the successful treatment of a disease or wound.

Cyanosis -- Cyanosis is a disordered circulatory condition due to inadequate oxygen supply in the blood.

Cyanotic -- Cyanotic is bluish in color due to cyanosis.

Cystic Fibrosis -- Cystic fibrosis clogs the lungs with an excess of mucus and eventually affects other parts of the body. Cystic fibrosis may be passed from parents to their offspring. 01 out of 20 adults unknowingly carries the gene which causes Cystic Fibrosis. Cystic Fibrosis is the #1 genetic killer of children and young adults.

Cystic Fibrosis is the most common fatal genetic disease in the United States, affecting approximately 30,000 children and young adults. Symptoms are bulky, foul smelling stools, clubbed fingers, excessive appetite, but poor weight gain, persistent coughing, salty-tasting skin and wheezing or pneumonia. If you suspect your child suffering from Cystic Fibrosis, see your doctor immediately. The sooner it is treated, the less damage it will have on the lungs and digestive system.

Cystitis -- Cystitis is a bacterial infection of the bladder characterized by a powerful desire to urinate. Symptoms include pain in the lower abdomen and back, frequent and painful urination, blood or pus in the urine and fever.

Debridement -- Debridement is the removal of foreign material or contaminated tissue from or adjacent to a traumatic or infected lesion until surrounding healthy tissue is exposed. See Insect Therapy in this section.

Decongestant -- A decongestant has the property of reducing congestion.

Decontamination -- Decontamination is the use of physical or chemical means to remove, inactivate or destroy bloodborne pathogens on a surface or item to the point where they are no longer capable of transmitting infectious particles and the surface or item is rendered safe.

Dehydration -- It is also called anhydration. Deprivation of water or reduction of water content. Prolonged dehydration dulls the mind. Simple math problems and loss of memory are just a few symptoms. Three days without consuming ample amounts of water can lead to serious health problems.

Dementia -- Dementia is an acquired, progressive impairment of intellectual function. Marked compromise exists in at least three of the following mental activity spheres: memory, language, personality, visuospatial skills and cognition (abstraction and calculation).

Depression -- Depression is a no-hope attitude and outlook and\or a feeling of despair. The three primary types of depression are major depression, chronic depression and manic depression. 01 in 20 Americans suffers from a depression severe enough to require medical treatment. 01 in 05 Americans will have a depression at some time in their life.

Dermatitis -- Dermatitis is the inflammation of the skin with itching, redness and various skin lesions.

Dermatologist -- A dermatologists is a skin specialist.

Desert Storm Syndrome In A Can -- During the Gulf War (Desert Shield & Desert Storm), Gulf War veterans drinking free diet sodas supplied by soft drink companies. Diet drinks contain aspartame!

When stored in temperatures above 85 degrees F, aspartame breaks down into the following neurotoxic substances: methanol, formaldehyde, formic acid and DKP (brain tumor agent). Aspartame may be found in meals Ready to Eat (MREs)! Aspartame is noted to change the DNA in lab tests (birth defects). Aspartame users complain of a wide variety of sickness as do Gulf War veterans.

Detoxification -- Detoxification is a process of removing toxins from the body. A universal agreement among natural healers both past and present, is detoxifying your body is probably the single most important thing you can do to restore or maintain good health. A detoxified system strengthens the immune system.

Dextrose -- Dextrose is a form of glucose. It is a dextrorotatory monosaccharide (hexose) found in the free state in fruits and other parts of plants.

DHA -- DHA which stands for docosahexaenoic acid. Omega-3 is noted to protect against heart disease and stroke. This is one of two nutrients found in Omega-3. The other nutrient that makes-up Omega-3 is called EPA. EPA stands for eicosapentaenoic acid. Omega-3 is noted to protect against heart disease and stroke.

Diabetes -- Diabetes is a metabolic disorder characterized by the decreased ability or complete inability of the body to utilize carbohydrates due to lower production of insulin. Major symptoms are excessive thirst, frequent urination, impaired vision, increased appetite with weight loss, muscle cramps and poor healing of wounds. Last year (1994), the complications from diabetes killed an estimated 300,000 people! There are three types of diabetes: Type I, Type II and Gestational diabetes. See this section for definitions. SOUND THE ALERT! The mission of the American Diabetes Association is to *"Prevent and cure diabetes and to improve the lives of all people affected by diabetes."*

Nearly 14 million Americans have diabetes and HALF DO NOT KNOW IT. ARE YOU AT RISK? Diabetes IS a serious disease which can lead to amputations, blindness, heart attack, kidney failure and stroke. Diabetes is the fourth-leading cause of death by disease in the United States, killing more than 160,000 Americans each year. Look up American Diabetes Association in Section 25 right now and call the Toll Free 800 number and ask for your free *"American Diabetes Alert"* brochure to see if you're at risk for diabetes. I scored '6' on my test which was passing for right now!

Diabetic Retinopathy -- Retinal changes occurring in diabetes of long duration, marked by hemorrhages, microaneurysms and sharply defined waxy deposits, or by proliferative retinopathy.

Diagnosis -- A diagnosis is a determination of the nature of a disease.

Diarrhea -- Diarrhea is an abnormally frequent discharge of fluid fecal matter from the bowel.

Diastolic Pressure -- Diastolic pressure is the period of least pressure in the arterial vascular system. It is the second number given in a blood pressure measurement, which is the point or phase of the greatest cardiac relaxation.

Diet -- A prescribed course of eating and drinking, in which the amount and kind of food, as well as the times at which it is to be taken, are regulated for therapeutic purposes. Reduction of the caloric intake so as to lose weight.

Dietary Fiber -- Dietary fiber is material from plant cells that humans cannot digest or can only partially digest. It helps move food through the intestine and out of the body, promoting a healthy digestive tract. A diet high in fiber and low in fat may reduce the risk of cancers of the colon and rectum.

Digestive System -- The process in which food enters your mouth, stomach and intestines so that it can be absorbed into your bloodstream.

Digitalis -- Digitalis, an important heart medication, is derived from the leaves of the foxglove plant. The main systemic effects are manifested in the strength of the heart beat while decreasing its rate.

Diphtheria -- Diphtheria is a respiratory bacterial disease marked by the formation of a false membrane that obstructs breathing.

Disability -- Disability is a general term used for a functional limitation that interferes with a person's ability (hear, learn, lift, talk, walk...).

Disease -- A disease is a morbus, illness, sickness, an interruption, cessation, or disorder of the body functions, systems or organs. It is any deviation from or interruption of the normal structure or function of any part, organ or system any combination, of the body that is manifested by a characteristic set of symptoms and signs and whose etiology, pathology and prognosis may be known or unknown.

Disorders -- A disorder is an imperfect functioning of part of the body or mind.

Diuretic -- A diuretic is a substance that promotes the excretion of urine. It increases urine flow, causing the kidneys to excrete more than the usual amount of sodium, potassium and water.

DNA -- DNA stands for deoxyribonucleic Acid (DNA). In 1953, geneticists James Watson and Francis Crick decipher DNA's structure. DNA is the substance in the cell nucleus that genetically codes amino acids and their peptide chain pattern and determines the type of life form into which a cell will develop.

Dose -- A dose is the quantity of a drug or other remedy to be taken or applied within a given period.

Drugs -- See *Prescription Drugs*.

Duodenal Ulcers -- They are ulcers of the duodenum of the small intestine.

Duodenum -- The duodenum is the portion of the small intestine starting in the lower end of the stomach and extending to the jejunum.

Dysentery -- Dysentery is a disease marked by frequent watery stools, often with blood and mucus, abdominal pain, tenesmus, fever and dehydration.

Dysfunction -- Dysfunction is difficult to abnormal function.

Eating Disorders -- Each year millions of people in the United States develop serious and sometimes life-threatening eating disorders. Approximately 90 percent are adolescent and young adult women.

E. Coli (Escherichia) -- A genus of gram-negative, facultatively anaerobic, rod-shaped bacteria found in the large intestine of humans and other warm-blooded animals. The organisms are nonpathogenic or opportunistic pathogens. Some strains are pathogenic and cause urinary tract infections, abscesses, conjunctivitis and sometimes septicemia, as well as diarrheal diseases, especially in children.

Insure raw meats (chicken, red meat...) do not come in direct or indirect contact with other foods you're preparing. The USDA recommends cooking hamburgers medium, to an internal temperature of at least 160 degrees to avoid E. Coli and Salmonella bacteria. To prevent the spread of E. Coli and Salmonella bacteria, Clorox Bleach recommends sanitizing all surfaces (cutting boards, cooking utensils, dish towel...) which come in contact with raw foods that may carry E. Coli and Salmonella bacteria like chicken, red meat... Knives, cutlery and other utensils should be washed and rinsed the follow through with the Clorox Bleach Sanitizing Solution*, then drain and air dry. Other items like dish towels and kitchen linen should be laundered according to the directions on the Clorox Bleach bottle.

Clorox Bleach Sanitizing Solution: After washing and rinsing all cookware, mix one tablespoon of regular Clorox Bleach with 01 gallon of water. Soak cookware in the solution for two minutes, drain and air dry. For cutting boards use three (03) tablespoons of Clorox bleach instead of two.

Edema -- Edema is fluid retention in the body resulting in swelling.

EDTA -- EDTA stands for Ethylene Diamine Tetraacetic Acid. It is an organic molecule used in Chelation Therapy.

EEG -- EEG stands for Electroencephalogram. It is a test measuring brain wave activity.

Efficacious -- Efficacious means capable of producing the desired effect. It also means having the potential to do it.

EKG or ECG -- EKG or ECG stands for Electrocardiogram. It is a test that shows a tracing of the electrical conduction of the heart.

Electrodes -- Electrodes are small devices containing wires that conduct electrical waves from the brain to a machine that records them.

Electrolyte -- Electrolytes are ionized salts in blood, tissue fluids and cells including salts of sodium and potassium. A substance that can conduct electricity when it is in solution.

ELISA -- ELISA stands for Enzyme-Linked Immunosorbent Assay. It is a test that detects the presence of the AIDS virus antibody.

Elixir -- An elixir is a clear, sweetened, hydroalcoholic liquid intended for oral use. It is used either as vehicles or for the therapeutic effects of the active medicinal agents.

Embolism -- An embolism occurs when some part of the circulatory system is either partially or completely blocked by some obstructing mass that has traveled through the system. The most common cause of embolism is from blood clots from within the heart or blood vessels. Emboli resulting from blood clots are often treated with a variety of anticoagulants which are agents that inhibit normal clotting mechanisms in the blood. Common anticoagulants, like heparin and warfarin prevent additional clots from forming.

Embryo -- An embryo is the developing human individual from the time of implantation to the end of the eighth week after conception. It is characterized by the development of tissues and primary organs and organ tissues.

Empathy -- Empathy means understanding so intimate that the feelings, thoughts, and motives of one person are readily comprehended by another.

Emphysema -- Emphysema is also called chronic obstructive lung disease. Swelling and destruction of the lung and sacks of the lungs leads to a loss of their elasticity which causes a decreased ability to use life giving oxygen. Causes of emphysema are asbestos (work related), asthma, bronchitis, dust, other respiratory diseases, polluted air and smoking.

Endocrine System -- The hormones that are responsible for regulating your basic drives and emotions, controls growth and temperature...

Endocrinologist -- An endocrinologist is a specialist in disorders of the glands of internal secretion, such as diabetes.

Enureseis -- Urinary incontinence, may be intentional or involuntary but not due to a physical disorder.

Enzyme -- See *Enzymes* and *Enzyme Therapy*.

EPA -- EPA stands for Environmental Protection Agency.

EPA -- EPA stands for eicosapentaenoic acid. This is one of two nutrients found in Omega-3. The other nutrient that makes-up Omega-3 is called DHA, which stands for docosahexaenoic acid. Omega-3 is noted to protect against heart disease and stroke.

Epidemic -- An epidemic occurs suddenly in numbers clearly in excess of normal expectancy, especially of infectious diseases but applied to any disease, injury or other health-related event occurring in such outbreaks. See *Pandemic* and *Flu*.

Epidermis -- The epidermis is the outer, protective layer of the skin in vertebrates.

Epilepsy -- Epilepsi is a disease characterized by seizures. There are two types of seizures: Simple partial - sensory, where a change in sensation occurs. May be a loss of consciousness. Convulsive seizures which are characterized by abnormal muscular behavior, unconsciousness, convulsions and sometimes loss of bladder control.

Esophagus -- The esophagus is a tube that leads from the throat to the stomach.

Essential Fatty Acids -- They are substances that the body cannot manufacture and therefore must be supplied in the diet. SEE *Flax Seed*.

Essential Nutrients -- They are any single substance of the forty-five different nutrients needed by the body for building and repairing.

Excessive Compulsive Disorder -- Approximately 5 million Americans suffer from this affliction. See *Obsessive Compulsive Disorder (OCD)* in this section.

Exercise -- Exercise is bodily exertion for the sake of restoring the organs and functions to a healthy state or keeping them healthy.

Fat -- A body is composed of body fat and fat-free mass. Fat-free mass includes bone, body fluids, muscles and organs. Body fat is classified as essential fat or storage fat. Essential fat is needed for body function. This essential fat is stored in major body organs and tissues like bones, heart, intestines, kidneys, liver, lungs, muscles, spleen and throughout the central nervous system. Females have additional fat in the breast and pelvic region for child-bearing and other hormone-related functions.

The Bad Fat is excessive storage fat brought on by an unhealthy diet. Storage fat is the extra fat that accumulates in adipose cells (fat cells) around internal organs and beneath the skin surface. Fat cells are with you forever. They expand (2 to 3 times) and contract as energy is stored and burned. Each fat gram consumed has twice the calories of a carbohydrate.

Fat calories are harder to burn off than the same amount of calories from carbohydrates. Dietary fat is easily converted to body fat. On the other hand, only a small amount complex carbohydrates are converted to body fat. Saturated fats are high in cholesterol and increase blood cholesterol. Fat has 09 calories per gram compared to protein with 04 calories per gram and starches with 04 calories per gram. Want to lose weight? Reduce the fat in your diet.

FBS -- FBS stands for Fasting Blood Sugar (FBS). Blood is drawn before breakfast\after fasting, to get a accurate measurement of glucose (sugar) in the blood.

Fiber -- Fiber comes from plant foods. There is no fiber in foods like eggs, beef, cheese, chicken, pork... Fiber is not digested. It provides no calories. Fiber speeds up the elimination of waste and combats constipation. Fiber helps remove cholesterol (lowers cholesterol) and cancer-causing chemicals out of bodies system. Nutritionists recommend at least 35 grams and up to 70 grams of daily fiber.

Fiber helps food pass through the intestines faster and lowers the absorption of fat. So if you eat any fatty foods insure that fiber is consumed during your meal. A diet high in fiber can be a factor in lowering cholesterol levels.

Remember, fiber comes from plant foods. Read the Nutritional Facts on all food products that you purchase. Stay away from the foods that are high in saturated fats, sodium and cholesterol. Choose foods that are have little or no fats, sodium and cholesterol but have ample protein, carbohydrates, fiber, Vitamins...

According to Dr. Elaine Fox, (Chief Nutritionist and the Executive Director of the North Nassau Health Center, New york -- The Guide to a Healthier Diet -- Eat Well Be Well VIDEO), fiber is the undigestible portion of food (fruits, vegetables & whole grains).

Fiber draws water to it thus increasing the health of the gastrointestinal system. If food stays in the lower bowel (colon) for too long, bacteria breaks down residues of fat that cause cancer producing chemicals. Fiber increases the transit time (time between when the food is consumed to when it is eliminated), so that the residue of food doesn't stay in the lower bowel too long which may cause bacteria that could break down residues of fat causing cancer producing chemicals.

Transit time should be between 24 to 36 hours. Good nutrition balances the transit time. If transit time is beyond 36 hours, gradually increase your fiber. Fiber also helps to bind cholesterol. Consuming fiber seems to lower cholesterol as well as being nutritious. Any whole grain has fiber as well brown rice (versus white rice), oat bran, wheat bran, fruits and vegetables (especially carrots).

Five Deadly Whites -- The five deadly whites are (listed in order as the most dangerous threat to your health): Meat, Dairy, Salt, Sugar and White Flour. See *The Five Deadly Whites*.

Flavonoid -- One family of phytochemicals, these antioxidants are natural compounds found in red wine, and in almost all fruits and vegetables. Flavonoids have been noted to help protect against heart disease and possibly cancer.

Flu -- The flu is the popular name for influenza. It is an acute viral infection involving the respiratory tract, occurring in isolated cases, in epidemics or in pandemics striking continents simultaneously or in sequence. The incubation period is 01 to 03 days and the disease usually lasts 03 to 10 days. There are a variety of influenzas.

Folic Acid -- Folic acid is considered brain food and needed for energy production and formation of red blood cells. It helps with protein metabolism. In addition to protecting against adult diseases, folic acid reduces the risk of birth defects in a fetus's developing nervous system by 50 percent!

The evidence is so strong that the Centers for Disease Control and Prevention (CDC) recommends that all women who may become pregnant consume 400mcg of folic acid a day. Folic Acid helps regulate embryonic and fetal development of nerve cells, vital for normal growth and development. Folic Acid works best with Vitamin B12. A sore, red tongue may be one sign of Folic Acid deficiency.

Significant sources of Folic Acid are barley, beans, beef, bran, brown rice, cheese, chicken, dates, green leafy vegetables, lamb, lentils, liver, milk, oranges, organ meats, split peas, pork, root vegetables, tuna, wheat germ, whole grains, whole wheat and yeast.

WARNING: Oral contraceptives may increase the need for Folic Acid. High doses of Folic Acid for extended periods should be avoided by anyone with a hormone-related cancer or convulsive disorder.

Food Poisoning -- Food poisoning refers to an illness caused by the ingestion of food that is either poisonous itself, such as wild poisonous mushrooms or that has been contaminated, usually by bacteria or their toxic by-products. The Food and Drug Administration estimates that 1 out of 10 people get sick every year from food poisoning. To prevent illness from food, it's important to know that microbes pose the biggest threat of food-borne illness. Powerful toxins produced by the microbes that have been introduced into the food by the fingernails area of someone who has handled the food as it travels from the factory to the table.

Everyone handling food must wash their hands as well as clean their fingernails. Also, keep juices from poultry or meat away from other food. Food poisoning can be caused by bacteria, bacterial toxins or poisons and by poisonous berries, fungi and insecticides or other harmful chemicals. Symptoms of food poisoning usually begin within 24 hours of eating contaminated foods and commonly include abdominal pain, chills, diarrhea, fever, nausea and vomiting.

Fracture -- A fracture is a break in a bone or cartilage. Some consequences of a fracture are infection; damage to blood vessels, internal organs and nerves.

Free Radical -- A free radical is an atom or group of atoms that has at least one unpaired electron. Because another element can easily pick up this free electron and cause a chemical reaction, these free radicals can affect dramatic and destructive changes in the body. Free radicals are activated in heated and rancid oils and by radiation in the atmosphere, among other things.

Free Radical Scavenger -- A free radical scavenger is a substance that removes or destroys free radicals.

Fructose -- D-Fructose, a ketohexose C6H12O6 occurring in honey and many sweet fruits.

Functional Electrical Stimulation (FES) -- FES devices have been used in Europe for over 20 years. A FES device is designed to cure incontinence by building strength of the weak involuntary muscles that control the flow of urine from the bladder through the urethra. The FES device is designed for women and can be obtained by prescription.

Fungus -- Fungus is a general term used to denote a group of eukaryotic protitis (cell types except bacteria) including molds, mushrooms, rusts, smuts, yeast... which are characterized by the absence of chlorophyll.

Gallstones -- Gallstones are an accumulation of crystallized cholesterol and bile that forms stones. The condition is most common in women over 40 who are overweight and have had children. Gallstones are often found in diabetics, the obese and elderly. Symptoms include jaundice (yellowish skin), clay colored stools and dark urine.

Severe right upper abdominal pain that may radiate to the shoulder and back and nausea and or vomiting are other symptoms after ingesting heavy fat or fried foods. Approximately 1/2 the population with gallstones do not have symptoms.

Gastric Ulcer -- A gastric ulcer is an ulcer in the mucous membrane lining the stomach.

Gastritis -- Gastritis is the inflammation of the stomach lining.

Gastroenteritis -- Gastroenteritis is the inflammation of the stomach and the intestines.

Gastroenterologist -- A gastroenterologist is a specialist in disease of the digestive tract.

Gastrointestinal System -- The gastrointestinal system pertains to the stomach, small and large intestines, colon, rectum, liver, pancreas and gallbladder.

Gelotology -- Gelotology is the study of humor and its effects on the body. Studies have indicated that laughter and other positive emotions boost the body's natural defenses against disease, pain and stress.

Genes -- Genes are sections of a chromosome. Each gene contains specific information that directs cellular purposes and controls the development of an individual.

Genetics -- Austrian monk, Gregor Johann Mendel discovered natural laws governing direct inheritance by offspring of certain traits or characteristics from one or the other parent. The modern study genetics derives from his work. Genetics is the branch of science concerned with hereditary.

Genitourinary System -- The urinary and reproductive organs and the difference between men and women.

Genus -- A taxonomic category (taxon) subordinate to a tribe (or sub-tribe) and superior to a species (or subgenus).

GERD -- More than 60 million Americans experience heartburn at least once a month and some 15 million Americans experience heartburn symptoms each day. Frequent heartburn (02 or more times a week), food sticking, blood or weight loss may be associated with a more severe gastroesophageal reflux disease (GERD).

Germ -- A germ is a microorganism such as a bacterium or virus, especially one causing disease.

Germanium -- Germanium is a substance that promotes healing by alerting the immune system, reducing harmful deposits and destroying free radicals, dangerous by products that float throughout the body causing a decline in health.

Gerontologist -- A gerontologist is one involved in the scientific study of the aging process and the problems and disease associated with it.

Gestational Diabetes -- Carbohydrate intolerance during pregnancy usually resolving after delivery.

Ghee -- Ghee is a form of butter. Milk solids have been removed to form clarified butter. It's noted to have healing properties. So don't sludge-up your arteries, look into this product! Go to your local health food store and ask for Ghee available from Purity Farms. See Purity Farms.

Gingivitis -- Gingivitis is inflammation of the gums surrounding the teeth.

GI Tract -- Gastrointestinal tract consists of the stomach, intestines and colon.

Gland -- A gland is an organ that excretes materials and manufactures substances not needed for its own metabolic function.

Glaucoma -- Glaucoma is a disease of the eye characterized by high intraocular pressure, damaged optic disk, hardening of the eyeball and partial or complete loss of vision. Glaucoma is the second leading cause of blindness. Symptoms include discomfort, halos around lights, impaired vision, inability to adjust from light to dark areas, loss of peripheral vision and pain.

Glucose -- Glucose is a dextrorotatory monosaccharide (hexose) found in the free state in fruits and other parts of plants.

Glycogen -- Glycogen is the form in which carbohydrates are stored in the human body for future conversion into sugar and for use in performing muscular work and distributing heat through the body. Glycogen is formed from sugar and is transformed into glucose as needed.

Gout – Gout is caused when there's a build-up of uric acid in the blood which eventually leads to a painful arthritis-like condition in a joint(s).

Gram -- A gram is a unit of weight. Many Nutritional Fact labels address   fat, cholesterol, sodium, carbohydrates, protein and sugar, in grams. Thirty grams is equal to one ounce or two tablespoons, or 1/8th cup. So when you see a Nutritional Fact label that states 03 grams of saturated fat and there are 10 servings and you ate all 10 servings you just ate 30 grams of fat, or two tablespoons of fat, or 1/8th cup of fat. Doesn't seem like much but it surely is a great deal of fat, especially if you eat like this from day to day.

Gulf War Syndrome -- A term used to denote many debilitating medical problems of soldiers involved in the Gulf War (January - February 1991). As of 1996, the Department of Defense (DOD) dedicated $15 million to research the possible effects of chemical exposure to Gulf War veterans. Approximately 30,000 Gulf War veterans have been plagued by mysterious symptoms, which include joint pain, rashes, sleep disorders and stomach disorders. According to the DOD, as of December 1996, the Veteran's Administration has approved more than 26,000 disability claims for Gulf War Veterans with diagnosed and undiagnosed illnesses. In January of 1997, President Clinton is scheduled to review the findings of the White House Advisory Committee on Gulf War veteran illnesses. The Veterans Affairs Committee has established a HELPLINE for Gulf War Veterans: 1-800-749-8387 who have questions pertaining to this subject.

Gynecologist -- A gynecologist is a specialist in the female reproductive system.

Handicap -- Mental or physical defect that may or may not be congenital that prevents the individual from participating in normal life activities - implies disadvantage.

Hantavirus -- A genus of Bunyaviridae responsible for pneumonia and hemorrhagic fevers. An outbreak of hantavirus infection, the Hantavirus Pulmonary Syndrome (HAS), causing severe and often fatal pulmonary symptoms was identified in the Four-Corners region of the U.S. in 1993.

Hard Water -- Hard water is caused by minerals like calcium and magnesium dissolved in the water. Safe for drinking and showering, hard water is noted to make your water taste good. Showering with regular soap reacts with the minerals in the hard water to form soap scum that leaves a drying film on your skin.

Headache -- A headache is a pain and pressure in different areas of the head. Headaches are not a disease. Sinus Headaches are caused by overproduction of mucous in the membranes. Vascular Headaches are caused by the tightening and contraction of muscles in the area of the neck, forehead and scalp. Migraine Headaches are caused by the alternating constriction and dilation of blood vessels in the brain.

Healing -- Healing means curing or restoring to health.

Heart -- The heart is a hollow, muscular organ that maintains blood circulation throughout your entire body every second of every day. The heart has four chambers, through which blood passes. Valves control the movement of the blood through these compartments. The blood flows from two large veins into the upper right chamber. The blood continues down to the lower chamber. From the right lower chamber, blood is pumped to the lungs, where carbon dioxide (waste product from the cells) is exchanged for oxygen. The rejuvenated blood then returns to the upper left chamber, where it then passes through the left lower chamber which forces the blood away from the heart through the main artery which extends through the chest and abdomen to other arteries and to all tissues of your body.

Heart Attack -- A heart attack (myocardial infarction) occurs when one or more of the coronary arteries is partially blocked by atherosclerosis and a blood clot plugs the remaining opening. The part of the heart muscle beyond the blockage is deprived of oxygen which results in injury or death of that part of the heart muscle.

If that part of the heart muscle is large enough or vital area of the heart, the casualty may die. A symptom of a heart attack is a crushing pain in the middle of the chest, behind the breastbone. The pain may also extend down one or both arms and into the neck, back, teeth or jaws. Fatigue, heavy perspiration, dizziness, difficulty in breathing and fever may also be present.

The immediate treatment for a heart attack is cardiopulmonary resuscitation (CPR). Professional medical help should be called immediately. Prevention of heart attacks begins with reading this entire book, EATING THE RIGHT STUFF and periodic check-ups with your doctor. **WARNING:** Symptoms or signs of a heart attack may differ between men and women.

Heartburn -- Heartburn is an esophageal symptom consisting of a retrosternal sensation of warmth or burning that rises in the chest. If severe, it may include the neck and head. Avoid lying down and seek medical attention.

Heart Murmurs -- Heart murmurs are the extra whishing sounds in addition to the regular "lub-dub" sounds of the heart beat that are made as blood flows through the chambers and valves of the heart. In most cases, heart murmurs are harmless. In other cases, heart murmurs may be an indicator of heart disease or a structural abnormality in the heart.

Heat Stroke -- Heat stroke is an exposure to intense heat which overwhelms the body's internal heat regulating system. The protective sweating reflex ceases to function. The body's temperature rises dangerously too high to temperatures of 104 degrees and above. Shock, coma, brain damage, kidney failure or even death may result. Heat stroke claims approximately 200 lives each year in the United States. When weather is hot and humid, pay close attention to the heat index. However, try doing this.

When the temperature and humidity add up to more than 180, stay inside, in an airconditioned building. Monitor the weather reports for humidity and heat readings as well as the heat index. Most weather reports will give advice on outdoor activities during heat waves. Drink plenty of water.

Heimlich Maneuver -- The Heimlich Maneuver is a method invented by Dr. Henry Heimlich for dislodging food or other material from the throat of a choking victim.

Hemorrhage -- A hemorrhage is the escape of blood from the vessels; bleeding.

Hemorrhagic Strokes -- Hemorrhagic strokes produce bleeding into the brain.

Hemorrhoid -- Hemorrhoids, often called piles, are enlarged veins inside or just outside the anal canal, which is the opening at the end of the large intestine. As the veins swell, they cause severe inflammation and discomfort. Causes of hemorrhoids are the result of habitual postponement of bowel movements and undesirable straining during elimination.

Another source of hemorrhoid irritation comes from pressure on the veins due to diseases of the liver or heart or from a tumor. Pregnancy may also contribute in the development of hemorrhoids, due to the enlarged uterus increases pressure on the veins. A poor diet plays a role in the development of hemorrhoids.

A diet containing a high proportion of refined foods rather than natural roughage increases the likelihood of constipation, reflecting the likelihood of hemorrhoids. Hemorrhoids can be treated by taking a warm sitz bath (sitting in a tub of warm water), over-the-counter preparations and prescriptions from your doctor. If hemorrhoids become a serious problem a surgical procedure called hemorrhoidectomy, removes the dilated portions of the affected vein and ties off the remaining parts of the vein. Newer procedures called cryosurgery and laser surgery, remove the hemorrhoid, but with less pain and fewer postoperative complications.

HEPA -- HEPA stands for High Efficiency Particulate Air. HEPA filters are recognized as the most efficient media for removing sub-micron size particles from the air (bacteria, dust, harmful fibers, house dust mites, mold spores, pollen, smoke particles....).

How HEPA filters work without going into great detail, it's like trying to blow a grain of sand through a stack of hay!

Hepatitis -- Hepatitis is the inflammation of the liver usually resulting in jaundice (yellowing of the skin and the whites of the eyes). Caused by a viral infection. Approximately 5 million Americans have hepatitis! Hepatitis is caused by several viruses. The most common are:

- **Hepatitis A** - Transmitted from person to person through contaminated food or water or contact with the stools of an infected person. May be epidemic where the water supply is contaminated and sanitation is poor. Hepatitis A virus can be more infectious than the AIDS virus.

- **Hepatitis B** - Virus enters the bloodstream through contact with contaminated blood, semen, stools or contaminated hypodermic needles. Hepatitis B virus can be more infectious than the AIDS virus.

- **Hepatitis C** - Virus is presumed to be a major cause of what was previously known as "non-A, non-B hepatitis." Transmission is similar to Hepatitis B. Frequently causes chronic hepatitis (more than 6 months). Hepatitis C virus can be more infectious than the AIDS virus.

Untreated hepatitis may lead to scarring of the liver and liver cancer. You may be at risk for hepatitis if exposed to infected blood or body fluids via body piercing, sharing razors, sharing toothbrushes and tattooing. Unprotected sex with many partners or experimentation with intravenous drugs also puts you at high risk! See your chosen physician for hepatitis testing and diagnosis. In many cases, hepatitis can be treated. Call the American Liver Foundation at 1-800-223-0179 for free information.

Herbal Therapy -- Various herbal combinations are used for healing as well as cleansing purposes. Herbs are utilized in the form of tablets, capsules, extracts, tinctures and herbal baths with poultices. Herbs are a valuable compliment to many therapies.

Herbs -- Herbs are any leafy plant without a woody stem, especially one used as a household remedy or as a flavoring.

Heredity -- Heredity is the genetic transmission of a particular quality or trait from parent to offspring.

Herpes -- Herpes is any inflammatory skin disease caused by a herpes virus characterized by the formation of clusters of small vesicles (small sacs containing liquid).

High Blood Pressure -- Blood pressure is pressure of your blood against your artery walls. Your blood pressure fluctuates between a high reading (when you first wake-up, nervous or excited) or low when you're sleeping or resting. A blood pressure reading may have to be taken twice to determine your normal reading. High blood pressure is also called hypertension. When your blood pressure stays up no matter what time of day, your activity or your mood this is good indicator that you have high blood pressure/hypertension!

Approximately 125 million Americans have high blood pressure! Many have no idea their blood pressure is dangerously high!

High blood pressure may increase with age, it tends to run in the family, twice as common in blacks than in whites, more common in men than in women and overweight people are more apt to have hypertension than non-obese people. If one or both of your parents have high blood pressure, you should have your blood pressure checked as soon as possible and several times a year. Many clinics, hospitals and medical mobile vans offer free checkups.

There really are no symptoms for high blood pressure, meaning you can't feel it, taste it or notice signs directly indicating that you have high blood pressure. That is why high blood pressure is called *"THE SILENT KILLER"*. If you have high blood pressure you can feel just fine, just great one moment then POW!!!

High-Density Lipoprotein (HDL) -- HDL is called the "GOOD CHOLESTEROL". HDL's job is to find LDL\bad cholesterol that is stuck to your blood vessels, liberates the LDL from the blood vessel and takes it back to the liver to be reprocessed to new VLDL or broken down and excreted as waste.

Histamine -- A histamine is a substance produced by the body during an allergic reaction.

HMO -- Health Maintenance Organization offers comprehensive health care to its members for a set fee each month. Check-ups, physical exams, visits, surgery hospital services, emergency care and other health care are covered.

Hodgkin's Disease -- It is cancer of the lymphatic system and lymph nodes. The job of the lymphatic system is to help fight disease and infection. Hodgkin's disease is rare. It accounts for approximately 01 percent of all cases of cancer in the U.S. Hodgkin's Disease is most often seen in young people aged 15 to 34 and in people over the age of 55. The most common symptoms of Hodgkin's disease is a painless swelling in the lymph nodes in the neck, underarm, or groin. Other symptoms of Hodgkin's Disease could include fevers, night sweats, tiredness, weight loss or itching skin.

Now, because of conventional treatment such as radiation therapy and combination chemotherapy, more than 75 percent of all newly diagnosed Hodgkin's disease patients are curable (see remission in this section). Recover chances improve as scientists find new and effective treatments.

Holistic -- Holistic pertains to holism (the theory that reality is made up of organic or unified wholes that are greater than the simple sum of their parts).

Homeopathy -- Homeopathy is a system of medicine based on the belief that the cure of disease can be affected by minute doses of substances that, if given to a healthy person in large doses, would produce the same symptoms as are present in the disease being treated. Homeopath employs natural substances in small doses to stimulate the body's reactive process to remove toxic waste and bring the body back into balance.

Homeopathy is a scientific teaching that is based on using specifically prepared, natural remedies to stimulate YOUR BODY'S INHERENT ABILITY TO HEAL ITSELF!
 Homeopathy was first discovered in the late 18th century by German physician-chemist Christian Hahnemann. Homeopathy is based on the premise known as the *"Law of Simulars"* which means whatever symptoms a substance will cause in a healthy person, it will create a healing response in an ill person. In the United States, Europe and in many other countries, homeopathic physicians are fully licensed M.D.'s.

Homocysteine -- Homocysteine attacks the heart muscle and allows the deposition of cholesterol around the heart muscle.

Hospice -- Hospice is an institution that specializes in the care of the terminally ill.

Hospital -- A hospital is an institution providing medical or surgical care and treatment for people who are ill, injured, obstetric treatment for women, psychiatric treatment for the mentally ill...

Is your hospital safe? Approximately 180,000 Americans die from mistakes (medical malpractice) in hospitals throughout the U.S. each year! How can you avoid a bad hospital?
- Word of mouth.
- Referral.
- Ask plenty of questions to your doctor.
- Have a family member with you or a patient advocate.
- Request a "Hospital Effectiveness Report" (report card).

As of 1995, by state law, Pennsylvania is the only state that has this report available to the public. The National Practitioner Data Bank has computer records of hospital discipline against doctors but this information is not available to the public!

Host -- A host is an organism in which another microorganism lives and obtains nourishment.

Hot Flash -- A hot flash is a transient vasomotor symptom of the menopause, resulting in from hormone imbalance, that involves dilation of the skin capillaries and the sensation of heat over all or part of the body.

Human Immunodeficiency Virus (HIV) -- HIV is a virus which is carried in the blood, semen and other body fluids, invades and destroys a specific type of white blood cell - T4 lymphocyte - a main component of the body's immune system. The virus multiplies over a period of several months producing fever, fatigue, sore throat, skin rash... Increasing numbers of T4 lymphocytes are destroyed by the virus causing symptoms of fever, swollen glands, night sweats, diarrhea, weight loss... Full blown AIDS may be diagnosed at a later time.

Huntington's Disease -- This is a relatively common autosomal dominant disease characterized by chronic progressive chorea and mental deterioration terminating in dementia. The age of onset is variable but occurs in the fourth decade of life. Death usually follows within 15 years. See chorea in this section.

Hydration -- Clinically, hydration is the taking in of water to correct a deficit, as in dehydration. See *Forced Hydration*.

Hyaluronic Acid -- This is an organic acid known as the most effective natural moisturizer. It is present in your skin and is able to hold 500 times its weight in water.

Hyperactivity -- Hyperactivity is a malfunction of the mechanism in the central nervous system which causes an excessive amount of energy. This demonstrated high level of energy leads to aggressive behavior, clumsiness, frustrations, poor concentration and poor sleeping patterns. Another name for hyperactivity is minimal brain dysfunction syndrome or attention deficit disorder (ADD). See *ADD* in this section.

Hypercholesterolemia -- This is elevated blood cholesterol. It is an excessive amount of cholesterol in the blood.

Hyperlipidemia -- This is elevated blood fats.

Hyperpyrexia -- This is abnormally high fever, with a body temperature of 106 degrees or above.

Hypertension -- Hypertension is high blood pressure.

Hyperthermia -- Hyperthermia is unusually high fever often artificially induced for therapeutic purposes.

Hyperventilation -- This is excessive or overbreathing resulting in a loss of carbon dioxide from the blood. It is frequently found in diseases such as asthma or in induced states of anxiety.

Hypnotherapy -- See *Hypnotherapy*.

Hypoglycemia -- Hypoglycemia is an abnormally low level of blood sugar causing the body and brain's energy levels to become incapacitated. This may lead to extreme fatigue and possibly coma or death.

Hypotension -- Hypotension is low blood pressure.

Hypotensive -- Hypotensive is any remedies that lower abnormally elevated blood pressure.

Hypothalamus -- The hypothalmus is a gland which contains neurosecretions that are of importance in the control of certain metabolic activities, such as water balance, sugar and fat metabolism, regulation of body temperature and secretion of releasing and inhibiting hormones.

Hypothyroidism -- Hypothyroidism is an underactive thyroid. Your thyroid regulates your body's basic rate of activity. Symptoms of an underactive thyroid are: chronic fatigue, depression, dysfunctional uterine bleeding, edema, fatigue, fibrocystic disease, hair loss, infertility, irregular menstrual bleeding, obesity, reduced immune function (leading to chronic colds, allergic diseases like chronic sinusitis).... Self-test:

If your underarm temperature is below 97.4 (early morning), you may have hypothyroidism. Seek out a doctor that is knowledgeable about the treatment of hypothyroidism using *"desiccated bovine thyroid"* - (most common brand is Armour thyroid).

Idiopathic -- Denoting a disease of unknown cause.

Illness -- An illness is a morbus, illness, sickness, an interruption, cessation, or disorder of the body functions, systems or organs.

Imaging -- Imaging is the production of images of internal organs of the body. Imaging techniques include x-ray, nuclear medicine procedures, CT scans and Magnetic Resonance Imaging (MRI).

Immune Reaction -- An immune reaction results in a antibody production.

Immune System -- The immune system is a combination of cells and proteins that assist in the host's ability to fight, resist foreign substances such as viruses and harmful bacteria. The liver, spleen, thymus, bone marrow and lymphatic system are interrelated in the immune system's normal function.

Immunity -- Immunity is the condition that enables a living organism to resist and overcome disease or infection.

Immunization -- An immunization's purpose is to render unaffected or resistant to disease. If you plan on traveling outside the borders of the United States, there are two kinds of immunizations:
* Recommended vaccinations which are optional for the traveler's own protection.
* Required vaccinations which are for the host country's protection and to prevent diseases between countries.

Immunodeficiency -- This is any immune reaction deficiency involving antibody or cell-mediated immunity.

Immunology -- Immunology is the science dealing with the specific mechanism by which living tissues react to foreign biological material in a way which may enhance resistance or immunity.

Immunosuppressive -- This is a substance which suppresses the body's natural immune response to an antigen.

Immunotherapy -- This is a technique used to stimulate or strengthen a person's own immune system.

Impotence -- Impotence is an inability to maintain an erection of the penis.

Incontinence -- Incontinence means incapable of controlling the passage of urine or feces. Approximately 40 million Americans have incontinence. Besides surgery, one effective treatment for incontinence is known as Kegel exercises. Kegel exercises strengthen the pelvic-floor muscles. To do them, tense the muscles you would tense if you were trying to hold back urine. Kegel exercises can be done anywhere and as often as you like.

Infarct -- Infarct is the death of part of a tissue due to lack of blood.

Infection -- An infection is multiplication of parasitic organisms within the body. Multiplication of the normal flora of the intestinal tract is not considered an infection.

Infectious Disease -- This is a disease which has the capability to spread or affect others. Do you want to take the first step in cutting down infectious diseases? WASH YOUR HANDS! Always wash your hands prior, in-between, and after preparing any meal. Wash your hands after using the bathroom, or doing any work. When in doubt wash your hands! See *Antibacterial*, *Salmonella* and *E. Coli* in this section.

Inflammation -- Inflammation is an immune reaction that occurs in response to any type of bodily injury. It may include heat, pain, redness and swelling.

Influenza -- See *Flu* in this section.

Infusion(s) -- The introduction of a solution into a vein by slow injection.

Inorganic -- Inorganic pertains to substances not of organic origin.

Inositol -- Inositol is vital for hair growth as well as preventing hardening of the arteries. Inositol is important in lecithin formation as well as fat and cholesterol metabolism. It also helps remove fat from the liver. Sources of Inositol are fruits, meats, milk, vegetables and whole grains.
WARNING: Drinking heavy amounts of caffeine may cause a shortage of inositol in the body.

Inpatient -- An inpatient is a patient who comes to the hospital, clinic, or dispensary for diagnosis and\or treatment and requires a bed for an extended time while under care of their respective doctor and medical staff.

Insoluble Fiber -- Insoluble fibers are able to add bulk to food mass - moving food through the digestive system thus reducing transit time.

Insomnia -- Insomnia is the inability to fall asleep within a normal amount of time, which is about five to ten minutes. It is also the inability to stay asleep without awakening two to three hours after going to sleep.

Insulin -- Insulin is an essential hormone produced by the pancreas. It regulates the metabolism of carbohydrates\sugar in the body. It is used in the treatment and control of diabetes.

Intelligence Quotient (IQ) -- IQ is an index of an individual's tested mental ability as compared to the rest of the population, usually arrived at by dividing an individual's mental age by his chronological age and multiplying by 100.

Interstitial Cystitis -- Interstitial cystitis is an inflammatory condition of the bladder.

Intestinal Flora -- Intestinal flora are all the harmless and beneficial bacteria that live in the intestinal tract.

Intestine(s) -- The intestines are the digestive tract passing from the stomach to the anus.

Intravenously -- This means to introduce, usually injected, into a vein.

IRISAP -- Intensive Research Information Services And Products. See *IRISAP* in the POC Section.

Ischemia -- Ischemia is the reduced blood supply to the heart due to atherosclerosis.

IU -- International Unit is equal to approximately a milligram.

Juicer Machines -- See *Juice Therapy*.

Kidney Disease -- Millions of Americans are afflicted with kidney disease. Each year, thousands of Americans die from these diseases. The following are brief descriptions of various kidney diseases.

- **Infection** - The most common disorder of the kidneys and of the urinary tract. Cystitis is a bladder infection. Symptoms include urgent, frequent and painful urination. Pyelonephritis is a kidney infection. It may cause fever, back pain and chills or possibly no symptoms.

- **Obstructions** - Kidney stones are hard deposits in the urinary tract can block drainage and cause damage or infection. Cysts are hollow spaces in kidney tissue. The cysts displace healthy tissue and can become infected, harming surrounding tissue.

- **Hypertension** - High blood pressure often accompanies many cases of kidney disease. Prolonged high blood pressure damages small arteries in the kidneys. This may start an unhealthy cycle, since damaged kidneys may cause more serious hypertension and further kidney damage.

- **Glomerulonephritis** - Also called nephritis or Bright's Disease. This kidney disease is an inflammation of the glomeruli (small blood vessels in the nephrons). This disease frequently occurs in children and young adults. Patients with the chronic form suffer slow progressive damage. Eventually the patient may need dialysis (artificial kidney treatment), and\or transplantation.

- **Nephrosis** - Also called nephrotic syndrome, it involves an abnormal leakage of protein into the urine. The most obvious symptom is generalized swelling, especially under eyes upon weakening.

Other diseases like diabetes may damage kidney function. Some drugs, solvents and insecticides may harm the kidneys. Approximately 20 million Americans suffer from urinary and kidney diseases.

Kidney Failure -- This is also called renal failure\uremia. When the kidneys are so diseased or damaged from injury they longer can clean waste products from the blood.

- Acute Kidney Failure is a sudden, usually short-term loss of kidney function. Dialysis may help the patient through this period of kidney failure.

- End-Stage Renal Disease is permanent, irreversible damage to both kidneys. It requires a dialysis or a kidney transplant.

According to the National Kidney Foundation, 40,000 Americans are currently awaiting a life-saving heart, kidney, liver, lung, pancreas or bone-marrow transplant. The National Kidney Foundation is urging all Americans to sign Uniform Organ Donor cards and to discuss their decision with family members. To request a free donor card call 1-800-622-9010. Simply follow the recorded instructions.

Kidneys -- The kidneys are bean-shaped and located in back of the abdomen. The kidneys chief functions are to filter waste from the blood (15 gallons of blood per hour) and to insure reabsorption of essential chemicals back into the bloodstream. Kidneys also help in blood pressure regulation and the production of red blood cells.

Blood enters the kidneys through the artery from the heart. The blood is cleaned by passing through millions of nephrons (blood filters - 02 1/2 million). Waste material that is filtered out by the nephrons passes through ureter and is stored in the bladder as urine. Once the bladder becomes full, urine passes out of the body through the urethra. Newly cleaned blood returns to the bloodstream via veins.

Kidney Stones -- Kidney stones are an abnormal accumulation of mineral salts that are formulated in the kidneys. There are three types of kidney stones: Stones that are formed from calcium oxalic acid are most typical. Oxalic acids are derived from dairy products, dark green leafy vegetables like spinach and kale, nuts, rhubarb and tea. Stones formed in uric acid. Stones formed from cystine, the result of too much protein in the diet.

Lactic Acid -- Lactic acid is an inorganic acid present in skin and human tissue that is natural moisturizing agent.

Lactose Intolerance -- A condition that results in abnormal cramps, nausea, bloating or diarrhea when milk is consumed.

Laxative -- A laxative is a substance which promotes bowel movements.

LDL -- LDL stands for Low-Density Lipoprotein. Once VLDL drops-off the fat throughout your body it becomes empty VLDL or better yet LDL. LDL becomes *"BAD CHOLESTEROL"* because pieces of LDL become stuck along blood vessel walls on its way back to the liver to be reprocessed to new VLDL or broken down and excreted as waste.

These pieces of LDL become stuck narrowing the blood vessel walls. This leads to high blood pressure and possibly heart disease. You already read the section on Blood Pressure so you know the consequences of high blood pressure.

Lead Poisoning -- Lead is undoubtedly, one of the most toxic metal contaminants. It is a poison that is retained in the bones, brain, central nervous system, glands and hair. Sources of lead are: bone meal, canned fruit (lead soldered cans leaches out and absorbed by the fruit), ceramic glazes, some domestic and imported wines, garden vegetables, insecticides, lead-acid batteries used in autos, lead-based paint, leaded gasoline, lead pipes, piping with solder, tobacco and water.

Lethargy -- Lethargy is abnormal drowsiness.

Leukemia -- Leukemia is cancer of the lymph glands and bone marrow resulting in overproduction of white blood cells (related to Hodgkin's Disease).

Ligament -- A ligament is a band of fibrous tissue that connects bones or cartilages, serving to support and strengthen the joints.

Limbic System -- The limbic system is a part of the brain governing basic activities, such as self-preservation, reproduction and the expression of fear & rage.

Lipid -- A lipid is a liquid fat or fatty substance.

Lipoprotein - These are packages of cholesterol, protein and triglycerides which circulate through the bloodstream.

Liver -- The liver is the largest organ of the body. The liver secretes bile and acts in the formation of blood and in the metabolism of carbohydrates, fats, proteins, minerals and Vitamins. The liver also removes worn-out cells from the blood and reprocesses their red pigment hemoglobin.

Liver Disease -- See cirrhosis (common disease) in this section.

Lobectomy -- A lobectomy is the surgical removal of an entire lobe of the lung.

Low Blood Pressure -- Low blood pressure is also called hypotension.

Lungs -- Your lungs are part of the respiratory system. They are cone-shaped organs composed of soft, spongy, pinkish-gray tissue. The function of the lungs is to exchange gases between the body and the atmosphere. Your lungs alternately take in oxygen, which is vitally required by your body's cells and expel carbon dioxide, a cellular waste product.

Lupus -- Lupus is a chronic, autoimmune disease which causes inflammation of various parts of the body, especially the skin, joints, blood and kidneys. The body's immune system normally makes proteins called antibodies to protect the body against viruses, bacteria and other foreign materials. Theses foreign materials are called antigens.

In an autoimmune disorder like lupus, the immune system loses its ability to differentiate between foreign substances (antigens) and its own cells and tissues. These antibodies are called *"auto-antibodies,"* react with the self-antigens to form immune complexes. The immune complexes build up tissue and can cause inflammation, injury to tissues and pain. According to the Lupus Foundation of America market research data (Bruskin\Goldring Research, 1994), between 1,400,000 and 2,000,000 people have been diagnosed with lupus.

On 30 October 1995, the division of Rheumatology at the St. Luke's-Roosevelt Hospital Center in Manhattan is participating in several clinical trials. One of the clinical trials "A new drug (DHEA) for patients with lupus."

Lyme Disease -- Lyme disease is an infection caused by a bacterial spirochete spread by a bite from an infected tick. Lyme Disease may affect several organ systems months or years after the bite. Untreated, the infection may affect the brain, heart and joints. Lyme Disease is more common in the Northeastern states and to a lesser extent in the Midwest. Signs and symptoms of lyme disease include chill, fever, fatigue, headache, muscle & joint pain, swollen lymph nodes and a skin rash called erythema migrans.

Erythema migrans is a red circular patch that appears at the site of the bite, usually 3 to 30 days after the bite of the infected tick. Lyme Disease got its name from Old Lyme, Connecticut where the disease was identified.

Lymph -- Lymph is a clear, transparent, watery sometimes faintly yellowish liquid, derived from body tissues that contain mainly white blood cells and travels through the lymphatic system to return to the venous bloodstream through the thoracic duct.

Lymph Glands -- Lymph glands are located in the lymph vessels of the body. These glands trap foreign material and produce lymphocytes. These glands act as filters in the lymph system and contain and form lymphocytes and permit lymphatic cells to destroy certain foreign agents.

Lymphangiogram -- This is an x-ray of the lymphatic system. A special dye is injected in order to outline the lymphatic vessels and organs.

Lymphatic System -- The lymphatic system is the interconnected system of spaces and vessels between tissues and organs by which lymph is circulated throughout the body and returned to the venous system. The duties of the lymphatic system are to fight diseases and infection. The lymphatic system includes a network of thin tubes that branch into the tissues throughout the body. Lymphatic vessels carry lymph, a colorless, watery fluid that contains infection-fighting cells called lymphocytes. Along the network of thin tubes are groups of small, bean-shaped organs called lymph nodes that filter the lymph as it passes through the nodes. Clusters of these lymph nodes are found in the abdomen, groin, neck and underarm. Other important parts of the lymphatic system are bone marrow, spleen, thymus and tonsils.

Lymphocytes -- Lymphocytes are a type of white blood cell found in lymph, blood, and other specialized tissue such as bone marrow and tonsils. B-and T-lymphocytes are crucial components of the immune system. The B-lymphocytes are primarily responsible for antibody production. The T-lymphocytes are involved in the direct attack against invading organisms. The helper T-lymphocyte, a subtype, is the main cell infected and destroyed by the AIDS virus. See T-Cell in this section.

Lymph Node -- A lymph node is one of the rounded masses of lymphoid tissue surrounded by a capsule of connective tissue.

Lymphoma -- A general term applied to any neoplastic disorder (cancer) of the lymphoid tissue.

Macular Degeneration -- Macular Degeneration is the deterioration of the macula (the yellowish depression in the central part of retina of the eye). The macula is the part of the eye with the greatest density of visual receptor cells. As light enters your eye, the image that is focused in the macula is the one most clearly perceived by your brain. The macula distinguishes fine detail in the central visual field. Degeneration of the macula leads to blurring of the central vision while peripheral vision remains intact. The exact cause of macular degeneration is unknown. Laser beam therapy may help the wet form of macular degeneration if treated early. At the time of this writing, there is no known treatment for the dry form of macular degeneration.

Magnetic Resonance Imaging (MRI) -- An MRI is a procedure in which a magnet linked to a computer is used to create detailed pictures of areas inside the body.

Malabsorption -- Malabsorption is a lack of nutrient absorption from the intestinal tract into the blood stream.

Malignant -- Malignant is mainly used to describe a cancerous growth. When used this way, it means that the growth is cancerous and inclined to spreading. See *Benign*.

Malignant Tumor -- Malignant tumors are cancer. Cancer cells can invade and damage nearby tissues and organs. Also, cancer cells can break away from a malignant tumor and enter the bloodstream or the lymphatic system. This is how cancer spreads (metastasis) from the original (primary) tumor to form new tumors in other parts of the body.

Mal-Practice -- Mal-practice is improper or negligent treatment of a patient by a physician, resulting in damage or injury.

Mammograms -- Mammograms are x-rays of the breast. A mammogram can often show tumors or changes in the breast BEFORE they can be felt or cause symptoms. However, mammograms cannot find every abnormal area of the breast. This is especially true in the breast of young women.

Measles -- The measles are also called rubeola. A contagious disease that mainly affects the respiratory system, skin and eyes. It was once considered a dangerous childhood disease because of its serious complications. Development of a vaccine to prevent measles has drastically reduced its occurrence.

Meat -- You must read about The FIVE DEADLY WHITES.

Medical Foods -- Specially formulated nutrient mixtures for use under medical supervision for treatment of various metalbolic diseases.

Mediterranean Diet -- See *Mediterranean Diet*.

Medium Chain Triglycerides (MCT) -- MCT's have been used in medicine for almost 40 years for patients who have difficulty digesting or absorbing nutrients or who need a rapidly available source of energy.

MCT's are 1/3 to 1/2 the size of long chain triglycerides (LCT's) which are found in virtually all oils in the foods we eat like butter, margarine, animal fats and vegetable oils. MCT's are much more water-soluble than LCT's meaning there are rapidly burned for energy!

LCT's (fat) on the other hand, may be stored in the body and utilized at a later time. MCT's may be a great diet replacement for LCT's.

Megavitamin -- A megavitamin is a large dose of a Vitamin in comparison to the RDA.

Melanoma -- A melanoma is a malignant tumor originating from pigment cells in the deep layers of the skin. It is a type of skin cancer which is extremely deadly if it isn't detected early. Melanoma skin cancer is increasing faster than any other cancer. Approximately 34,100 new cases and 7,200 deaths are anticipated for 1995.

Menopause -- Menopause is a decrease in the production of female hormones and the cessation of menstruation. It usually occurs after the age of forty-five or when female organs are removed.

Menses -- Menses is the monthly flow of blood from the genital tract of women.

Metabolism -- Metabolism is a general term for the physical and chemical processes, and reactions to them, taking place in the body. These processes primarily deal with the way the body uses nutrients. It is the chemical process of living cells in which energy is produced in order to replace and repair tissues and maintain a healthy body. Responsible for the production of energy, biosynthesis of important substances and degradation of various compounds.

Metastasis -- Metastasis is the shifting of disease, or its local manifestations, from one part of the body to another. In cancer, it is the appearance of neoplasms in parts of the body remote from the seat of the primary tumor. It is the transportation of bacteria from one part of the body to another, through the bloodstream or lymph channels.

Microorganisms -- Bacteria or protozoan of microscopic size.

Microscopic -- Microscopic means too small to be seen by the unaided eye, but large enough to be studied under a microscope.

Milligram -- A milligram is 1/1,000 of a gram by weight. Less than ten-thousandth of an ounce.

Minerals – Macro (large amounts) and trace (small amount) minerals are needed for building strong bones, transmitting nerve impulses, produce hormones,… Macro minerals include calcium, phosphorus, potassium, sodium,… Trace minerals include cobalt, copper, fluoride, iron, manganese, selenium, zinc,… See Indium.

Miracle -- A miracle is a marvelous event occurring within human experience that goes beyond the laws of nature.

Modality -- Modality is a method of therapy, usually physical, such as massage.

Monounsaturated Fat -- Monounsaturated fats (good fat) help lower bad LDL cholesterol, blood pressure and protect the arteries from arteriosclerosis (clogging of the arteries). Monounsaturated fats are found in foods like avocadoes, canola oil, olives, olive oil, peanuts and peanut oil.

Morbidly Obese -- Overweight to the point where the risk of death is high. Morbidly obese is associated with high risks of heart disease, hypertension, stroke, diabetes, cancer,...

MRI -- MRI stands for Magnetic Resonance Imaging. It is a technique used in diagnosis that combines radio waves and magnetic forces to produce detailed images of the internal structures of the body.

MSG -- MSG stands for Monosodium L-Glutamate. It is a white crystalline salt, with a meat-like taste, used extensively as a food additive. MSG is noted to cause or is a contributing factor to *"Chinese Restaurant Syndrome."* See *Chinese Restaurant Syndrome* in this section.

Mucilage -- Mucilage is a naturally formed viscous or sticky fiber which consist of a gum dissolved in the juices of a plant.

Mucocutaneous -- Mucocutaneous pertains to or affecting the mucous membrane and the skin.

Mucopolysaccharides -- Mucopolysaccharides are beneficial ingredients in Aloe Vera.

Mucous Membranes -- Mucous membranes are the membranes, such as the anus, mouth, nose, vagina, that line the cavities and canals of the body which communicate with the air.

Multi-Infarct Dementia -- It is dementia brought on by a series of strokes.

Muscle -- Muscle is a tissue composed of fibers capable of contracting and relaxing to effect bodily movement. There are three types of muscle: cardiac, smooth and striated. Cardiac muscle is the muscle of your heart with the job of pumping blood. Smooth or organic muscles are present in several of the internal organs, including the intestines, the bladder and large blood vessels.

This type of muscle functions under involuntary control by the autonomic nervous system. Functions of smooth muscle include blood circulation, glandular secretions, moving material through the digestive tract and regulate breathing. Striated or striped muscles consist of layers of tissue divided into bundles of interwoven fibers that run parallel to one another. Striated muscles aid your body in voluntary movement.

Muscular System -- Muscular System has more than 650 muscles that are attached to your skeleton that power all your actions from moving your tongue to lifting heavy weights. See *Skeletal System* in this section.

Myocardial -- Myocardial refers to the heart muscle.

Myocardial Infarction -- This is a medical term for heart attack.

Myocardiopathy -- This is any disease of the heart muscle.

Myopathy -- Myopathy is any disease of the muscle.

Natural Anticoagulant -- An anticoagulant is a substance that retards or prevents blood clots or coagulation which could be life-threatening. Noted natural anticoagulants are garlic, onions, ginkgo biloba...

Nausea -- Nausea is a strong disturbance characterized by a feeling of the need to vomit.

Nervous System -- The nervous system is a coordinating mechanism in all multicellular animals, except sponges, that regulates internal body functions and responses to external stimuli. Three systems working together that control your five senses, regulate your breathing and relay information to your brain.

Neurologist -- A neurologist is a specialist in disorders of the nervous system.

Neuropathy -- Neuropathy is a group of symptoms caused by abnormalities in motor or sensory nerves. Symptoms include tingling or numbness in hands or feet followed by gradual, progressive muscular weakness. Any disease or abnormality of the nervous system.

Neurotransmitters -- Neurotransmitters are substances that transmit nerve impulses to the brain.

Niacin -- Niacin is a Vitamin. In high doses, niacin is a drug and used to lower cholesterol levels. Side effects from high doses of niacin are glucose intolerance, gout, headaches, itching, liver damage and skin flushing. Endur-acin which is a sustained-release niacin is explained in The *Eight-Week Cholesterol Cure* by Robert E. Kowalski. Endur-acin is a drug which lowers cholesterol levels with less side effects.

Nicotine -- Nicotine is a poisonous, addictive substance derived from tobacco. In small doses, nicotine has a stimulating effect on your nervous system, which increases blood pressure and pulse rate.

Nutrients -- Nutrients are substances needed by all living cells to maintain life, including carbohydrates, fats, minerals, proteins and Vitamins.

Nutrition -- Nutrition is the study of the food and drink requirements of human beings for maintenance, growth, activity, reproduction and lactation.

Obesity -- Obesity is the state of having an excessive amount of fat on the body. Twenty percent over your maximum healthy weight according to your height and build is considered obese.

Obsessive-Compulsive Disorder (OCD) -- OCD is characterized by anxious thoughts or rituals you feel you can't control. If you have OCD, you may be plagued by persistent, unwelcome thoughts or images or by the urgent need to engage in certain rituals. You may be obsessed with germs or dirt, so you wash your hands over and over.

You may be filled with doubt and feel the need to check things repeatedly. You might be preoccupied by thoughts of violence and fear that you will harm people close to you. You may spend long periods of time touching things or counting... See *Anxiety Disorder* and *Post-Traumatic Disorder* in this section.

Occult Blood Test -- An occult blood test is a test used in screening for cancer that identifies bodily excretion of blood (stool sputum, urine).

Omega-E -- Omega-3 is made from two nutrients called EPA which stands for eicosapentaenoic acid. The other nutrient that makes-up Omega-3 is called DHA, which stands for docosahexaenoic acid. Omega-3 was initially noted to protect against heart disease and stroke. Other benefits from Omega-3 have also surfaced through several studies.

Oncologist -- An oncologist is a specialist in tumors and cancer.

Oncology -- Oncology is the study of cancer.

Ophthalmoscope -- An ophthalmoscope is a lighted instrument used in eye examinations. It enables a doctor to look through the pupil and see the retina and optic nerve.

Optic Nerve -- The optic nerve is the nerve that conducts visual stimuli from the retina to the brain.

Organically Grown -- This means pertaining to or cultivated by the use of animal or vegetable fertilizers rather than synthetic chemicals.

Organochlorines -- Organochlorines are used by the chemical industry in the production of everything from plastic and paper to pesticides and pharmaceuticals. Most organochlorines are harmless, however others are some of the most dangerous substances known to mankind! Some include pesticides like DDT, industrial compounds such as PCB and toxic byproducts like dioxin which have been proven to cause cancer. Your body has no way of excreting synthetic compounds so they accumulate in your body. More than 177 different organochlorines have been found in the tissues of people living in the United States and Canada.

Osteoporosis -- Osteoporosis develops silently over a period of years. It is a condition in which bone mass is low (softening of the bones). Over 24 million Americans are afflicted with osteoporosis and 80 percent are post-menopausal women. An early sign of osteoporosis is loss of height, caused by weakened bones in the spine become compressed. As the vertebrae fracture and collapse, a curvature of the spine may occur. Dietary and exercise habits may help prevent osteoporosis. According to research at Washington University of Medicine, researchers found that female hormone estrogen replacement therapy combined with exercise can effectively prevent bone loss on post-menopausal women.

OTC -- OTC stands for Over-The-Counter. This is commonly used to identify with non-prescription drugs.

Out-Patient -- An out-patient is a patient who comes to the hospital, clinic, or dispensary for diagnosis and\or treatment but does not occupy a bed. See *In-Patient* in this section.

Oxidation -- Oxidation is a chemical reaction that occurs when oxygen is added, resulting in a chemical transformation.

Oxygen -- Oxygen is a gaseous element existing free in the air.

p53 -- In 1979, p53 was independently discovered by David Lane of the University of Dundee in Scotland and Arnold Levine of Princeton University. In 1989 Levine and Dr. Bert Volgelstein of the Howard Hughes Institute, discovered that p53 was a tumor killer. With more than 5,200 published studies on p53, it promises to be a new weapon in the war of deadly cancers. p53 is a gene and works like a clerk who stops the continuous typos on a document (cancer) and corrects them!

PABA -- PABA (Para-Aminobenzoic Acid) is constituent of folic acid and helps in the utilization of Vitamin B5 (Pantothenic Acid).

Pacemakers -- Pacemakers are a scientific electrical instrument that controls the normal rhythm of the heart beat when the physiological mechanisms fail. The pacemaker is implanted in the chest and attached to the ventricle by a wire passed through the connecting veins. The heart rate is maintained at a steady number of beats per minute according to what is normal for the individual.

Pain -- Pain is an unpleasant sensation, occurring in varying degrees of severity, especially as a consequence of injury, disease, or emotional disorder. An estimated $80 billion in pain killers are among the best selling drugs. Is this an indicator that convention treatments aren't effective?

Panacea -- Panacea is a term to mean a remedy for all diseases, evils, or difficulties; a cure-all.

Pancreas -- The pancreas is the organ that produces insulin.

Pancreatitis -- Inflammation of the pancreas by either disease or injury.

Pandemic -- A panademic is an epidemic occurring over a very large area or worldwide.

Panic Disorder -- Panic disorder strikes at least 01.6 percent of the American population. In other words, approximately 02.4 million Americans suffer this disorder. People with panic disorder have feelings of terror that strike suddenly and repeatedly with no warning. A panic attack can't be predicted and many with this disorder develop intense anxiety between episodes, worrying when and where the next one will strike. Thirty percent of those Americans that suffer this disorder will develop agoraphobia.

Pap Test -- For a Pap test, a sample of cells is collected from the upper vagina and cervix with a small brush or a flat wooden stick. This is placed on a glass slide and checked under a microscope for cancer or other abnormal cells. Pap test should be scheduled every year after the 18th birthday or becoming sexually active.

Paralysis -- Paralysis is a loss of power of voluntary movement in a muscle through injury or disease of its nerve supply. The condition may vary in severity and degree from paralysis of one muscle to paralysis of almost the entire body.

Paraplegic -- This is paralysis of the lower half of the body.

Parasite -- A parasite is an organism that lives off of another organism.

Parasomnia -- Any dysfunction associated with sleep, e.g., somnambulism, pavor nocturnus, enureseis or nocturnal seizures.

Parkinson's Disease -- This is a progressive neurological disease of the later years, characterized by muscular tremor, slowing of movement, partial facial paralysis, peculiarity of gait and posture, and weakness.

The cause of Parkinson's Disease is unknown at the time of this writing. Approximately 1 million Americans are afflicted with Parkinson's Disease.

Pathogenic -- Pathogenic means capable of causing a disease.

Pathologist -- A pathologist is a doctor who specializes in identifying diseases by studying cells and tissues under a microscope.

Pathology -- Pathology is the scientific study of the nature of disease and its causes, processes, development and consequences.

Patient -- A patient is a person or animal receiving medical treatment.

Pectin -- Pectin is any of a group of complex colloidal substances of higher molecular weight found in ripe fruits, such as apples.

Pediatrician -- A pediatrician is a doctor who specializes in the treatment of children and childhood development and illnesses.

Pelvic Exam -- In a pelvic exam, your doctor feels the uterus, vagina, ovaries, fallopian tubes, bladder and rectum for any change in size or shape (cancer or less serious medical problems).

Penicillin -- In 1928, British bacteriologist Alexander Flemming discovers the first antibiotic - penicillin! Originally, this was an antibiotic substance obtained from cultures of the molds.

Peptic Ulcer -- A peptic ulcer is a sore on the lining of the stomach or duodenum (small intestine just below the stomach). An ulcer occurs when the lining is unable to resist the damaging effects of acid and pepsin (produced by the stomach to digest food).

Percentage of Hydrogen (pH) -- pH is used to describe the acidity or alkalinity of a liquid or a solution. pH is measured on a scale running from 0 to 14. Zero being extremely acidic and 14 being extremely alkaline. One unique characteristic of a high pH is that bacteria cannot live in it!

Percutaneous Needle Biopsy -- This is removal of a sampling of lung tissue through a needle inserted through the skin.

Periodontal Disease -- This is also known as periodontitis or pyorrhea. Periodontal Disease is a progressive deterioration of the gums, bones and other tissues around the teeth. Diagnosis may be based on swollen gums and deposits of plaque around the teeth. Oral hygiene such as brushing the teeth with a soft-bristled toothbrush after each meal, flossing and using mouthwash are standard hygiene procedures. Regular dental checkups are highly recommended.

pH -- See percentage of hydrogen in this section.

Pharmaceutical -- This pertaining to legal drugs, where they are scientifically prepared and dispensed by a licensed pharmacist.

Pharmaceutical Grade -- Meeting the standards of compounds or drugs by which licensed pharmacists prepare and dispense supplements.

Phlebotomy -- Phlebotomy is the practice of opening a vein to draw blood.

Physiatry -- Physiatry is the branch of medicine using physical therapy in diagnosis, prevention and treatment of bodily disorders.

Phytochemicals -- See Phytochemicals throughout this Survival Book.

Pica -- Pica is a craving for unnatural food such as mud, cloth, cigarette ashes... as occurs occasionally in hysteria and pregnancy.

Placebo -- A placebo is an indifferent substance, in the form of a medicine, given for the suggestive effect. An inert pill used in controlled studies to simulate real medication.

Plaque -- Plaque is a localized abnormal patch on a body part or surface. With respect to cardiovascular disease, a patch or lesion in a blood vessel. It is often described incorrectly as a deposit, but it is an eruption of cells from the middle layers of an artery through the wall into the artery interior. Plaques can continue to grow after they break through the artery wall.

Plasma -- Plasma is the clear fluid portion of the blood. It is 90 percent water and enables your body to carry out most of the transportation tasks assigned to it (red blood cells, white cells and platelets).

P.M.S. -- P.M.S. stands for pre-menstrual syndrome. P.M.S. affects some women one or two weeks before their menstrual period begins. Symptoms include bloating, breast tenderness, cramping, depression, personality changes, undue anxiety, unusual cravings and weight gain. The average woman spends six years of her life in P.M.S.

Pneumonectomy -- Pneumonectomy is the surgical removal of an entire lung.

Pneumonia -- Pneumonia is an infection of the lungs which the one or more sections of the lungs become inflamed and filled with fluid and white blood cells, which try to fight off the infection. There are several types of pneumonia, depending on the location, causative agent and extent of infection.

Lobar pneumonia is an infection in only one lobe (a section of the lungs) whereas double pneumonia is an infection in all parts of the lungs. Bronchial pneumonia is an infection in the areas of the lungs near the main airways connecting the windpipe and the lungs.

Walking pneumonia is a form of pneumonia where an individual may have for a week or more without no serious symptoms except for a cough. Viral pneumonia is indicated by coughing, other cold symptoms and general fatigue.

Bacterial pneumonia generally comes on suddenly with shaking chills, a rapid rise in temperature, shallow breathing, and a cough that brings up bloody, dark yellow or rust-colored sputum. Symptoms of pneumonia are characterized by four major symptoms: chest pain, sudden rise in temperature, coughing and difficulty in breathing. Pneumonia is diagnosed by listening to the chest with a stethoscope to detect the presence of fluid in the lungs. Pneumonia may be fatal, especially to the very young and the very old. Vaccines help prevent some types of pneumonia. If you suspect you may be suffering from pneumonia, see your doctor immediately.

Pneumonitis -- Pneumonitis is inflammation of the lungs.

Poison -- A poison is any substance that causes injury, illness or death, especially by chemical means.

Polyunsaturated Fat -- Polyunsaturated fats may lower the cholesterol in the blood. Sources of polyunsaturated fats are corn, safflower, soybean and sunflower seed oils.

Post-Traumatic Stress Disorder (PTSD) -- PTSD is a debilitating condition that follows a terrifying event. Often, people with PTSD have persistent frightening thoughts and memories of their ordeal and feel emotionally numb, especially with people they were once close to. PTSD, once referred to as shell shock or battle fatigue, was first brought to public attention by war veterans, but it can result from any number of traumatic incidents to include car accidents, kidnapping, natural disasters, train accidents, violent attacks (mugging, held captive, rape, torture...).

Prescribe -- Prescribe means to designate in writing a remedy for administration.

Preservative(s) -- A preservative is a substance added to food products or to organic solution to prevent chemical change or bacterial action.

Prescription Drugs -- This is a controlled drug that is available only by the order of a physician's prescription. Did you know that approximately 146,000 Americans die every year from prescription drugs, FDA-approved drugs! That's about 400 people per day, each and every day. This information product may provide you with an alternative.

Processed Food -- Food that is altered from its original state in order to enhance the taste, shelf-life and other factors so to sell the product. Most processed foods contain additives that may be harmful to your health. Over 70 percent of the food we eat, is processed food. See The FIVE DEADLY WHITES.

Prognosis -- Prognosis means the foretelling of the probable course of a disease. A forecast of the outcome of a disease and the prospect of recovery.

Prophylactic -- A prophylactic is intended to prevent disease.

Prophylaxis -- Prophylaxis is the prevention of or the protective treatment for disease.

Prostate Specific Antigen (PSA) -- PSA is a test that indicates the presence of either malignant cancer cells or abnormal prostate stimulation.

Protease Inhibitor -- Protease inhibitors are thought to help reduce the activation of both certain viruses and chemical carcinogens in the intestine, thus helping to prevent certain infections and cancers.

Protein -- Protein is three-fourths of the dry weight of most cell matter and is involved in structures, hormones, enzymes, muscle contraction, immunological response and other essential life functions. Protein has 04 calories per gram compared to fat with 09 calories per gram and starches with 04 calories per gram.

Protein-Calorie Malnutrition (PCM) -- PCM is consumption of too little protein is a health hazard to children all over the world. PCM may be found in affluent homes in which the parents are following a fad diet. Pure protein deficiency, which is rare, is called kwashiorkor. Prolonged protein deficiency will impair a child's growth, the production of hormones and enzymes, the body's ability to heal itself and the actions of the immune system. More than 300 million adult survivors of PCM worldwide remain impaired in one way or another.

Psoriasis -- Psoriasis is a chronic skin disorder. The cause is unknown. It is not contagious. There is no cure, but there are many treatments. There are several forms of psoriasis, but the most common form is plaque psoriasis or psoriasis vulgaris. It is characterized by raised, inflamed red lesions covered with a silvery white buildup of dead skin cells called scale.

Other forms of psoriasis are erythrodermic psoriasis, guttate, inverse, and pustular. Psoriasis affects approximately 5 million people in the U.S., with 150,000 to 260,000 new cases of psoriasis each year. Approximately 400 people die each year from psoriasis-related causes. Nail psoriasis occurs more frequently than previously thought.

Psychosomatic -- Psychosomatic pertains to phenomena that exhibit an interaction of the physiological and the psychological, especially disorders, such as high blood pressure that may be initiated or aggravated by mental stress.

Psychotherapy -- Psychotherapy is treatment of emotional and psychosomatic disorders based on the application of psychological knowledge, rather than exclusively on the use of drugs, surgery or other physical treatment.

Public Health -- Public health is the art and science of protecting and improving community health by means of preventive medicine, health education, communicable disease control and the application of the social & sanitary sciences.

Pulmonary -- Pulmonary means relating to the lungs.

Pulmonary Edema -- The accumulation of fluid in tissues of the lung(s).

Pus -- Pus is a liquid inflammation product made up of cells (leukocytes) and a thin fluid called liquor puris.

Pycnogenol -- Pycnogenol is an extract from the maritime pine consist of proanthocyanidins and water-soluble nutrients. Pycnogenol, a specific blend of bioflavonoids (patented), a "super protector nutrient" is a made up of powerful antioxidant nutrients for use to scavenge free radicals.

This mixture of nutrients can help you live better longer, stay healthier and appear more youthful! Pycnogenol is noted to protect you from approximately eighty diseases, including arthritis, cancer, heart disease and most non-germ diseases which are linked to the deleterious chemical action of free radicals.

It is well known that antioxidant nutrients protect the body's cells from attack free radicals. Free radicals form during normal metabolism and are multiplied by environmental pollutants and radiation. Pycnogenol slows the damage associated with aging, restores elasticity and smoothness to skin because of its influence on skin protein, nourishes blood cells and blood vessels. This amazing antioxidant alleviates hay fever, other allergies, strengthens capillaries to reduce edema, bruising, varicose veins...

Quackery -- Quackery is the promotion of a misleading and fraudulent health claims that is unproven.

Quadriplegic -- A person of quadriplegia, has a complete paralysis of the body from the neck down.

Rabies -- Rabies is a viral infection of the central nervous system caused (in most cases) by an RNA Rhabdovirus. The virus is contained in the saliva and certain body materials (brain tissue, cerebral spinal fluid) of rabid animals and humans. Transmission is mostly by skin penetration via bites by rabid animals.

Radiation -- Radiation is the emission and transmission of energy. It is often used to refer to what is actually radioactivity, which is, basically, the release of energy and particles by unstable isotopes.

Radiation Therapy -- This usually refers to treatment of cancer with ionizing radiation, including Roentgen rays, radium or other radioactivity substances.

Radioactive -- Radioactive is the property possessed by some chemicals of spontaneous emitting radiation.

Radioimmunotherapy -- This is treatment with monoclonal antibodies that have been chemically linked to radioactive molecules. These antibodies can selectively deliver radiation to cancer cells.

Radiosensitizers -- These are substances that increase cancer cells' sensitivity to radiation.

Raynaud's Disease -- Raynaud's Disease is a condition characterized by spasms of small blood vessels when exposed to cold, especially the fingers and toes, which become cyanotic.

RDA -- RDA is Recommended Dietary Allowance of Vitamins and minerals to meet most healthy peoples' needs as determined by the FDA. See U.S. RDA.

Red Blood Cells -- They are cells that transport oxygen from the lungs to all tissues of the body.

Reflexology -- See *Reflexology Weight-Loss Points* and *Reflexology Blues Killer*.

Refractory -- Refractory means not responding to treatment.

Remedy -- A remedy is anything that cures, palliates or prevents disease.

Remission -- Remission is abatement of disease. Many doctors often use the terminology of *"surviving"* cancer, or they may use the word "remission" instead of "cure."

Renal Care -- Renal care pertaining to, resembling or in the region of the kidneys.

Rescue Breathing -- This is the process of breathing air into the lungs of a person who has stopped breathing. Mouth-to-Nose and mouth-to-mouth breathing are types of rescue breathing. Also called *Artificial Respiration*.

Resection -- Resection is the surgical removal of a portion of an organ or structure, such as a lung.

Respiratory System -- The system responsible for transporting oxygen from your lungs to your blood as well as expelling carbon dioxide from your body.

Restenosis -- Restenosis means to unclog arteries, one medical procedure being conducted is called angioplasty. The drawback with angioplasty is patient's arteries often reclog with scar tissue. This is called restenosis.

Retina -- The retina is the sensory membrane that lines the eye and receives the image formed by the lens of the eye. The retina is the instrument of vision. The retina is connected with the brain by the optic nerve.

Retinopathy -- Noninflammatory degenerative disease of the retina.

RFIR -- Requires Further Intensive Research.

Rheumatic Fever -- Rheumatic fever is the result of a bacterial disease characterized by inflammation, soreness of the joints (especially ankles, knees, wrist), swelling and inflammation of the heart. Most common in children and adolescents, it may result in permanent damage to the heart.

Rheumatism -- Rheumatism is any variety of disorders marked by inflammation, degeneration or metabolic derangement of the connective tissue structures of the body, especially the joints and related structures, including muscles, bursae, tendons and fibrous tissue.

Rheumatoid Arthritis -- This is a chronic disease marked by stiffness and inflammation of the membranes of the joints, weakness, loss of mobility and deformity.

Rheumatologist -- A rheumatologist is a specialist in arthritis and rheumatism.

Rickets -- Rickets is an early childhood disease characterized by softening of the bones and consequent deformity, caused by deficiency of Vitamin D.

Ringworm -- Ringworm is a skin infection caused by a fungus and not a worm. There are several types of ringworm and each is caused by a different type of fungus. Two very common ringworms are tinea cruris also known as jock itch and tinea pedis also known as athlete's foot. Ringworm spreads by direct contact with an infected person or pet or by contact with contaminated objects, like combs, pillows, towels, and clothing. Antifungal ointment and special medicated shampoos are available to treat ringworm.

Risk Factors -- Risk factors are agents or conditions that increase a person's chance of developing a disease.

RNA -- RNA stands for Ribonucleic Acid. A ribonucleic acid is found in plant and animal cells; a complex protein chemical. It is important in the coding of genetic information with DNA carrying information from the nucleus of the cell into the cytoplasm.

Saccharin -- Saccharin is a white crystalline powder, having a taste about 500 times sweeter than cane sugar, used as a calorie-free sweetener. If you use this product, read and reread the WARNING till it sinks in! See *The FIVE DEADLY WHITES*.

Salmonella -- Salmonella is any of various rod-shaped bacteria of the genus Salmonella, many of which are pathogenic. Food poisoning is caused by salmonella. Insure raw meats (chicken, red meat...) do not come in direct or indirect contact with other foods you're preparing. The USDA recommends cooking hamburgers medium, to an internal temperature of at least 160 degrees to avoid Salmonella and E. Coli bacteria. To prevent the spread of Salmonella and E. Coli bacteria, Clorox Bleach recommends sanitizing all surfaces (cutting boards, cooking utensils, dish towel...) which come in contact with raw foods that may carry Salmonella and E. Coli bacteria like chicken, red meat...

Knives, cutlery and other utensils should be washed and rinsed with the Clorox Bleach Sanitizing Solution*, then drain and air dry. Other items like dish towels and kitchen linen should be laundered according to the directions on the Clorox Bleach bottle.

- **Clorox Bleach Sanitizing Solution:** After washing and rinsing all cookware, mix one tablespoon of regular Clorox Bleach with 1 gallon of water. Soak cookware in the solution for two minutes, drain and air dry. For cutting boards use three (03) tablespoons of Clorox bleach instead of two.

Salt -- See *Sodium Chloride* in this section and see *The FIVE DEADLY WHITES.*

Saponin -- Saponin is the scientific name for yucca juice. Over 1,000 years ago, American Indians learned that the juice of the yucca plant helped relieve arthritic pain. Today, research has revealed that saponin protects friendly intestinal bacteria that compete with harmful microorganisms and prevent these microorganisms from causing allergic reactions associated with arthritis.

Sarcoma -- A tumor, usually malignant, arising from connective tissue.
Saturated Fat -- Saturated fats are fats that harden at room temperature and may raise blood cholesterol levels. Saturated fats are found in most animal and some vegetable products like butter, coconut oil, cream, palm oil and whole milk products.

Saturates -- Saturates are solid fats of animal origin.

Seasonal Affective Disorder (SAD) -- SAD is a depression which surfaces during the reduction of exposure to sunlight during the winter months (November to February). During the summer months, we are exposed to 100,000 lux. During the winter months, we are exposed to only 5,000 lux! SAD is linked to weight gain, lethargy, reclusiveness...

Studies have demonstrated that an increase in light exposure through the eyes, SAD patients improved significantly. Light Therapy may be the solution too those suffering from SAD. Call 1-800-705-5559 for a product called Nutralux (artificial light).

Sedentary -- Sedentary means accustomed to sitting or to taking little exercise. It is as equally unhealthy as saturated fat is to your diet and your health!!

Seizures -- Seizures are convulsions. They are sudden violent disturbances characterized by involuntary contractions of the muscles.

Selenium -- It is an essential mineral, being a constituent of the enzyme glutathione peroxidase and believed to be closely associated with Vitamin E in its function, but it occurs in toxic levels in several kinds of plants growing in soils with high levels, causing disease in grazing animals.

Sensory Organs -- Every available sensory to experience the world around you (sight, smell, hearing, feeling, smelling, tasting, skin, hair...).

Serological Analysis -- This is the medical study of serums or blood.

Serotonin -- Serotonin is a mood enhancing chemical.

Serum -- Serum is the clear yellowish fluid obtained upon separating blood into its solid and liquid components. It is also called blood serum.

Serving -- Use the following as a serving guide: 1/2 cup of cut fruit or vegetables which is about 03-04 ounces. One average piece of fruit, 3/4 cup of juice, one cup of salad greens, or 1/4 cup dried fruit.

Shock -- A condition of profound hemodynamic and metabolic disturbances characterized by failure of the circulatory system to maintain adequate perfusion of vital organs.

Sickle-Cell Anemia -- Hereditary disease occurring mostly among Negro men and women, in which many or a majority of the red blood cells are sickle-shaped, producing chronic anemia.

Sickness -- Morbus; illness; sickness; an interruption, cessation, or disorder of the body functions, systems or organs.

Sigmoidoscopy -- During a sigmoidoscopy, your doctor uses a thin, flexible tube with a light to look inside the rectum and colon for abnormal areas which may indicate cancer or a lesser medical problem.

Simple Carbohydrate -- A simple form of sugar (glucose, lactose, fructose...). This type of sugar is rapidly absorbed into the bloodstream.

Sinusitis -- Inflammation of the sinus. Sinusitis is an infection, usually bacterial, of one or more of the sinuses. Sinusitis occurs more often in adults than children.

Skeletal System -- The framework of your body consisting of 206 bones.

Skim Milk -- Milk from which the cream has been removed.

Skin -- The tissue forming the external, protective covering of the body of a vertebrate. Consisting of an outer epidermis and an inner dermis.

Skin Graft -- A surgical graft of skin from one part of the body to another or from one individual to another.

Skull -- The skeleton of the head that encloses and protects the brain and chief sense organs. The skull also supports the jaws.

Sleep Apnea -- Snoring could be a potentially life-threatening condition called sleep apnea. Sleep apnea is a condition in which the throat relaxes and closes during sleep. Sleep apnea affects nearly 01 out of every 10 Americans, usually middle-aged to older men who are usually overweight. The difference between sleep apnea and snoring is with sleep apnea, you actually STOP breathing from 10 seconds to up to 03 minutes!

These breathing stops are frequent, approximately 15 times per hour. People with sleep apnea may have a much higher risk of heart attack (see *Coenzyme Q10*). The usual cause of apnea in infants is immaturity of the brain centers that regulate breathing. An infant with sleep apnea suddenly stops breathing completely and turns blue. A flick of the finger on the bottom of the foot will usually have the baby breathing again.

Parents of high-risk infants may want to consider equipment that sounds an alarm when your baby stops breathing. If you feel you are afflicted with sleep apnea or someone in your family has this condition, see your doctor immediately.

Sleepwalking -- Sleepwalking is walking while asleep or in a sleep-like condition. It is also called noctambulation, noctambulism and somnambulism. As much as 15% of the population, as many as 30 million Americans are sleepwalkers. Sleepwalking is prevalent between the ages of 06 and 12 and usually ends by the 14 years of age. If sleepwalking continues after 18 years of age, professional help is recommended. According to Peter Hauri, Ph. D, co-director of the Mayo Clinic Sleep Disorders Center in Rochester, Minnesota, in adults, sleepwalking is associated with excessive stress.

Slipped Disk -- A slipped disk is a back problem, which involves the disks of soft elastic tissue located between the vertebrae (bones of the spinal column). The vertebrae are loosely connected together by bands of ligaments which allow flexibility.

The primary function of each disk is to prevent friction and trauma between adjacent vertebrae as you move your body. If the spinal structure experiences strain or overexertion, the rim of the disk may weaken and tear, which may cause part of the gelatinous center of the disk to be forced out of position (slip or herniate). The protrusion of the disk often presses against an adjacent nerve, causing pain along the path of the affected nerve. Mild or disabling pain and tenderness may result.

Avoid movement and lifting objects. Initial treatment may require bed rest on a firm mattress and possibly back support during movement. Professional medical care for diagnosis and treatment is strongly advised.

Smell -- Smell means to perceive the scent of (something) by means of olfactory nerves. To have or emit an odor.

Smoking -- Smoking is an act of smoking a form of tobacco. Smoking is noted to constrict all arteries and capillaries which causes the heart to pump harder to force blood through them. Read about other health problems associated with smoking throughout this book. See *Smoker's Body Starts Healing Itself* and other *Smoking POCs* in the POC Section.

Snake Oil -- Plains settlers adopted the echinacea herb plant, but it remained a folk remedy until 1870, when a patent-medicine purveyor, Dr. H.C.F. Meyer of Pawnee City, Nebraska, used echinacea herb in his *"Meyer's Blood Purifier."* Dr. Meyer's, promoted the echinacea concoction as *"an absolute cure"* for rattlesnake bite, blood poisoning and a host of other maladies. Claims like Dr. Meyer's gave patent-medicines the name "snake oil." However, he was on the right track for the great potential of this amazing herb.

Snore -- Snore means to breathe through both nose and mouth while sleeping, making snorting noises caused by the vibration of the soft palate.

Social Security -- This is the provision by the government of financial and other assistance to those in need, such as the unemployed, the elderly and the disabled.

Sodium Chloride -- See *The Five Deadly Whites*.

Soft Tissue -- Soft tissue is the connective tissue other than bone. Soft tissue includes muscles, tendons, fibrous tissue, fat, blood & lymph vessels and nerves.

Soluble Fiber -- It is fiber susceptible of being dissolved. While insoluble fibers are able to add bulk to food mass - moving food through the digestive system thus reducing transit time, soluble fibers like in oat bran are noted to help lower cholesterol and regulating blood-sugar levels.

Somnambulism -- This is a disorder of sleep involving complex motor acts which occur primarily during the first third of the night but not during rapid eye movement sleep.

Sorbic Acid -- Sorbic Acid is an organic acid and food preservative.

SPF -- SPF stands for Sun Protection Factor and indicates how long a person can be exposed to the sun without burning. For example, if a sunscreen has an SPF of 04, it means a person can be exposed to the sun four times longer than without the sunscreen without being burned. Anyone with lighter skin need a higher SPF than those with darker skin. SPF values range from 02 to 15 and are usually numbered 02, 04, 06, 08, 15 and higher. A quality SPF lotion should be applied 30 minutes prior to exposure to allow good skin penetration. Reapply every two hours. Follow the instruction on the bottle! SPF's selectively screen out redness-producing rays whereas sunblocks screen out everything.

Spina Bifida -- Congenital defect in the fetal closing of the neural tube to form a portion of the lower spine, leaving the spine unclosed and the spinal cord open to various degrees of exposure and damage. SEE *Folic Acid*.

Spleen -- The spleen is a highly vascular ductless organ near the stomach concerned with the final destruction of blood cells, storage of blood and production of lymphocytes.

Stevia – A South American herb that's used as a sweetener. Noted to be 30-times sweeter than sugar.

Stigmata -- Stigmata means the crucifixion wounds of Christ appear on a living person. See *The National Centre for Padre Pio*.

Stinking Rose -- Stinking Rose may be used in reference to garlic. Stinking Rose was the name of a British Social Club where club members enjoyed eating garlic and drinking. It is unknown if the club still exist.

Strep Throat -- Strep throat is a sore throat caused by infection with bacteria of the genus Streptococcus.

Stress -- Stress is a physical or psychological stimulus which, when impinging upon an individual, produces strain or disequilibrium.

Stroke -- A stroke occurs when the flow of blood going to the brain is blocked by a blood clot. Brain cells can die from decreased blood flow and the resulting lack of oxygen.

Substance-P -- This is a neuropeptide produced by the nerves that carry pain sensation.

Sugar -- See *The Five Deadly Whites*.

Sulfa Drugs -- Sulfa drugs are any of a group of sulfonamide compounds, such as sulfathiazole and sulfadiazine, capable of inhibiting bacterial growth and activity and used to treat a wide variety of infections.

Sunblock -- Sunblocks are designed to screen out everything. If you can't tolerate exposure to the sun, a quality sunblock product may be beneficial. A zinc-oxide paste or a sunscreen with PABA with titanium-dioxide paste may be effective depending on your intentions. See SPF in this section.

Sunburn -- Sunburn is an inflammation of the cells of the skin caused by overexposure to the ultraviolet radiation of the sun or a sunlamp. Damage to the skin may vary from insignificant to serious. The best prevention is avoiding prolonged exposure to direct rays of the sun or sunlamp. The second best defense is to cover all exposed skin with loose-fitting clothes as well as wearing a wide-brimmed hat and appropriate eye wear. A quality sunscreen is also recommended. See *SPF* and *Sunblock* in this section.

Superoxide Dismutase (SOD) -- SOD is a very important enzyme which revitalizes the cells and reduces the rate of cell destruction. SOD removes the most common free radical, superoxide. During aging, free radicals production increases while SOD decreases. SOD can be obtained naturally from barley grass*, broccoli, Brussels sprouts, cabbage, wheatgrass and most green plants. See *Pycnogenol*.

Suppuration -- Suppuration means becoming converted into and discharging pus.

Supplement -- A supplement is an addition.

Surgery -- Surgery is the branch of medicine concerned with the treatment of injury, deformity and disease by manual and instrumental operations.

Suture -- Suture means the process of joining two surfaces or edges together along a line by or as if by sewing.

Symptom -- A symptom is a reaction to a bodily disorder.

Symptomatology -- Symptomatology is the study of the symptoms of disease.

Systolic -- Systolic is the first number given in blood-pressure measurements. It pertains to the heart cycle in which the heart is in contraction. It is the high or top reading which measures the pressure in the blood vessels at the time of a heartbeat.

Tachycardia -- Tachycardia is a very rapid heartbeat above normal.

Tachypnea -- Tachypnea is rapid breathing.

T-Cell -- A T-cell is a type of lymphocyte crucial to the immune system and involved in the direct attack upon invading organisms. An average healthy human being has a T-cell count of approximately 1,000 per cubic milliliter of blood. A low T-cell count of 200 is considered borderline and life-threatening. See *Lymphocytes*.

TDD -- TDD stands for Telecommunication Device for Deaf.

Tendons -- Tendons are bands of connective tissue attaching bones to muscles.

Tenosynovitis -- See *Carpal Tunnel Syndrome* in this section.

Terminally Ill -- Those diagnosed with a disease or sickness which may end in death. If you are diagnosed as Terminally Ill or you know someone that is terminally ill.

Tetracycline -- Tetracycline is a yellow crystalline compound, synthesized from chlortetracycline or derived from bacteria of the genus Streptomyces and used as an antibiotic.

Thermal Pollution -- Thermal pollution is caused principally by high temperatures of such heating systems as forced air furnaces, resistance electric heaters, light bulbs, etc.

Therapeutic -- Therapeutic is the treatment of disease.

Therapy, Alternative -- This is the treatment of disease using techniques supplementing surgery, radiation and chemotherapy.

Thermogenic -- Science of heat production.

Thrush -- Thrush is a fungal infection from Candida albicans. Occurs more often in infants, immunocompromised patients and AIDS victims. It is characterized by whitish spots on the tongue and inside of the cheeks.

Thymus -- The thymus gland is an organ in which lymphocytes mature and multiply. Its location is behind the breastbone.

Thyroid Gland -- The function of the thyroid gland is to supply thyroxin, the thyroxine hormone, to individual cells for the purpose of metabolism. Oxygen is used in this procedure. The oxygen content is regulated in the cells by thyroxine. When insufficient oxygen is supplied, the person is a slow oxidizer and hypothyroidism, an underactive thyroid occurs.

If an overabundance of oxygen is supplied, the person is a fast oxidizer and has hyperthyroidism (also called Grave's Disease), an overactive thyroid. Insufficient thyroxin thickens blood, causing clotting which can lead to heart attacks. An overabundance of thyroxin thins blood and can cause hemorrhaging.

Tinnitus -- Tinnitus is abnormal sounds in the inner ear such as buzzing, hissing, ringing, roaring or thumping.

TMJ -- TMJ stands for temporomandibular joint. TMJ is a jaw disorder that is linked to numerous symptoms like pain in the jaw, neck, headaches... TMJ may be accompanied by stiffness and locking or clicking of the jaw joint. According to the American Dental Association, almost 60 million people are affected by T.M.J. Dysfunction.

Tonsillitis -- Tonsillitis is an inflammation or infection of the tonsils which are two small, almond-shaped lumps of specialized lymph node tissues located in the back of the mouth. It is most common in children from 05 to 15. It is caused by many infectious agents. Bed rest, reduced activity and the use of antibiotics (penicillin) may be recommended. Seek professional medical attention.

Toxic Shock Syndrome -- TSS is a rare infection that is characterized by vomiting, fever, a rash and a sharp drop in blood pressure. Most known cases have occurred in women using vaginal tampons.

Toxicity -- Toxicity is a poisonous reaction in the body that impairs bodily functions and or damages cells. It is caused from ingesting an amount of a substance that is higher than one's level of tolerance.

Toxin -- A toxin is a poison to the body that impairs bodily functions.

Trace Elements -- Trace is an amount too small to measure. Trace minerals are essential for normal body functioning and health. Most people do not get the trace minerals required for health due to processed foods, where the foods are grown (poor soil)...

Trachea -- The trachea is the tube connecting the larynx and the bronchi. It is also called the windpipe.

Trans Fatty Acids -- Trans fatty acids are created when liquid vegetable oils are hydrogenated, a process where bubbling hydrogen through the oil. This is done to make the oils more solid and increase their shelf life. It is noted that processed foods containing *"hydrogenated oils"* should be avoided.

Transient Ischemic Attack (TIA) -- One warning sign of impending stroke, at times, the only warning is Transient Ischemic Attack (TIA).

A temporary deficiency of blood in the brain is caused by a blockage of blood flow or by a piece of artery plaque or a blood clot that lodges in a blood vessel inside the brain. Symptoms include weakness, numbness, dizziness, blurred vision and difficulty in speaking.

Triglycerides - They are the most common fat molecule found in fatty tissue. The body turns dietary fats into triglycerides, which are a storage form of fat. Triglycerides can be broken down for energy in times of need. Triglycerides in excess team up with cholesterol and other substances to clog the arteries and cause heart attacks and strokes.

Tryptophan -- Tryptophan is an amino acid existing in proteins. It is essential for optimum growth in infants and for nitrogen equilibrium in human adults. It is a precursor of serotonin.

Tuberculosis (TB) -- IT'S BACK, AND THIS TIME IT'S BACK WITH A VENGEANCE!! Also called Consumption, TB is an infectious disease of humans and animals caused by microorganisms, Mycobacterium Tuberculosis, manifesting itself in lesions of the lung, bone and other parts of the body. A tuberculosis vaccine was developed by French physicians Leon Calmette and Camille Guerin thus giving the vaccine name Bacillus Calmette Guerin (BCG). American health officials use skin-testing to test for exposure to the TB germ. Treatment is followed-up by proper medication.

Officials feel mass vaccination was not necessary since many who came in contact with the germ were not infected and vaccinations also lead to false positives during the skin-test.

- 10 to 15 million Americans carry the germ that cause TB and 25,000 new cases of active TB occur each year.

- 09 out of 10 people that carry the TB bacterium never develop symptoms.

- Worldwide, more than 03 million people die of TB every year!

- Outbreaks occur in detention centers, homeless shelters, hospitals, offices, schools...

- If a TB skin test is positive, a 06 to 09 month course of anti-TB drugs may be prescribed by your doctor.

Tumor -- A tumor is a new growth of tissue in which the multiplication of cells is uncontrolled and progressive. It is also called neoplasm. Tumors perform no useful body function. They may be either benign (not cancerous) or malignant (cancerous).

Tumor Markers -- Tumor markers are substances in blood or other body fluids that may serve as indicators for the presence of cancer.

Tumor Suppressor Gene -- This is a gene whose function is to stop the cancer process at the earliest stages.

Type I Diabetes -- Insulin-dependent diabetes mellitus.

Type II Diabetes -- Non-insulin-dependent diabetes mellitus.

Typhoid Fever -- Typhoid fever is an acute, highly infectious disease caused by the typhoid bacillus, Salmonella Typhosa, transmitted by contaminated food or water and characterized by red rashed, high fever, and in severe cases, intestinal hemorrhaging.

Tyramine -- A sympathomimetic amine having an action in some respects resembling that of epinerphrine. Migraine headaches can be activated by tyramine type foods, like aged cheese, bananas, nuts, pork, shell fish and wine.

Ulcer -- An ulcer is a local defect or excavation, of the surface of an organ or tissue, which is produced by the sloughing of inflammatory necrotic tissue.

Ultrasonography -- An ultrasonography is the utilization of sound waves to produce pictures of internal organs. It is used to find abnormal growths.

Universal Precautions -- This is an approach to infection control. All human potentially infectious materials are treated as if known to be infectious for HIV, HBV or other bloodborne pathogens.

Uric Acid -- Uric acid is normally excreted in urine. High values are associated with arthritis, gout, kidney problems and the use of some diuretics. Low values of uric acid are probably not significant.

Urinalysis -- Urinalysis is the analysis of the urine for a multitude of things depending on the type and purpose of the test.

Urologist (M.D.) -- A urologist is a specialist in the urinary system, including the bladder and kidneys in both sexes and the male reproductive system.

U.S. RDA -- United States Recommended Daily Allowance is established by the Food and Drug Administration and is used to provide nutrient information on food and nutrition supplement labels. The U.S. RDA's express the food's nutrient value as a percentage of recommended levels and are a little higher than the RDA's in order to represent the nutrient needs of all healthy adults.

Vaccine -- A vaccine is a suspension of attenuated or killed disease-causing microorganisms, as of viruses or bacteria, incapable of inducing severe infection but capable, when inoculated, of stimulating the production of antibodies against the virulent microorganisms.

Vaginitis -- Vaginitis is the inflammation of the vagina.

Varicose Veins -- The vein valve acts like the canal locks that maintain water levels between bodies of water. In your "leg locks", traffic or blood flow is always up towards the heart. This prevents blood pooling. If valves weaken, pooled blood eventually stretches the veins themselves. If this happens in surface vessels, they become visible through the skin as unattractive bluish tangles or varicose-veins.

Vasodilator Drugs -- They are drugs which cause the blood vessels to widen.

Vasomotor -- Causing or regulating constriction of blood vessels or dilation of blood vessels.

VDL -- VDL stands for Very Low-Density Lipoprotein. The VDL, LDL and HDL each have their own special job. Once you eat fat, it is digested and absorbed in the small intestine and is then sent to the liver for processing into VLDL packaging and transportation throughout the body. VLDL carries the fat from the liver to all parts of your body. Again fat cannot travel through your blood vessels on its own because fat doesn't mix with water and water is a major ingredient in blood.

Veggie Burgers -- These are meatless burgers replacing beef or meat-type burgers. For meatless burger products, look for Moringstar Farms, Green Giant and The Original Gardenburger in your grocer's frozen foods section.

Veins -- Veins are tubular branching vessels that carry blood from the capillaries toward the heart.

Vinegar -- See *Apple Cider Vinegar*.

Virus -- A virus is an infectious agent that causes disease that multiplies in living cells.

Vision Therapy -- See *Vision Therapy*.

Vital Signs -- Vital signs include pulse, breathing, blood pressure and temperature. These vital signs are always taken for emergency and non-emergency casualties\patients in order to assess the patient's condition and initiate proper medical attention.

Vitiligo -- Vitiligo is an affliction in which areas of the skin completely lose their pigment. Treatments area available.

Vitamin -- Vitamins are organic (carbon-containing) substances required in small amounts for the normal functioning of the body. They are necessary for growth and maintaining life. Along with minerals, Vitamins are necessary for our bodies to utilize the carbohydrates, protein and fat in the food groups that we eat. Vitamins can be classified into two groups:

- Fat-soluble Vitamins which are found in the fat portion of the body cells and include Vitamins A, D, E and K.

- Water-Soluble Vitamins are found in the water portion of body cells and include the B Vitamins and Vitamin C.

Vita-Mix TNC -- I was so amazed by the Vita-Mix TNC (Total Nutrition Center), that I had to insure you read about it. No, I'm not getting a dime for it! Vita-Mix TNC is a *"whole food juicing"* machine that delivers nature's medicines to your body. According to Lancaster Laboratories (registered with the FDA), discarded pulp from juice extractors is 9.6 times more nutritious than the juice! The Vita-Mix TNC provides "total juice", which means it puree's whole fruits and vegetables (except for bitter parts and certain seeds) to a smooth, creamy texture. With the Vita-Mix TNC, you can make superior, and healthy soups, juices, ice cream, grains, sauces... in record time and it does even more to benefit your health. You're getting 9.6 times more nutrition than regular juice extracting machines! Call or write for free information. At least look into Vita-Mix TNC!

Vitro -- Vitro is a term pertaining to artificial environments. See *Vivo* below.

Vivo -- A term pertaining to - within the living body. See *Vitro* above.

Volatile Organic Compounds (VOCs) -- VOC's are a class of carbon-based chemicals that volatilize or evaporate at room temperature. Sources of VOC's are solvents, organochlorines and phenols. VOC's, through research, have indicated that they cause acute and chronic health effects which may include blurred vision, dizziness, euphoria, fatigue, headaches, irritations of the eyes, nose and throat, joint pain, numbness in extremities and weakness. The most common VOC found in indoor air is formaldehyde.

Warts -- Warts are infectious (can spread from person to person) growths in the outer layers of skin. Warts mostly appear on hands, fingers, and the soles of feet. Studies indicate that 02 out of every 03 warts disappear on their own within two years. There are over-the-counter preparations as well as surgery to remedy the problem.

Water -- Water is a clear, colorless, nearly odorless and tasteless liquid, essential for most plant and animal life and most widely used of all solvents.

Water Pollution -- Unsafe levels of hazardous substances are found in drinking water supplies across the country. On the waterways there are between 5,000 and 6,000 pollution incidents in US waters each year. Most are considered small (less than 1,000 gallons) and are never cleaned up. The National Wild Life Federation (NWF) is fighting to enhance federal clean water protection. Developing a comprehensive plan on reducing toxic pollution on the Great Lakes. Holding workshops and producing videos to promote awareness of the problem The NWF created *"Citizens Guide to Water Conservation."* The NWF needs your support.

Weight Loss -- Refers to weight lost during a period of time where a routine of exercise, diet and other factors are incorporated. SEE your doctor prior to initiating any weight-loss program.

Western Blot -- A test designed to detect the AIDS virus exposure by assessing the presence of the AIDS virus antibody.

Wetlands Protection -- More than half of America's original wetlands have been destroyed by development and conversion to agriculture uses. The rate of destruction is about 300,000 acres annually. The National Wild Life Federation is combatting attempts by Congress, developers and agricultural interests to reduce and all but eliminate wetlands protection laws.

Successfully used litigation to assure enforcement of critical wetlands laws. The NWF needs your support.

Whole Salt -- Table salt IS NOT Whole Salt, meaning it lacks over 80 minerals which protect the body from toxic effects of pure sodium chloride. Table salt (almost pure sodium chloride) is heated in an oven and stripped of its vital buffer minerals and may contribute to cardiovascular disease.

Everybody needs whole salt and not the refined salt you buy at the local grocery store. Whole salt is required for digestion, energy, regeneration of body cells and many other biological functions of the body. Whole salt, used in moderation, is not only harmless but a valuable nutrient. One type of whole salt contains over 80 buffer elements including magnesium is called Celtic Sea Salt. Celtic Sea Salt clean and unrefined is hand-harvested in Brittany near the Celtic Sea in northwest France. Natural Celtic Sea Salt is obtained from the evaporation of the ocean's water.

NO synthetic mineral supplement can equal the wealth of minerals that natural Celtic Seal Salt provides! Celtic Sea Salt is gathered after the ocean water is channeled daily into pristine ponds that is edged with natural waterways, wild grasses and other green plants. The wind and sun evaporate the ocean water, leaving rich brine. Within hours, the crystals are gathered by hand.

Natural Celtic Sea Salt has been noted to reverse many chronic type maladies. Why? Celtic Sea Salt's many beneficial minerals and bio-electronic power offers countless health benefits!
Celtic Sea Salt may help, prevent, heal or fight:
- Absorption to nutrients.
- Balances alkalinity\acidity levels.
- Banishes fatigue.
- Higher resistance to infections and bacterial diseases.
- Restores good digestion.
- Relieves allergies.
- Relieves skin diseases.
- Renewed energy.

Some health food stores may sell Celtic Sea Salt
WARNING: Some companies sell worthless whole salt products! Insure you purchase authentic Celtic Sea Salt products.
Follow the recommended dosage and instructions from the label and as per your doctor's instructions.

Wild Harvested -- The plants (herbs) were foraged in the wild in their native habitats.

Withdrawal -- Withdrawal is the termination of a habit-forming substance.

IRISAP (Joseph A. Laydon Jr.)
P.O. Box 48
Cutler, IL 62238-0048
USA
E-Mail: wwwsurvivalexpert@yahoo.com

More Survival Kindle E-Books And Survival Paperback Books For YOU!

Joseph A. Laydon Jr. (MSG Ret. Army) is the author and owner of Intensive Research Information Services And Products (IRISAP). Joseph has been writing "*self-reliance*" orientated data since 1991 and since July 2012 has been re-publishing his works via Kindle E-Books and Kindle Paperback Books. He has self-published more than **100+ Survival Books** (Kindle E-Books and Kinde Paperback Books). Below is a list of all his Survival Books and you can see these books by simply going to the website listed below for detailed descriptions and videos. See "*About The Author.*"

- **Kindle E-Books:**-----------www.survivalexpertblog.com/52-survival-books/

- **Kindle Paperback:**-------www.survivalexpertblog.com/52-survival-books/

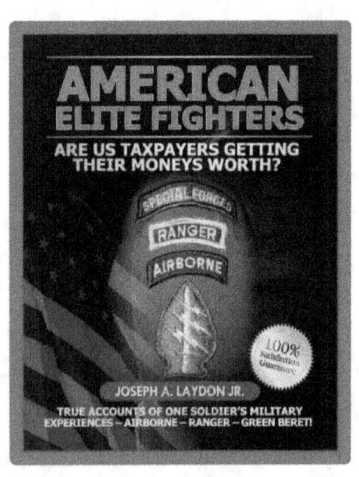 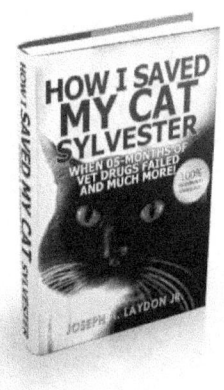 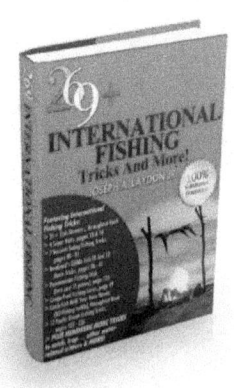

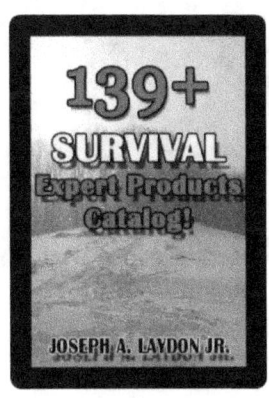 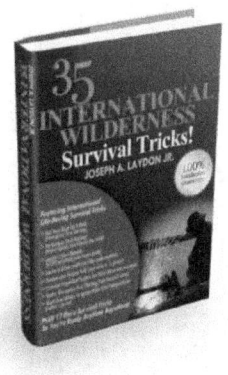 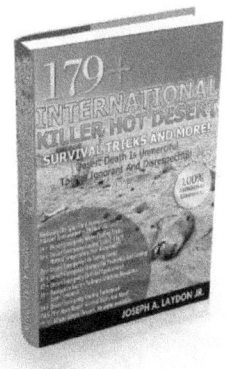

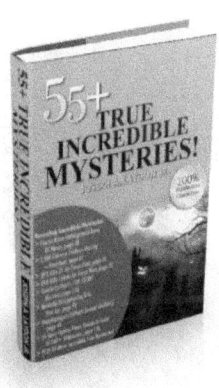 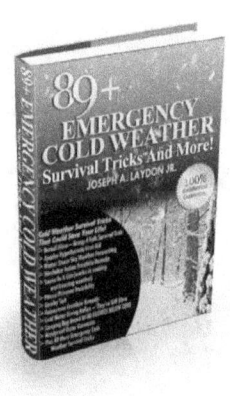 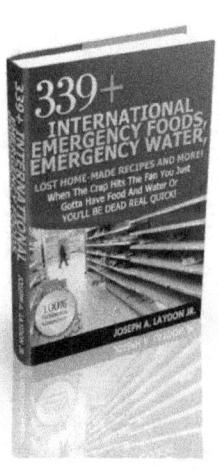

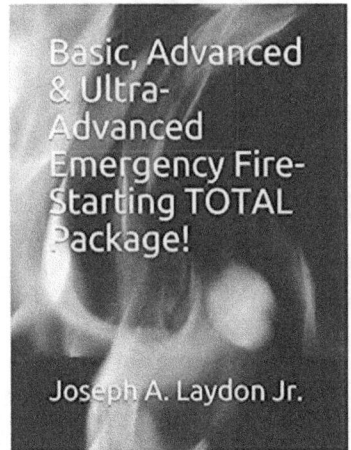 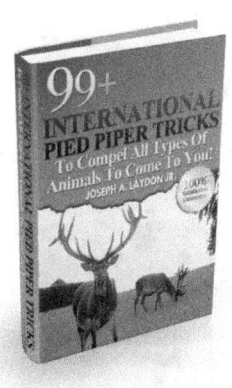 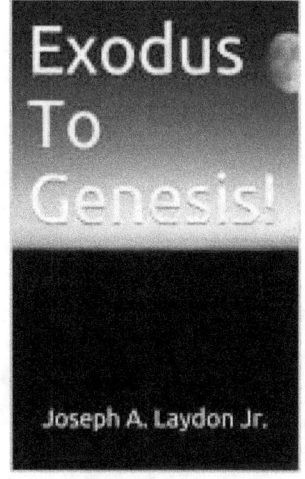

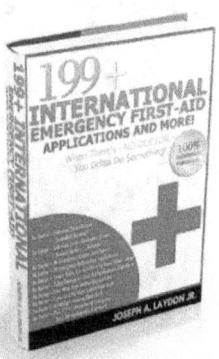

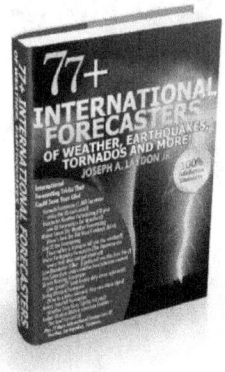

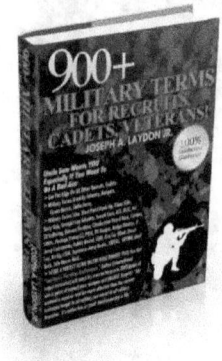

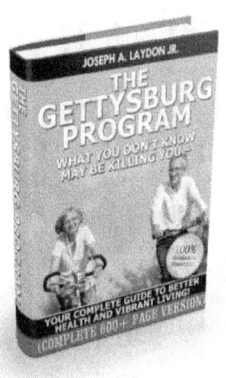

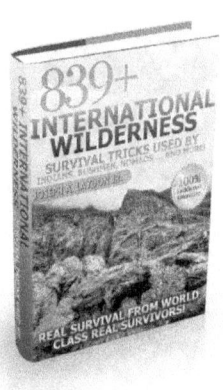

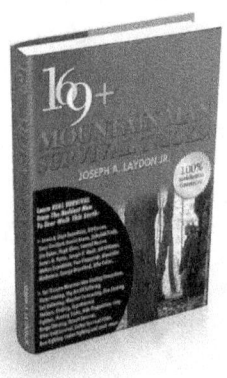

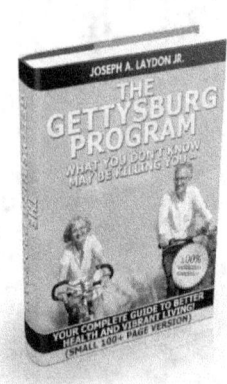

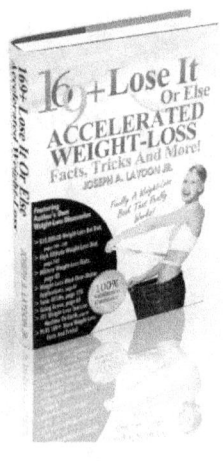

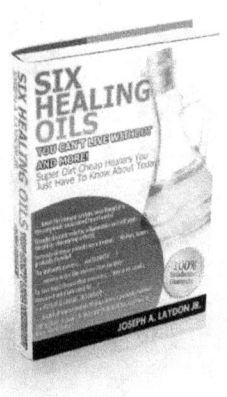

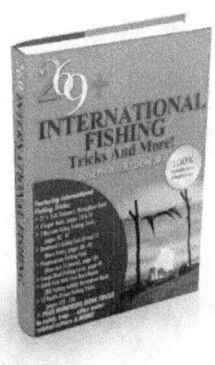

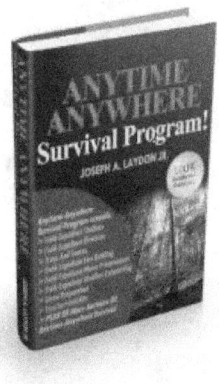

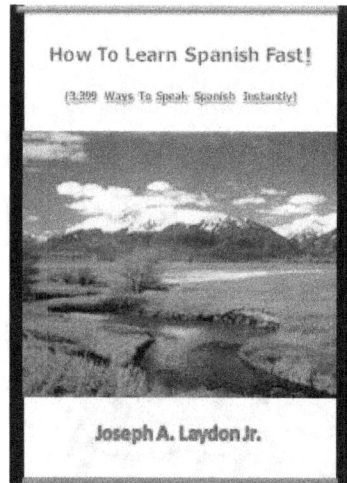

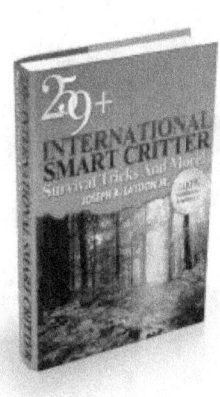

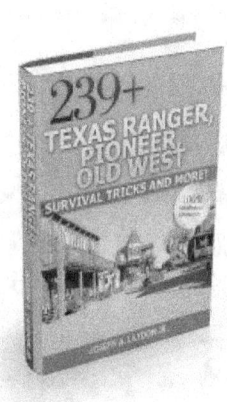

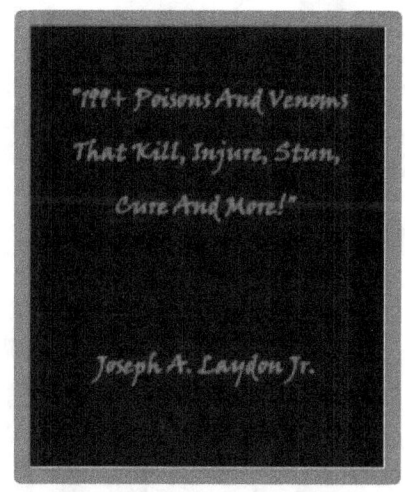

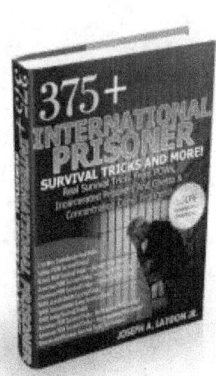

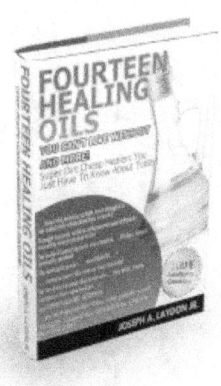

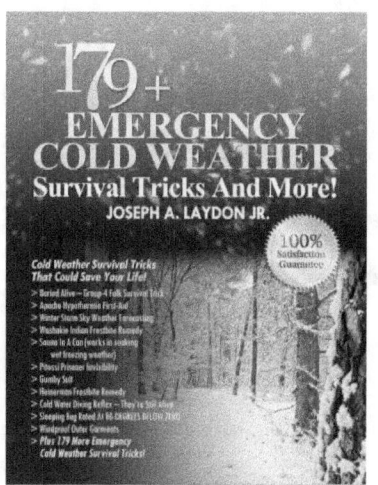

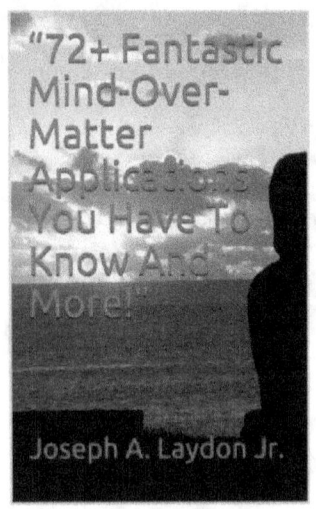

"72+ Fantastic Mind-Over-Matter Applications You Have To Know And More!"

Joseph A. Laydon Jr.

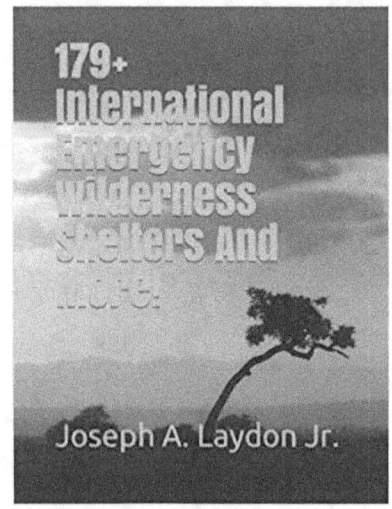

179+ International Emergency Wilderness Shelters And More!

Joseph A. Laydon Jr.

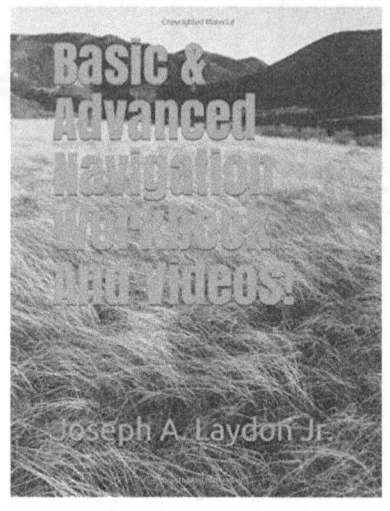

Basic & Advanced Navigation Methods And Videos!

Joseph A. Laydon Jr.

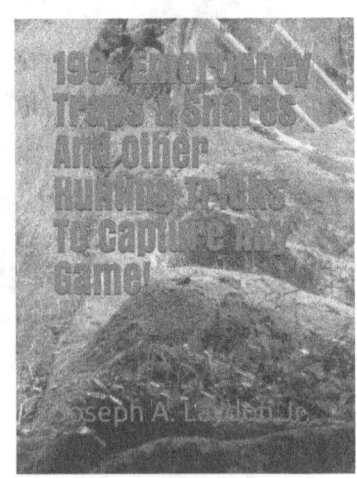

199+ Emergency Traps, Snares And Other Hunting Tools To Capture Wild Game!

Joseph A. Laydon Jr.

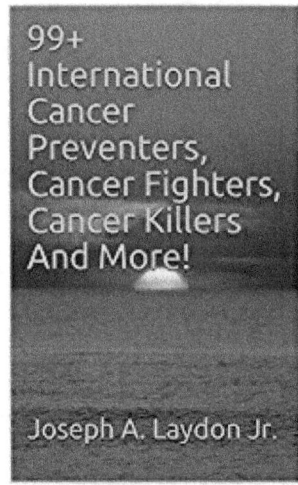

99+ International Cancer Preventers, Cancer Fighters, Cancer Killers And More!

Joseph A. Laydon Jr.

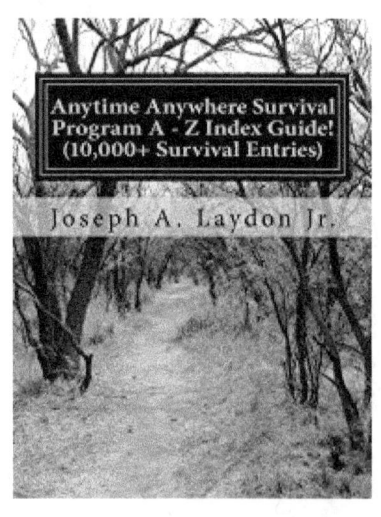

Anytime Anywhere Survival Program A - Z Index Guide! (10,000+ Survival Entries)

Joseph A. Laydon Jr.

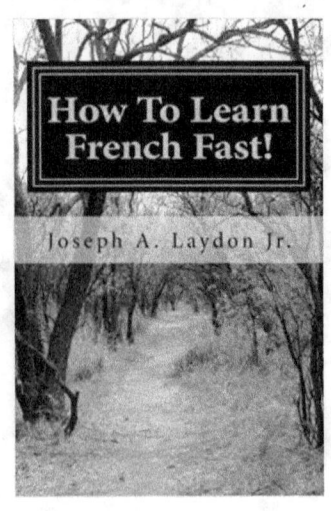

How To Learn French Fast!

Joseph A. Laydon Jr.

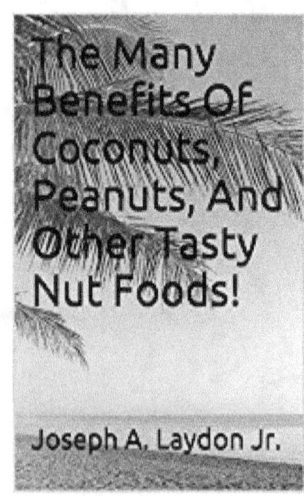

The Many Benefits Of Coconuts, Peanuts, And Other Tasty Nut Foods!

Joseph A. Laydon Jr.

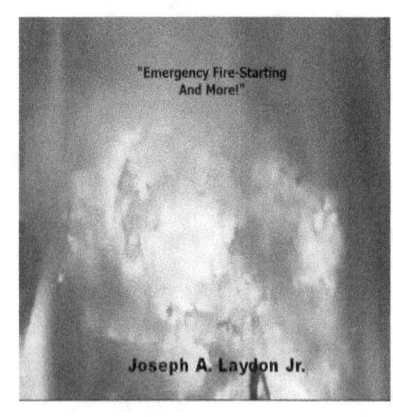

"Emergency Fire-Starting And More!"

Joseph A. Laydon Jr.

288

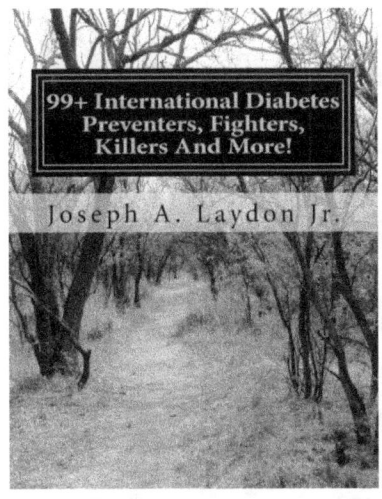

99+ International Diabetes Preventers, Fighters, Killers And More!

Joseph A. Laydon Jr.

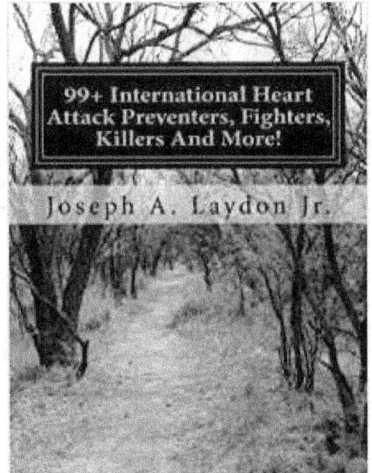

99+ International Heart Attack Preventers, Fighters, Killers And More!

Joseph A. Laydon Jr.

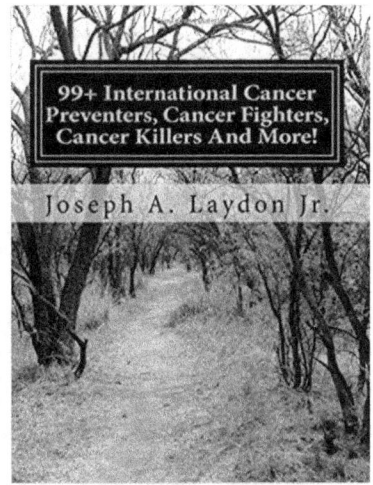

99+ International Cancer Preventers, Cancer Fighters, Cancer Killers And More!

Joseph A. Laydon Jr.

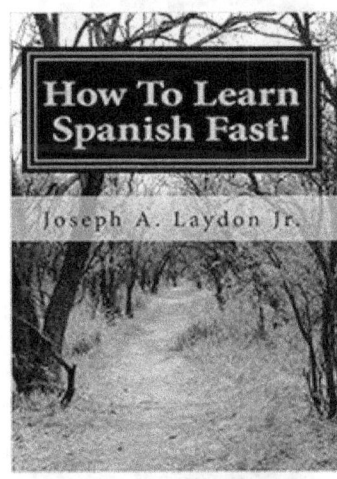

How To Learn Spanish Fast!

Joseph A. Laydon Jr.

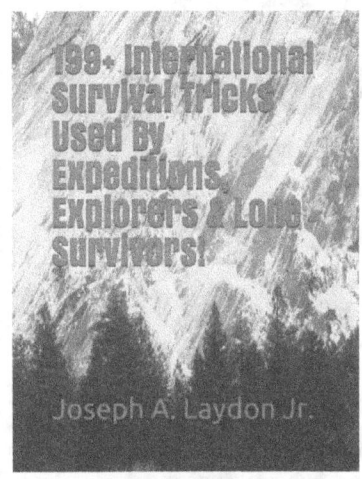

199+ International Survival Tricks Used By Expeditions, Explorers & Lone Survivors!

Joseph A. Laydon Jr.

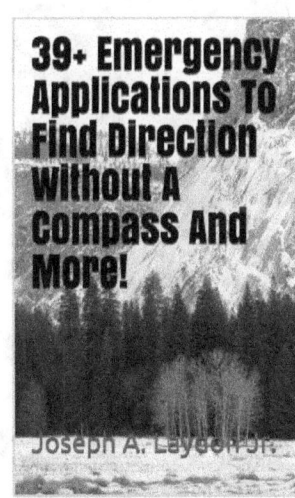

39+ Emergency Applications To Find Direction Without A Compass And More!

Joseph A. Laydon Jr.

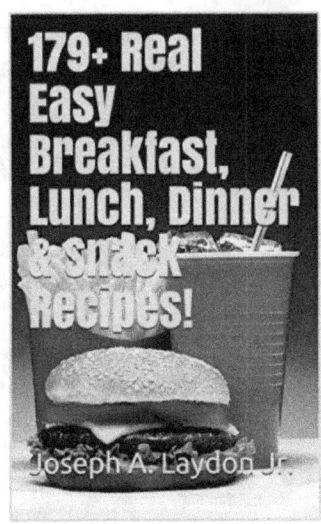

179+ Real Easy Breakfast, Lunch, Dinner & Snack Recipes!

Joseph A. Laydon Jr.

99+ Healings And Cures You Have To Know and More!

Joseph A. Laydon Jr.

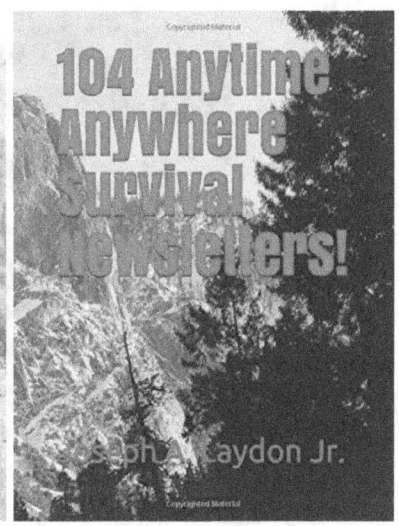

104 Anytime Anywhere Survival Newsletters!

Joseph A. Laydon Jr.

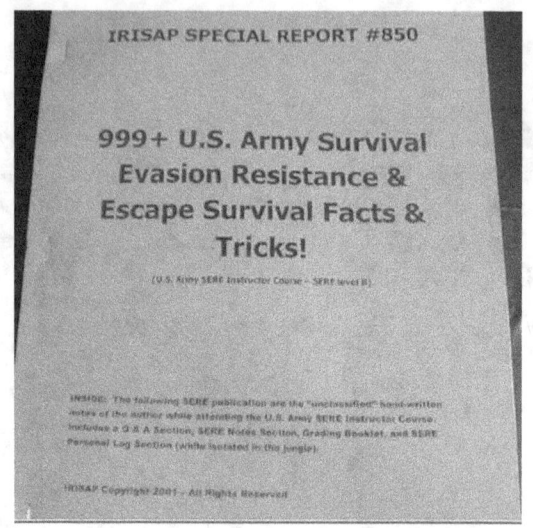

IRISAP SPECIAL REPORT #850

999+ U.S. Army Survival
Evasion Resistance &
Escape Survival Facts &
Tricks!

(U.S. Army SERE Instructor Course – SERE level II)

INSIDE: The following SERE publication are the "unclassified" hand-written notes of the author while attending the U.S. Army SERE Instructor Course. Includes a Q & A Section, SERE Notes Section, Grading Booklet, and SERE Personal Log Section (while isolated in the jungle).

IRISAP Copyright 2001 – All Rights Reserved

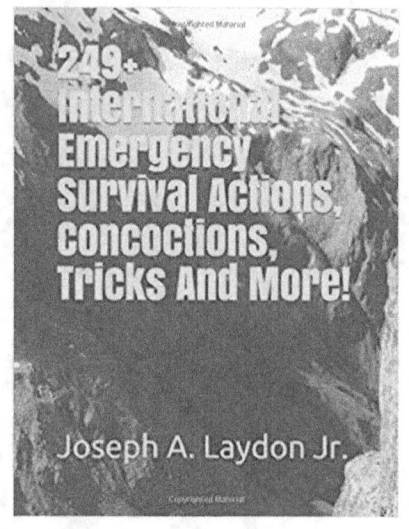

249+
International
Emergency
Survival Actions,
Concoctions,
Tricks And More!

Joseph A. Laydon Jr.

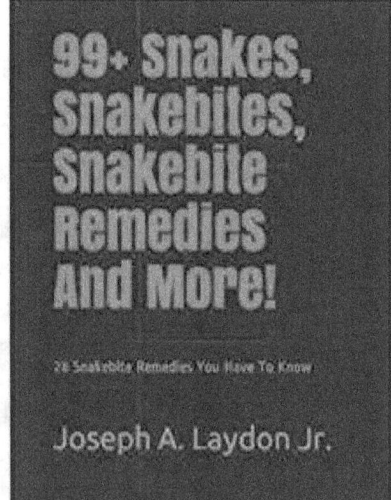

99+ Snakes,
Snakebites,
Snakebite
Remedies
And More!

28 Snakebite Remedies You Have To Know

Joseph A. Laydon Jr.

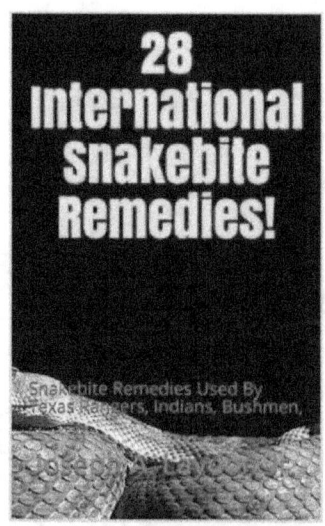

28
International
Snakebite
Remedies!

Snakebite Remedies Used By
Texas Rangers, Indians, Bushmen,

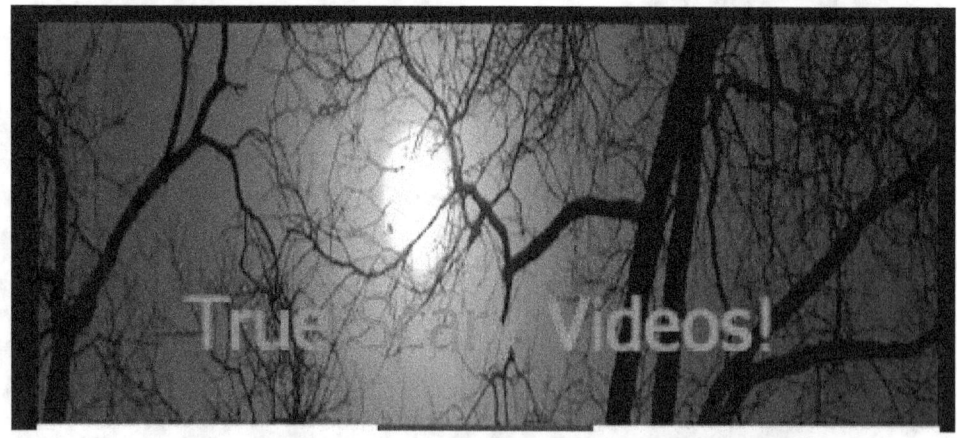

True Scary Videos!

www.patreon.com/truescaryvideos/

About The Author

Joseph A. Laydon Jr. (MSG (E-8) Retired United States Army - 18Z5V) is 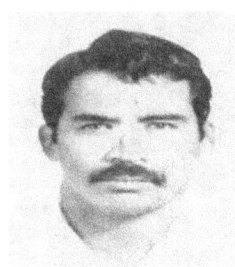 the author and owner of *Intensive Research Information Services And Products (IRISAP)*. Joseph is a well-qualified instructor in international wilderness survival and the other 03 Survivals he teaches (Health Survival, Crime Survival and Money Survival). He is a 20-year US Army veteran (Master Sergeant E-8 - 18Z5V) associated with all Special Operations units in the US military, as well as Special Ops units in the Mid-East and Central & South America.

He's a qualified SERE Instructor (Survival Evasion Resistance & Escape) and has **taught wilderness survival** at the college level for 03 years. He's a qualified instructor in basic & advanced pistol marksmanship, basic & advanced rifle marksmanship, CQB (Close Quarter Battle), basic & advanced cross-country navigation, basic mountaineering techniques, and self-defense. Since 1994, he's published many self-improvement Survival Programs, Survival Videos, SPECIAL Reports, Intelligence Reports, monthly Newsletters, **100+ Survival Books** (Kindle E-Books & Kindle Paperback Books) and more in the works.

He's an inventor, he *"sideways engineers"* new survival tricks that can SAVE YOUR LIFE! An example: On 17 August 2000 - 1417 hours, at Scott Lake, Scott AFB, IL, Joseph made international history! He is the 1st in the world to replicate the mysterious fires of Africa using a single drop of water! On 05 January 2001, he discovered how to start a life-saving fire in just 02-seconds using a beam of light from a flashlight in pitch black *"blind man"* darkness! On 06 April 2005 - 1810 hours, he invented delicious & tasty Solid Fuel Rolls and several Trail-Mix Cookies that are used as emergency foods and used as long-burning emergency fire-starting kindling.

And recently - **50+ MORE TOP SECRET INVENTIONS** of advanced & **ultra-advanced fire-starting** like starting EMERGENCY FIRE-STARTING using personal care products and first-aid products you already use like:

- Shampoo

Toothpastes
- Mouthwashes
- Breath Drops & Breath Sprays
- Salves
- Ointments
- Over-The-Counter Medicines
- Drink Enhancement Products
- Other ingredients like your spit (saliva), your urination,...

See **www.survivalexpert.com/fire**

He also teaches Advanced Navigation (*Basic & Advanced Navigation Workbook And Videos* [includes Workbook, Videos, maps, protractors,…]) so you're ready Anytime Anywhere! Only from IRISAP and only for privileged IRISAP subscribers - YOU! See *Basic & Advanced Navigation Workbook And Videos* at **www.survivalexpertbooks.com/navigation**

Below is a sample of his military achievements & qualifications (**not in chronological order**) which reflect his unique & superior ability to teach basic, advanced & ultra-advanced survival applications, techniques and "tricks" that could help you AVOID serious killer survival threats as well as SAVE YOUR LIFE when you get in life or death situations. His trade secrets, Programs, and Videos are only offered to IRISAP subscribers-YOU!

- US Army Airborne School
- US Army Special Forces Qualification Course - SFQC (Green Beret)
- US Army Master Parachutist Wings
- Uruguayan Parachutist Wings
- British Parachutist Wings
- Kingdom of Jordan Parachutist Wings
- Expert Infantry Badge – EIB
- 82nd Airborne Division Recondo Course
- Adverse Weather Aerial Delivery System Tests – AWADS (01 of 386 volunteer paratroopers)
- US Army Special Forces Weapons Course (US & foreign pistols, submachineguns, assault rifles, rifles, machineguns, mortars, anti-tank weapons, anti-aircraft weapons,…)

- Weapons Armorer Course
- Indirect Fire Course (60mm, 81mm, & 4.2 inch *"four deuce"* mortars)
- Jumpmaster Course
- Basic French Language Course
- Combat Infantry Badge - CIB
- US Army Ranger Course
- Advanced Navigation Course
- Special Forces Sniper Course (02)
- Survival Evasion Resistance and Escape Instructor Course (SERE Level B)
- Wilderness Survival Instructor (College level - 03 years / 1991 - 1994)
- Rappell Master
- Fast Rope Master
- International Sniper Instructor
- International Close Quarter Battle (CQB) Instructor
- Participated In Multiple Combat Actions
- Special Forces Operations And Intelligence Course (O&I)
- Good Conduct Medal (06)
- Army Commendation Medal
- Army Achievement Medal (02)
- Meritorious Service Medal (02)
- Armed Forces Expeditionary Medal
- Letters Of Commendation (13)
- Letters Of Appreciation (08)
- Infantry Advanced NCO Course (11B)**
- Infantry Officer Basic Course **
- Military Intelligence Officer Basic Course **
- Held **SECRET** and **TOP SECRET Clearances** for 20+ years

** = These are military home study correspondence courses which took years to complete. This demonstrates Mr. Laydon's dedication to duty and desire to go beyond the training standards set by the US Army Special Forces. You won't find too many soldiers completing years of military home study courses on their own time off. This reflects the author's many superior Survival Products like this Survival Product.

Featured on FOX-2 (24 August 2000). Joseph now resides in Illinois.
He offers products concerning Wilderness Survival, Health Survival,
Crime Survival and Money Survival so to greatly enhance the lives of
all IRISAP subscribers - YOU! Any questions, write to Joseph today.

Sincerely,
Joseph A. Laydon Jr. (IRISAP)
P.O. Box 48
Cutler, IL 62238-0048

You And Yours Have A Safe One
Anytime Anywhere,

Joseph A. Laydon Jr.

E-Mail: wwwsurvivalexpert@yahoo.com

E-Mail: josephlaydonjr@gmail.com

WEBSITES

- Main Website--------------------www.survivalexpert.com
- 45+ Survival Paperback Books-----www.survivalexpertbooks.com
- 45+ Survival Kindle E-Books------www.survivalexpertebooks.com
- Anytime Anywhere Survival--------www.anytimeanywheresurvival.com
- Weight-Loss----------------------www.loseitorelseweightloss.com
- True Scary Videos----------------www.patreon.com/truescaryvideos
- Exodus To Genesis (Fiction Book)-www.exodustogenesis.com
- **NEW** - 'Survival Expert Blog'--https://www.survivalexpertblog.com
- **NEW & IMPROVED** - *'Save My Life - Basic, Advanced And Ultra-Advanced Emergency Fire-Starting TOTAL Package'*
  https://www.survivalexpertblog.com/save-my-life-survival-program

Take Notes

Take Notes

Take Notes

Take Notes

Take Notes

Take Notes

Take Notes

Take Notes

More Super Healthy Survival Books Just For YOU!

Joseph A. Laydon Jr. (MSG Ret. Army) is the author and owner of Intensive Research Information Services And Products (IRISAP). Joseph has been writing *"self-reliance"* orientated data since 1991 and since July 2012 has been re-publishing his works via Kindle E-Books and CreateSpace Paperback Books. See *"About The Author."*

- **Kindle E-Books:**------**https://www.survivalexpertblog.com/52-survival-books/**

- **Paperback Books:**---https://www.survivalexpertblog.com/52-survival-books/

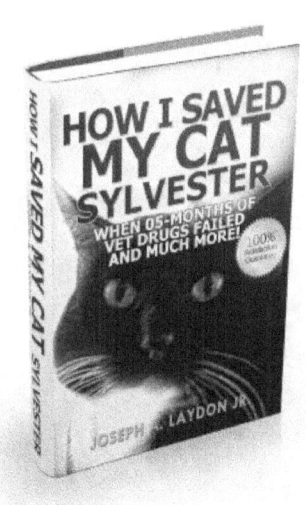
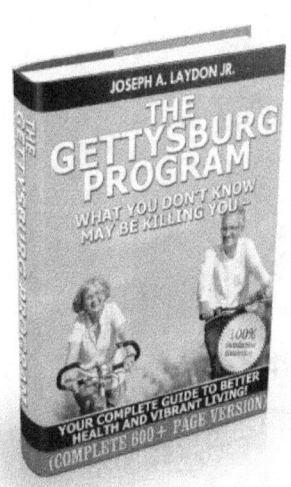

https://www.survivalexpertblog.com/52-survival-books/

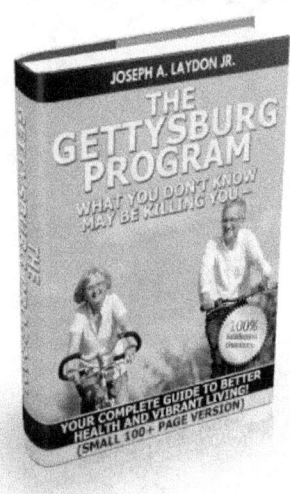

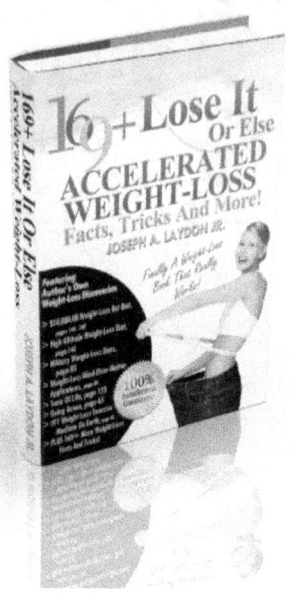

https://www.survivalexpertblog.com/52-survival-books/

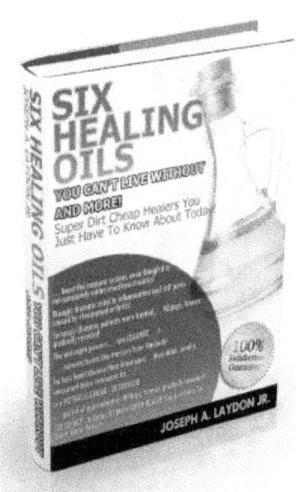

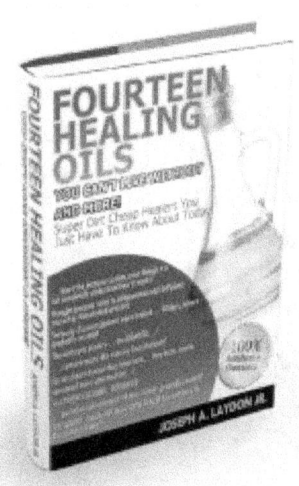

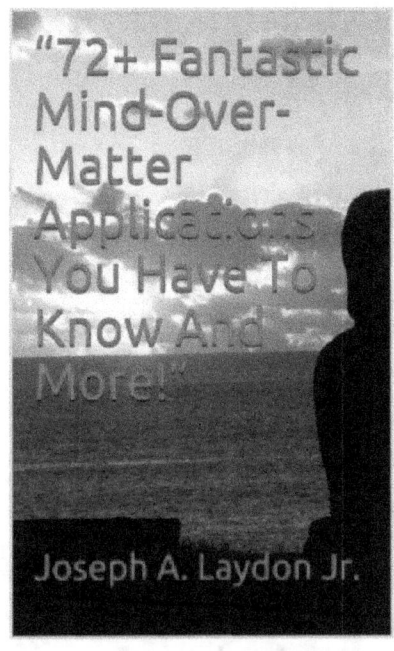

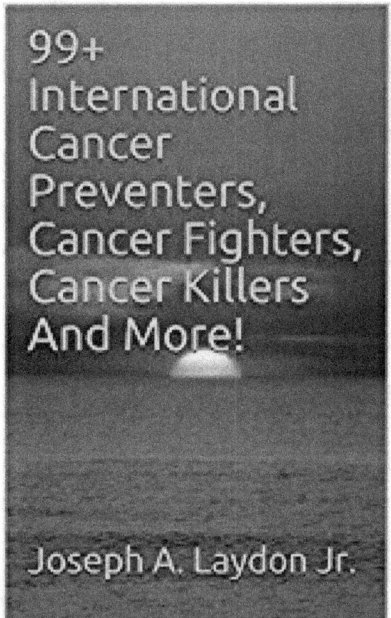

https://www.survivalexpertblog.com/52-survival-books/

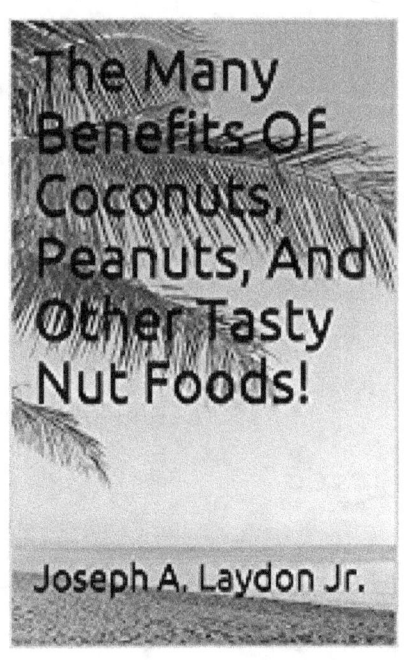

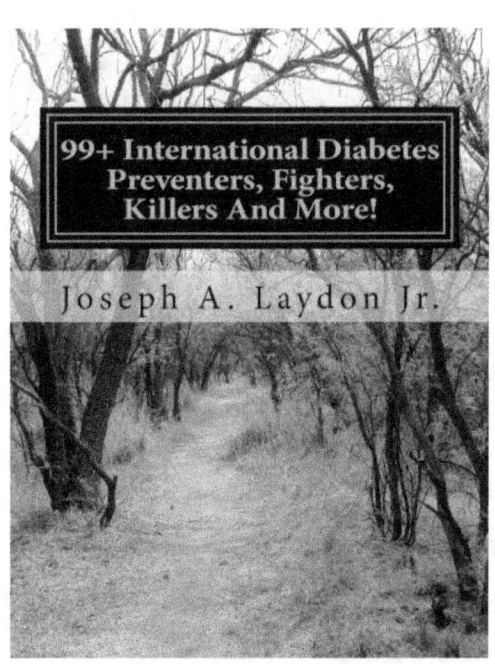

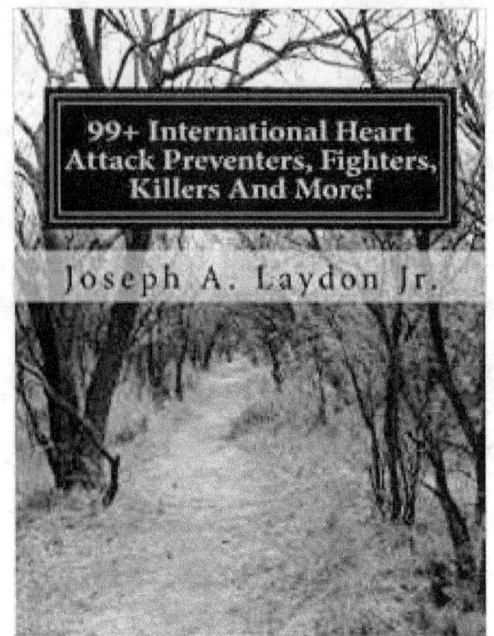
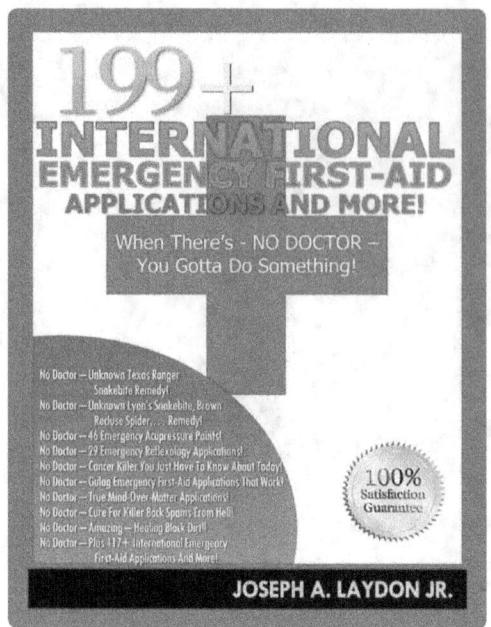

https://www.survivalexpertblog.com/52-survival-books/

IRISAP Copyright 2018 - All Rights Reserved

www.ingramcontent.com/pod-product-compliance
Lightning Source LLC
Chambersburg PA
CBHW080407290526
45791CB00008BA/2178